Prostate Cancer: Diagnosis, Therapy and Case Studies

Prostate Cancer: Diagnosis, Therapy and Case Studies

Edited by **Karl Meloni**

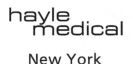

New York

Published by Hayle Medical,
30 West, 37th Street, Suite 612,
New York, NY 10018, USA
www.haylemedical.com

Prostate Cancer: Diagnosis, Therapy and Case Studies
Edited by Karl Meloni

© 2015 Hayle Medical

International Standard Book Number: 978-1-63241-330-7 (Hardback)

Contents

Preface

The main aim of this book is to educate learners and enhance their research focus by presenting diverse topics covering this vast field. This is an advanced book which compiles significant studies by distinguished experts in the area of analysis. This book addresses successive solutions to the challenges arising in the area of application, along with it; the book provides scope for future developments.

Prostate cancer is a serious health concern in men-related disorders across the globe. This book provides significant information regarding various crucial topics including diagnostic markers, therapeutic novelties, and cancer biology. It serves as an important resource for healthcare professionals and scientists devoted to the field of research on prostate cancer. It reflects important developments in this field over the past decade, serving as a facilitator for the removal of this potentially debilitating and fatal malignancy.

It was a great honour to edit this book, though there were challenges, as it involved a lot of communication and networking between me and the editorial team. However, the end result was this all-inclusive book covering diverse themes in the field.

Finally, it is important to acknowledge the efforts of the contributors for their excellent chapters, through which a wide variety of issues have been addressed. I would also like to thank my colleagues for their valuable feedback during the making of this book.

Editor

Part 1

Cancer Biology

Epidemiology of Prostate Cancer: The Case of Ethnic German Migrants from the Former Soviet Union

Volker Winkler and Heiko Becher
Institute of Public Health
University of Heidelberg
Germany

1. Introduction

1.1 Epidemiology of prostate cancer
1.1.1 Situation in Germany

In Germany, prostate cancer is the leading cause of cancer (26%) and the third leading cause of death from cancer in males (10%). The mean age of disease and of death due to prostate cancer is 70.1 years and 77.5 years, respectively (Ziegler et al., 2009). Few people are diagnosed before the age of 50 years. A 70-year old man has a 6% risk of developing prostate cancer within the next ten years, whereas, the risk for a 40-year-old man is 0.1% (RKI, 2010). In 2006, approximately 238,500 men were diagnosed with prostate cancer during the previous five years in Germany.

Currently, there is a statutory screening programme for prostate cancer in Germany. All men aged 45 years and over are asked once a year by their physician if they have any symptoms. This screening also includes an examination of the sexual organs, the lymph nodes, as well as a palpation examination of the prostate via the rectum. Presently, the prostate-specific antigen (PSA) blood test is not part of the statutory screening.

1.1.2 Longitudinal trends in Germany

During the 1970s incidence was stable around 50 per 100,000 persons (Ziegler et al., 2009). Since 1980, the incidence has increased (see Figure 1). The yearly number of new prostate cancer cases in Germany has risen by 200% (from 1980-2006), which may partly be due to the demographic change. During the same period the age-standardized incidence rate (standardized to the European standard population) also increased by 110%. In 2006, the age-standardized incidence rate was 110.1 per 100,000 men (RKI, 2010). This increase is mainly due the use of new diagnostic methods, e.g. testing for PSA. Earlier diagnosis, in terms of both the cancer's stage of development and the patient's age, has led to much higher incidence rates in the age group 50- to 69-years and lower rates among over-75-year-olds. Additionally, the mean age at onset fell from 73 years in 1980 to 70 years in 2006 (RKI, 2010).

On the other hand, age-standardized mortality rates have been more or less stable during the last decades and began to fall slightly since 1995. In 2006, the age-standardized mortality rate was 21.2 per 100,000 men. The 30% increase in the number of deaths since 1980 is a result of demographic change.

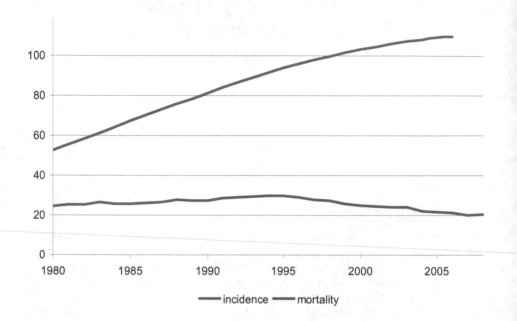

Fig. 1. Age-standardized prostate cancer incidence and mortality rates per 100,000 (European Standard) in Germany (RKI, 2011)

Between 1984 and 1998, the 5-year survival rate in Germany was 82% (RKI, 2008). Currently, relative 5-year survival rates are about 90% (Ziegler et al., 2009). However, whether this slight improvement in survival is a result of earlier diagnosis due to screening in the last years is not clear. With regards to prognosis, a distinction must be made between slowly progressing forms and aggressive metastasizing forms, which occur in greater proportions among younger men (under 60).

1.1.3 International comparison
An international comparison of German prostate cancer mortality and incidence to selected international countries is displayed in Figure 2. The cancer mortality rate in Germany is among the lowest in Europe, whereas the incidence is around the European average. Internationally, some of the lowest prostate cancer rates with regard to mortality and incidence are seen in Hong Kong. Scandinavian countries are among those with the highest prostate cancer mortality worldwide. Prostate cancer mortality rates are also estimated to be very high in some African and South American countries (Ferlay, 2010). A country-specific comparison shows that high prostate cancer mortality rates do not necessarily mean high incidence rates and vice versa (RKI, 2010).

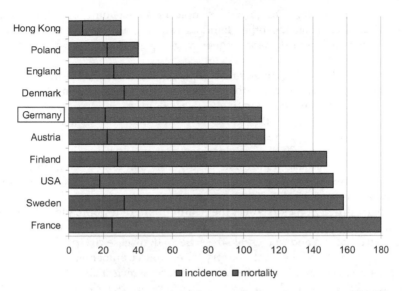

Fig. 2. Age-standardized prostate cancer incidence and mortality rates per 100,000 (European Standard) in Germany in 2006 compared internationally (except France in 2005) (RKI, 2010)

1.1.4 Risk factors

Risk factors and factors affecting disease progression are basically unknown. Clearly, male sex hormones play a role, without them prostate cancer would not develop. In addition, the aging process contributes to the development of prostate cancer as it does for all cancer sites. Cellular repair mechanisms become more and more error prone with age, which contributes to the development of malignancies.

A genetic predisposition has been discussed, because of a higher incidence in several ethnic groups and disease at a younger age. A clustering of the disease among close relatives has also been shown, although there is no consensus on which inheritable genetic defects are involved. In spite of extensive research, reliable findings on risk factors relating to lifestyle, diet or the environment remain elusive. Possible lifestyle risk factors are high intakes of α-linolenic acid (a polyunsaturated fatty acid in vegetables and dairy products) and calcium. Common risk factors for various cancer sites such as tobacco smoking, alcohol consumption and low physical activity do not seem to affect prostate cancer risk (Grönberg, 2003; Patel & Klein, 2009).

1.2 Migration and health
1.2.1 General aspects

Worldwide, there are many epidemiological studies of migrant populations that lead to new findings on the etiology of diseases (McCredie, 1998). Additionally, these studies help to develop targeted cancer prevention and early detection strategies for migrant groups.

In general, research on migrants focuses on topics that are related to selection. There are push and pull factors influencing the migration process. Push factors make people more willing to leave their country of origin, for example a poor economy, or political or religious persecution. Pull factors on the other hand attract migrants to a country like a good employment situation, labour demand, higher wages, higher living standards, political and religious freedom.

It has been suggested that migrants are not representative samples of their population of origin. Migrants are likely to be positively selected when they respond to pull factors in the country of destination and negatively selected in respond to push factors in the country of origin (Lee, 1966). With regards to health, this leads to the so called "healthy migrant effect". In general, people that are younger and healthier are more willing and able to migrate (Jasso et al., 2004). The elderly and people that are ill tend to stay in their country of origin. So, this selection results in migrants that tend to be healthier than their population of origin. It has been shown, that the healthy migrant effect diminishes dramatically with time (Fennelly, 2007).

In general, many different factors affect the health of migrant populations (Marmot et al., 1984): First, the migration itself can have an impact on health. This refers to positive or negative selective factors and to mental stress. Second, disease risk profiles in the country of origin may differ from the host country due to environmental factors for example, which may lead to disease. Third, destination effects which include physical and social environments, for example the integration politics in the destination country may influence migrant health strongly by making health care services easily accessible for migrant populations.

1.2.2 Migration and cancer incidence & mortality

Cancer is one of the leading causes of deaths in the industrialized world (World Health Organization [WHO], 2004) and the second leading cause of death in Germany (Federal Statistical Office of Germany [DeStatis], 2007). It has been demonstrated that migrant cancer incidence and mortality differs in general from cancer patterns in the respective host population.

Cancer is known to have a long latency period between exposure and disease onset. Important exposure factors can be traced back to childhood and young adulthood. This means short and medium term cancer mortality among first generation migrants is mainly influenced by country-of-origin factors (Parkin & Khlat, 1996).

The longer migrants live and adapt to their destination country, the more their cancer rates converge towards those in that country. This has been shown for stomach, colon and prostate cancer (McKay, 2003). Migrants from non-western countries to Europe were found to be more prone to cancers that are related to infections experienced in early life, such as liver, cervical and stomach cancer. In contrast, migrants of non-western origin were less likely to suffer from cancers related to a western lifestyle, e.g. colorectal and breast cancer (Arnold et al., 2010).

Evidence was found for a transition of cancer incidence and mortality patterns towards the host population among Turkish migrants in Germany (Zeeb et al., 2002). Convergence may occur due to diet acculturation, adaptation of new lifestyles or utilization of often superior health services. Higher mortality from cancers where incidence can be reduced by effective screening programs and those where survival depends on availability of treatment options, may decrease in a relatively shorter time. Another study analyzed differences in cancer rates between first and second generation migrants relative to the host country, stratified by country of origin, showing cancer site specific patterns for succeeding generations (Thomas & Karagas, 1987).

Results of an American study support the theory of a rather strong genetic influence on risk of prostate cancer. The study compared patterns of prostate cancer among black and white men (Chu et al., 2003). Black Americans had substantially higher prostate cancer rates than white Americans, but the longitudinal trends such as decreasing mortality, increasing incidence and survival were similar. Although this was not a typical migrant study, it compared different ethnic and thus genetic and lifestyle factors in a known risk pattern environment.

1.3 Ethnic German migrants in Germany - background on the study population

In the year 2005, only 2.9% of the global population were migrants, but migration is unequally distributed throughout the world. In past years, migration flows have shifted and in some cases, international migration is actually decreasing. Only two areas in the world have seen an increase in migration – North America and the Former Soviet Union (FSU) (International Organization for Migration, 2005).

Germany has long been a country of immigration. At present, there are two big groups of migrants, the Turks and ethnic Germans from countries of the FSU. We study disease patterns, focusing on cancer incidence and mortality, in the latter group.

The 'Aussiedler' are ethnic German migrants and represent a unique group of diaspora migrants. Since 1993, the officially correct term for Aussiedler is Spätaussiedler, however for ease of presentation we will use the term Aussiedler throughout the text.

The first Aussiedler came to Russia when Peter I (1689–1725) changed his politics towards Europe. They were the beginning of the urban German population in Russia. Tsarina Katharina II (1762–1796) promised the Aussiedler tax exemptions for 30 years, exoneration from military service, freedom of religion, autonomy and subsidy for resettlement. Many Germans living in regions still suffering from war migrated to Russia under these terms. During the first half of the 19th century approximately 55,000 German colonists settled in the Black Sea region. With time the Aussiedler lost several of the rights they were promised.

For centuries these ethnic Germans lived abroad and were a relatively closed group of people. After the start of World War I the laws of liquidation were implemented. On the basis of these laws more than 200,000 German colonists were driven away. In 1922, after the October-revolution and civil war the Union of Soviet Socialist Republics (USSR) was founded. When the Nazi Party came into power in Germany the situation of the Germans in the USSR worsened. Seen as an internal enemy, Stalin restricted their rights.

Soon after the German aggression against the USSR in 1941 the deportation of the German population started. Following Stalin's decree about 1,200,000 ethnic Germans were deported into the eastern parts of the Soviet Union, predominantly to Siberia, Kazakhstan and in the Urals. Their civil rights were disregarded; they were detained and forbidden to speak German. Most had to work in labour camps in inhumane conditions. An estimated 700,000 Germans died due to bad working and living conditions and inadequate medical treatment. In particular, the Stalinism destroyed the independent German culture in Russia. In 1955, the discrimination was subsided, and the ethnic Germans were allowed to change their residence, but not to their former colony areas. The Aussiedler became partly assimilated in the last decades of the USSR.

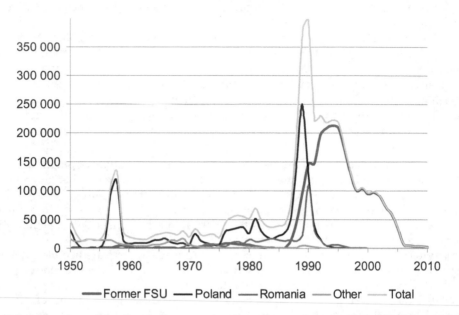

Fig. 3. Immigration of the Aussiedler over time by country of origin (Federal Ministry of the Interior, 2009; Federal Office of Administration, 2011)

When the iron curtain fell around 1990, a wave of migration to Germany started (see Figure 3). Since then more than two million Aussiedler migrated to Germany from countries of the FSU, with most coming from Kazakhstan and the Russian Federation. There are few examples of a large migration of one ethnic group from one country to another in a similarly short period of time.

In 1993, the German government began to restrict the immigration of Aussiedler by implementing annual quotas, which were further reduced in 1996. In parallel the government eliminated several benefits previously offered to Aussiedler, e.g. special credits and unemployment benefits.

The number of Aussiedler immigrating to Germany has fallen rapidly in recent years. In 2010, only 2,350 Aussiedler migrated to Germany (Federal Office of Administration, 2011). Today, the Aussiedler comprise about 2.5% of the German population, representing a relatively large group within German society (Destatis, 2008a; Destatis, 2008b).

More information on the history of the Aussiedler can be found elsewhere (Federal Central Office for Political Education, 2000; Bade & Olmert, 1999; Eisfeld, 1999; Pohl, 2001).

1.4 Comparing German incidence and mortality to the Former Soviet Union

The health situation in the FSU has changed dramatically during the last thirty years. Since the late 1980s the FSU has been experiencing a mortality crisis, in temporal association with massive social changes.

In Russia between 1987 and 1994, increases were observed for all major causes of death, except for cancer (Leon et al., 1997). Age-standardized mortality for all causes of death rose from 1140 in 1987 to 1600 per 100,000 persons in 1994 (adjusted to Segi). Development was very similar in Kazakhstan and in Ukraine. After a dip, the excess mortality increased sharply following the economic crisis of 1998. Mortality is largely due to vascular and external causes of death in adults (Men et al., 2003). In 2006, mortality was still high with about 1300 per 100,000 people. During the same period in Germany, all cause mortality declined continuously from around 850 to 650 per 100,000 people (WHO, 2011a).

In 2008, the age-standardised mortality rate per 100,000 males for all cancers was 181.3 in Kazakhstan and 180.7 in the Russian Federation (Ferlay, 2010). In Germany, mortality for all cancer sites combined in the respective year was much lower with 133.2 per 100,000 males. An important reason for the lower cancer mortality in Germany compared to countries of the FSU is better survival. However, longitudinal trends in mortality for all cancer sites developed in parallel between Germany and the FSU.

A comparison of cancer incidence rates between Germany and the Aussiedler's countries of origin show much lower rates in the Former Soviet Union. However, it is likely that incidence rates are underestimated in the FSU as evidenced by mortality patterns and differences in diagnosis and treatment.

Mortality from prostate cancer in FSU countries is lower compared to Germany, however, during recent years this difference has diminished (see Figure 4). In 2006, the age-standardised mortality rate per 100,000 males was 12.3 in Germany, 5.7 in Kazakhstan, 10.1 in the Russian Federation, and 9.3 in Ukraine (WHO, 2011b).

Incidence from prostate cancer is also much lower compared to Germany. In 2008, the age-standardised incidence rate was estimated to be 82.7 in Germany, 10.9 in Kazakhstan, 26.1 in the Russian Federation, and 20.3 in Ukraine (Ferlay, 2010). Low incidence in countries of the FSU is likely due to less prostate specific antigen (PSA) testing and may also represent a general underestimation of cancer incidence. This results in an incidence : mortality ratio of 7 in Germany and only 2 in Kazakhstan, 2.5 in the Russian Federation, and 2 in Ukraine.

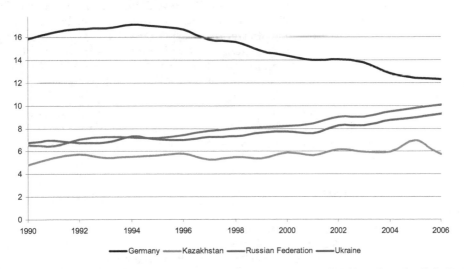

Fig. 4. Age-standardized prostate cancer mortality rates per 100,000 (Segi Standard) (WHO, 2011b)

1.5 Aims of the study and expected findings

Our studies focus on the health profile of ethnic German migrants from the Former Soviet Union in Germany. The presented work focuses on mortality and incidence of prostate cancer.

We compare two cohorts of Aussiedler to the autochthonous German population to investigate the Aussiedler's overall health status with regard to all cause mortality, and overall cancer and prostate cancer incidence and mortality. For prostate cancer we also consider the influence of age and length of stay in Germany in order to differentiate between the effects of genetic versus life-style dependent factors.

The two study cohorts are located in different Federal States of Germany. The Saarland cohort provides information on cancer incidence and mortality of the Aussiedler, whereas the North Rhine Westphalian cohort provides information on mortality only.

Aussiedler are exposed to different kinds of risk factors in different times of their lives. Before migration they are exposed to risk factors in their countries of origin, which have different disease patterns than Germany. Later, the Aussiedler are exposed to the migration process itself which can cause mental stress and, finally, they are exposed to the German pattern of risk factors.

Since most Aussiedler migrated to Germany at the beginning of the 1990s the mortality crisis in countries of the FSU could have influenced their health status. High mortality rates in their countries of origin and physical as well as psychological stress caused by migration was thought to negatively affect the general health of the Aussiedler. On the other hand, the better health care system in Germany may have improved their health status, if they have access to it. Additionally, social integration may also influence their health status.

A previous study confirmed the hypothesis that Aussiedler experienced higher mortality only for specific causes of death. In contrast, overall mortality of the Aussiedler was lower compared to the German population (Becher et al., 2007).

In general, few migrant studies assess cancer incidence and even fewer investigate both cancer incidence and mortality. Most investigations that do are occupational cancer studies, which describe health risks associated with workplace exposures only.

Aussiedler are likely to have higher mortality rates for all cancers due to country of origin effects. With regards to prostate cancer, a slighty lower mortality compared to Germany is expected, and incidence rates should confirm the observed mortality pattern. A previous study showed no differences in incidence and mortality for all cancers and confirmed expectations for prostate cancer, although it had incomplete follow up (Winkler et al., 2009). It is likely that incidence and mortality rates of the Aussiedler and the German population converge with time. This has already been shown for stomach cancer (Ronellenfitsch et al., 2009).

2. Materials and methods

2.1 Study population
2.1.1 North Rhine Westphalian cohort

In 2001, the North Rhine Westphalian (NRW) cohort was established (Ronellenfitsch et al., 2004). In brief, routine information from the Aussiedler reception centre of NRW was collected to setup a cohort. The original dataset included all Aussiedler from countries of the FSU who settled in NRW between 1990 and 2001.

The dataset contains information on name, date of birth, date of arrival in Germany, sex, country of origin, first city of residence and a unique code that identified members of the same family. After sample size calculation the cohort was restricted to a representative sample of 34,393 Aussiedler who were at least 15 years old when they migrated to Germany.

To ascertain vital status of each cohort member until the 31st December 2005 a follow up procedure was performed: Letters were sent to local registry offices in the cities of residence. In case of someone moving to another city, the registry provided the new city of residence and date of moving. The registry of the new city was then contacted until the individual was located. Changes of residence were recorded in a database with the exact date of moving. In the case of death, date and city of death were provided by the local registry office.

Cause of death was either ascertained through a record linkage system of the NRW regional statistical office or through the local health offices. The record linkage system has been described in detail by Klug and colleagues (2003). Local health offices provided an anonymous copy of the relevant death certificate. All copies of death certificates were then professionally coded at the Saarland Cancer Registry by International Classification of Diseases (ICD).

2.1.2 Saarland cohort

The Aussiedler reception centre of the Saarland could not provide a dataset with the standard information on the Aussiedler as in NRW. As an alternative, all local refugee offices of the Saarland were contacted to ask for access to their available data on the Aussiedler. In order to be eligible for the Saarland cohort, migrants must have arrived in Germany between 1990 and 2005 from countries of the FSU.

All together information on 26,384 Aussiedler (more than 90% of all Aussiedler who settled in the Saarland during the respective period) was available. The dataset contains name, date of birth, date of German passport as an approximation for date of migration, sex, country of birth for about 70% of the cohort, and first city of residence. The final cohort consisted of a sample of 18,619 individuals without missing data.

Follow up and cause of death ascertainment used the same method as for the NRW cohort. Follow up for cancer incidence was done directly by the Saarland cancer registry. Most individuals were identified by name, sex and date of birth. However, many Aussiedler change names during the first years of stay in Germany complicating simple identification by name. To minimize this problem the name matching procedure was done phonetically. For some individuals, city of residence was used as an additional variable to ensure correct identification. 43 cases were excluded from the analysis because they were already diagnosed in their country of origin.

All analyses were restricted to the first cancer diagnosis; multiple tumours per individual were not considered.

2.1.3 Data for comparison

For evaluation of the Aussiedler's cancer incidence and mortality in comparison to the autochthonous German population, rates for comparison are needed. To analyse mortality, rates of the German population were used. Although these rates include the

Aussiedler as a part of the German population, this should not bias the results of the comparison. For cardiovascular disease mortality it has been shown that the Aussiedler's influence on German mortality is limited to approximately 1% (Deckert et al., 2010). German mortality rates were calculated using the WHO mortality database (WHO, 2011b). Before 1998 causes of death are coded with 9th revision of ICD, thereafter the 10th is used in Germany.

A comparison to German incidence is not possible for the period between 1990 and 2005, since nation-wide information on cancer incidence is not available. For those years German incidence is estimated on basis of the Saarland Cancer Registry. Therefore, we directly compare cancer incidence of the Saarland Aussiedler cohort to the Saarland population. The Saarland Cancer Registry provided data on Saarland population figures and number of cancer cases (Saarland Cancer Registry, 2008). Cancer incidence data is coded in ICD9 only.

2.2 Statistical methods
2.2.1 Calculation of person-time

In most cohort studies it is necessary to calculate the actual time-at-risk for each individual as person-time. The person-time is used to either calculate mortality or incidence rates of the cohort or to perform indirect standardization or multivariate analysis.

Person-time was calculated in person-years (PY) by a SAS® macro. The macro uses the three time variables of age, length of stay in Germany and calendar-year. The macro calculates and distributes the person-years exactly to the day. Age and length of stay are categorized in one year intervals. Afterwards age is categorized into five year age groups up to 85 and older.

2.2.2 Indirect standardization

For comparing Aussiedler incidence and mortality with the German/Saarland population, indirect standardization was used. Compared to the method of direct standardization, the indirect method is advantageous when the stratum-specific rates of one of the populations to be compared are based on small numbers. In this case one can use the more stable rates of the larger population for the indirect standardization, thus gaining robustness with regard to sampling variation (Breslow and Day, 1987).

The standardized mortality ratio (SMR), and the standardized incidence ratio (SIR) are given by the observed number of events O (incident cases or number of deaths) divided by the number of events which one would expect E if the cohort had the mortality rate of the population used for standardization. Equation 1 shows the SMR as an example.

$$SMR = \frac{O}{E} = \frac{\sum_{i=1}^{i} O_i}{\sum_{i=1}^{i} py_i \lambda_i} \tag{1}$$

O_i gives the number of deaths in stratum i of the cohort. py_i gives the person-years in stratum i and λ_i the rate stratum j of the population used for standardization. All 95% confidence intervals (95% CI) were calculated using the exact method (Breslow and Day, 1987).

2.2.3 Multivariate analysis: Poisson regression

It is possible to measure effects of different covariables e.g. age, length of stay in Germany, etc. on the SMR and SIR by categorization, but this method is limited because of small sample sizes in subcategories. Another approach classically used in cohort studies is a Poisson regression model, which assesses the effects of different covariables simultaneously. It is based on the Poisson distribution, which is an approximation of the binomial distribution applied in large samples where the probability of the outcome is small.

After transformation, the Poisson model estimating the SMR and the SIR can be written as given in equation 2. α is the intercept, β_i is the regression coefficient, and x_i is the vector of covariable i.

$$\log(O_i) = \log(E_i) + \alpha + \beta_i x_i \tag{2}$$

The Poisson model is a generalized linear model characterized by the dependence of the outcome on a linear predictor through a non-linear link function. The predictors β_i can be estimated by maximum likelihood estimation.

More detailed information on the statistical methods can be found elsewhere (Breslow and Day, 1987). Data management was done by using Microsoft Access® and analysis was performed with SAS® version 9.2.

3. Results

3.1 Descriptive results

Descriptive characteristics of both cohorts and results of the follow up procedure are presented in Table 1. The Saarland cohort was approximately half the size of the cohort in NRW. Females were slightly overrepresented in both cohorts. The arrival period for entering the cohort was four years longer for the Saarland cohort. The NRW study population was restricted by age at migration of 15 years or older, whereas the Saarland cohort had no age restriction. Thus, the Saarland cohort was on average younger. Country of origin distribution was similar for both cohorts: around 55% of the Aussiedler came from Kazakhstan, 37% from the Russian Federation. Other countries of the FSU contributed each less than 5%.

Overall, the NRW cohort accumulated 344,486.1 PY and the Saarland cohort 147,165.2 PY. Follow up of the NRW cohort was complete for 96.7% of the cohort members with a mean follow up time of 10.1 years. Overall 2,580 (7.5%) cohort members died. Causes of death were known for 94.8% of deceased persons. 1,138 (3.3%) persons were lost to follow-up within the observation period, which means their last date of contact was censored. Individuals were lost follow-up due to different reasons, if they moved abroad or moved to an unknown destination.

Vital status was known for 77.4% of individuals in the Saarland cohort. Mean follow up time was 8 years. 87% of individuals lost to follow-up were censored on the day of leaving the study area because they moved to another Federal State. Since the Saarland is a relatively small state people are much more likely to move into another state than in the NRW. During the observation period 780 (4.2%) persons died. Cause of death is known for all types of cancer. Between 1990 and 2005, 448 members of the Saarland cohort were diagnosed with a malignant neoplasm (ICD-9: 140-208; except 173).

	Migrant cohort in the Federal State of NRW	Migrant cohort in the Federal State of Saarland
Number of cohort members	34,393	18,619
Males (%)	16,734 (48.7%)	8,977 (48.2%)
Females (%)	17,659 (51.3%)	9,642 (51.8%)
Immigration period	1990-2001	1990-2005
1990-1993	14,728	6,933
1994-1997	11,441	6,536
1998-2001/5	8,224	5,150
Age restriction	15+	-
Mean age at migration (standard deviation; range)	40.0 (17.0; 15-97)	32.4 (19.8; 0-103)
Males	38.4 (16.0; 15-93)	30.9 (19.0; 0-95)
Females	41.5 (17.7; 15-97)	33.8 (20.4; 0-103)
Descriptive results of the follow-up procedure		
End of follow-up date	31-12-2005	31-12-2005
Mean time of follow-up	10.1 years	8.0 years
Person-years	346,671.5	148,313.1
Males	167,882.0	71703.4
Females	178,789.4	76,609.6
Alive	89.2%	73.2%
Dead	7.5%	4.2%
Lost to follow-up	3.3%	22.6%

Table 1. Descriptive results of the two Aussiedler cohorts, from North-Rhine Westphalia and Saarland

During the observation period, 28 men died due to prostate cancer in both cohorts. Their mean age of deaths was 76.9 years (Range: 60.8 - 92.1). In the Saarland cohort 35 men were diagnosed with prostate cancer. Mean age of diagnosis was 67.6 years (Range: 45.3 - 85.8;). Figure 5 displays all 35 incident prostate cancer cases, starting with their migration to Germany, their age at diagnosis and their final status. Most cases were alive at the end of the observation period. Two cases moved out of the study area and nine died during the observation. Three of the deceased men died from prostate cancer, one case (no. 30) was not diagnosed before death, and the cause of death is known from the death certificate only (DCO).

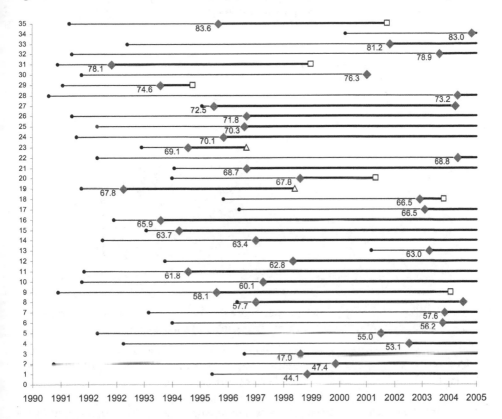

• migration to Germany ◆ date of diagnosis ◆ prostate cancer death □ non prostate cancer death △ moved out of study area

Fig. 5. Overview of all 35 incident prostate cancer cases with age at diagnosis from the Saarland cohort

3.2 Comparing mortality and incidence of the Aussiedler to Germany

This analysis of the Aussiedler in Germany focuses on prostate cancer. However, to place this in context of the Aussiedler's general health situation all cause mortality and mortality and incidence for all malignant neoplasms is presented. SMR is calculated for both cohorts together in comparison to the German population. SIR is based on the Saarland cohort in comparison to the Saarland population. Figure 6 shows SMR and SIR calculated for the whole observation period.

All cause mortality is significantly reduced for both sexes of the Aussiedler. In contrast, the mortality from all neoplasms is also reduced among females, but equal to the German population for males. Incidence of all cancer sites is somewhat lower for males compared to females, but not significantly reduced for either sex in comparison to the Saarland population.

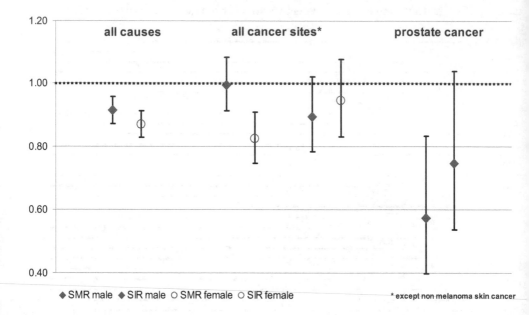

Fig. 6. Standardized mortality (SMR) and incidence (SIR) ratios for all causes, all cancer sites (except non melanoma skin cancer), and prostate cancer of the Aussiedler

Mortality from prostate cancer is strongly reduced among male Aussiedler with an SMR of 0.58 (95% CI: 0.40-0.83) for both cohorts combined. Cohort specific analysis shows a somewhat higher mortality among the NRW cohort compared to the Saarland cohort. In both cohorts mortality due to prostate cancer is significantly reduced.

Prostate cancer incidence is also reduced among the Aussiedler, however, the result is not significant with 0.75 (95% CI: 0.54-1.04).

3.3 Longitudinal effects on prostate cancer mortality and incidence of the Aussiedler

Results from the univariate analysis of prostate cancer mortality and incidence do not take into account the effect of different covariables, which might influence the SMR and SIR. Various covariables where considered to model longitudinal effects: age, calendar year, year of immigration, length of stay in Germany; cohort was considered for the analysis of mortality.

Multivariate Poisson regression did not show any significant effect of the considered covariables on mortality (data not shown). This is in contrast to the analysis of prostate cancer incidence. While the covariables length of stay and year of immigration did not reveal significant effects on the SIR, calendar year was nearly significant (estimate: -0.1213; p-value: 0.0650). Age, however, influenced the SIR. Table 2 shows the result of a model considering age as a dichotomised variable (age below 60 and over 60 years). The modelled SIR of Aussiedler being older than 60 years is 0.63 (exp(-0.47)). In contrast, the SIR of males aged below 60 years is 1.43 (exp(-0.46+0.83)).

	Estimate	p-value
intercept	-0.47	0.0165
age		
younger than 60 years	0.83	0.0401
older than 60 years*	0	-

*reference category

Table 2. Parameter estimates of the multivariable Poisson Model for the SIR function of prostate cancer

4. Discussion

The aim of the study was to analyse prostate cancer mortality and incidence among ethnic German migrants who came to Germany from the FSU after 1990. Additionally, we highlighted some general aspects of the Aussiedler's health profile to place prostate cancer incidence and mortality into a broader context. We analyzed two cohorts of migrants in terms of all cause mortality, overall cancer and prostate cancer mortality and incidence including longitudinal and age effects.

Methodological aspects of the cohorts and the statistical analysis have been discussed in detail elsewhere, they have been shown to be representative samples of the Aussiedler. representative (Klug et al., 2003; Ronellenfitsch et al., 2004; Becher et al., 2007; Winkler et al., 2009). In brief, both cohort studies have the pros and cons of historical cohort studies. It is possible to give valid estimates of Aussiedler mortality and incidence in terms of SMR and SIR. Indirect standardization is more appropriate for rare outcomes than direct standardization, resulting in the calculation of rates (McMichael and Giles, 1988). A limitation of this study is that we did not have access to information on potentially important risk factors such as lifestyle.

Results for all causes of deaths were significantly lower compared to the autochthon German population. Overall SMR is reduced for the Aussiedler, therefore, they seem to be healthier or more resistant than the Germans and therefore they are much healthier than populations of countries from the FSU.

Whether this is due to the healthy migrant effect is not immediately clear. For groups like the Aussiedler who have a legal right to migrate to Germany without fulfilling any prerequisites (at least in times when the majority immigrated), it may be assumed that the impact of self-selection on mortality trends is attenuated due to the small number of people staying in the country of origin. The assumption that almost all ethnic Germans migrated to Germany is supported by the continuously declining numbers of newly arriving Aussiedler. On the other hand, declining numbers of migrants may also be due to changes in German law. In addition, there are no official statistics about the number of ethnic Germans for the USSR nor for the FSU and estimations are highly controversial. There are estimates that approximately one million ethnic Germans live in the FSU (Ohliger, 1998). However, an analysis of family size in the NRW cohort shows that the Aussiedler tend to migrate with their whole complete family. Therefore, we think the healthy migrant theory is not applicable to this group of migrants.

The lower overall mortality is largely due to lower cardiovascular disease mortality, which is the predominant cause of death. Reasons for the reduced mortality remain unclear, but may be the result of genetic selection. For centuries the Aussiedler lived as a relatively closed group of people, which was only partly assimilated in the last decades of the USSR.

Among males, incidence and mortality due to all malignant neoplasms is neither different from the autochthon population nor different from each other. However, male cancer incidence is lower compared to mortality and to female cancer incidence. A possible explanation may be that in general males do not utilize health services as well as females. This may also lead to lower mortality among females.

Additionally, smaller differences between SIR and SMR may be explained by differences in the underlying populations for comparison. SMR was calculated on the basis of German rates and SIR on the basis of rates from the Saarland population.

Overall cancer incidence and mortality of the Aussiedler is comparable to the German population. Although there are larger differences for specific cancer sites (data not shown). Mortality for all cancer sites among females is lower, which is largely due to low mortality due to breast and lung cancer

The analysis of prostate cancer mortality and incidence revealed several interesting points. First, there was no difference between the mean age of death from prostate cancer in the Aussiedler and the Saarland population, at 76.9 and 77.5 years of age, respectively. However, mean age of diagnosis was 2.5 years earlier among Aussiedler, but this difference was not significant, which might be due to the limited number of observations.

Overall evaluation of prostate cancer shows lower mortality in Aussiedler than in the German population. Multivariate analysis did not reveal any longitudinal trends or differences in age patterns of dying from prostate cancer. However, this could be due to the relatively small number of observed deaths.

Prostate cancer diagnosis is lower among Aussiedler, but clearly higher than mortality. Poisson regression also revealed that Aussiedler below 60 have significantly more prostate cancer diagnoses than the Saarland population of this age. Longitudinal covariables had no significant effect on the SIR.

5. Conclusion

The Aussiedler are a unique group of diaspora migrants. There are few examples in the world of the migration of a large ethnic group from one country to another in a similarly short time period. Kazakhstan and Russia, the main countries of origin, have very different disease patterns than Germany, which may influence the risk profile of the Aussiedler. Studying the health risks of the Aussiedler not only helps to improve the health care they receive in Germany but also has wider implications for understanding the etiology of disease. The strength of this study is its cohort design. However, the retrospective cohort design relies on data from public registries and does not include information on individual risk factors such as lifestyle, which may also be important.

Results were in contrast to expectations based on country of origin data. Aussiedler have a lower mortality due to all causes of death, which cannot yet be explained completely. Cancer mortality and cancer incidence also differ from FSU countries, but are relatively equal to German rates, however, there are big differences in cancer site specific rates.

Prostate cancer mortality and incidence is lower among the Aussiedler and somehow reflects the situation in the FSU. Analysis did not reveal any short-term convergence of the Aussiedler's prostate cancer to German rates as would be expected in lifestyle driven cancer sites. Therefore, our results support the hypothesis of a relatively strong genetic influence on the development of prostate cancer.

6. Acknowledgment

Many thanks to Robin Nesbitt for language editing and critical thoughts on the manuscript.

7. References

Arnold, M.; Razum, O. & Coebergh, JW. (2010). Cancer risk diversity in non-western migrants to Europe: An overview of the literature. *Eur J Cancer*, 46, 14, (September 2010), pp. 2647-59, ISSN 1879-0852

Bade, KJ. & Oltmer, J. (1999). *Aussiedler: deutsche Einwanderer aus Osteuropa* (Volume 8), IMIS, ISBN 978-3-89971-120-2, Osnabrück

Becher, H.; Razum, O.; Kyobutungi, C.; Laki, J.; Ott, JJ.; Ronellenfitsch, U. & Winkler, V. (2007). Mortalität von Aussiedlern aus der ehemaligen Sovietunion: Ergebnisse einer Kohortenstudie. *Deutsches Ärzteblatt*, 104, 23, (June 2007), pp. A-1655-62

Breslow, NE. & Day, NE. (1987). *Statistical Methods in Cancer Research. The Design and Analysis of Cohort Studies* (Volume II), International Agency for Research on Cancer, ISBN 978-9-28320-182-3, Lyon

Chu, KC.; Tarone, RE. & Freeman, HP. (2003). Trends in prostate cancer mortality among black men and white men in the United States. *Cancer*, 97, 6, (March 2003), pp. 1507-16, ISSN 0008-543X

Deckert, A.; Winkler, V.; Paltiel, A.; Razum, O. & Becher, H. (2010). Time trends in cardiovascular disease mortality in Russia and Germany from 1980 to 2007 - are there migration effects? *BMC Public Health*, 10, 488, (August 2010), ISSN 1471 2458

Destatis. (2008). Bevölkerung, In: *Auszug aus dem Datenreport 2008*, 19.05.2011, Available from
http://www.destatis.de/jetspeed/portal/cms/Sites/destatis/Internet/DE/Conte nt/Publikationen/Querschnittsveroeffentlichungen/Datenreport/Downloads/Dat enreport2008Bevoelkerung,property=file.pdf

Destatis. (2008). Bevölkerungsentwicklung 2008, In: *Wirtschaft und Statistik*, 03.04.2011, Available from:
http://www.destatis.de/jetspeed/portal/cms/Sites/destatis/Internet/DE/Conte nt/Publikationen/Querschnittsveroeffentlichungen/WirtschaftStatistik/Bevoelker ung/Bevoelkentwicklung042010,property=file.pdf

Eisfeld A. (1999). *Die Russlanddeutschen* (Volume 2.2), Stiftung Ostdeutscher Kulturrat, ISBN 978-3784423821, München

Federal Central Office for Political Education. (2000). *Aussiedler* (Volume 267), Informationen zur politischen Bildung, Bonn

Federal Ministry of the Interior. (2009). *Migrationsbericht 2009*, 02.03.2011, Available from: http://www.bmi.bund.de/SharedDocs/Downloads/DE/Broschueren/2011/Migrationsbericht_2009_de.pdf?__blob=publicationFile

Federal Office of Administration. (2011). *Spätaussiedler und ihre Angehörigen Jahresstatistik 2010*, 12.05.2011, Available from: http://www.bva.bund.de/cln_180/DE/Aufgaben/Abt__III/Spaetaussiedler/statistik/Jahre/J__Jahresstatistik2010,templateId=raw,property=publicationFile.pdf/J_J ahresstatistik2010.pdf

Fennelly, K. (2007). The "healthy migrant" effect. *Minn Med*, 90, 3, (March 2007), pp. 51-3, ISSN 0026-556X

Ferlay, J.; Shin, HR.;, Bray, F.; Forman, D.; Mathers, C. & Parkin, DM. (2010). *GLOBOCAN 2008 Cancer Incidence and Mortality Worldwide*, 08.01.2011, Available from: http://globocan.iarc.fr

Grönberg, H. (2003). Prostate cancer epidemiology. *Lancet*, 361, 9360, (March 2003), pp. 859-64, ISSN 0140-6736

IOM. (2005). *Costs and Benefits of International Migration* (Volume 882), International Organization for Migration, Geneva

Jasso, G.; Massey, DS.; Rosenzweig, MR. & Smith, JP. (2004). *Immigrant Health: Selectivity And Acculturation*, 21.04.2011, Available from: http://129.3.20.41/eps/lab/papers/0412/0412002.pdf

Klug, SJ.; Zeeb, H. & Blettner, M. (2003). New research avenues in exploring causes of death in Germany via regional statistical offices as exemplified by a retrospective cohort study. *Gesundheitswesen*, 65, 4, (April 2003), pp. 243-9, ISSN 0941-3790

Lee, ES. (1966). A Theory of Migration. *Demography* 3, 1, (n.d.), pp. 47-57

Leon, DA.; Chenet, L.; Shkolnikov, VM.; Zakharov, S.; Shapiro, J. & Rakhmanova, G. (1997). Huge variation in Russian mortality rates 1984-94: artefact. alcohol. or what? *Lancet*, 350, 9075, (August 1997), pp. 383-8, ISSN 0140-6736

Marmot, MG.; Adelstein, AM. & Bulusu, L. (1984). Lessons from the study of immigrant mortality. *Lancet*, 1, 8392, (June 1984), pp. 1455-7, ISSN 0140-6736

McCredie, M. (1998). Cancer epidemiology in migrant populations. *Recent Results Cancer Res*, 154, (February 1998), pp. 298-305, ISSN 0080-0015

McKay, L.; Macintyre, S. & Ellaway, A. (2003). *Migration and Health: a review of the International literature*, MRC Social and Public Health Sciences Unit, ISBN 1-901519-05-8, Glasgow

McMichael, AJ. & Giles. GG. (1988). Cancer in migrants to Australia: extending the descriptive epidemiological data. *Cancer Res*, 48, 3, (February 1988), pp. 751-6, ISSN 0008-5472

Men, T.; Brennan, P.; Boffetta, P. & Zaridze, D. (2003). Russian mortality trends for 1991-2001: analysis by cause and region. *Br Med J*, 327, 721, (October 2003), pp. 964, ISSN 1468-5833

Ohliger, R. (1998). *Deutschland: Rückgang des Zuzugs von Ausländern*, 01.02.2011, Available from: http://www.unics.uni-hannover.de/bollm/wandel/aussiedl.htm

Parkin, DM. & Khlat, M. (1996). Studies of cancer in migrants: rationale and methodology. *Eur J Cancer*, 32A, 5 (May 1996), pp. 761-71, ISSN 0959-8049

Patel, AR. & Klein, EA. (2009). Risk factors for prostate cancer. *Nat Clin Pract Urol*, 6, 2, (February 209), pp. 87-95, ISSN 1743-4289

Pohl, OJ. (2001). *The deportation and destruction of the German minority in the USSR*, 12.02.2011, Available from: http://www.odessa3.org/journal/pohl.pdf

Robert Koch Institute. (2011). Prostata (C61), In: *Excel-Tabellen zu Inzidenz und Mortalität*, 05.04.2011, Availaible from:
http://www.rki.de/cln_169/nn_203956/DE/Content/GBE/DachdokKrebs/KID /Lokalisationen__Tabellen/C61,templateId=raw,property=publicationFile.xls/C 61.xls

Robert Koch Institute (Ed.) und Gesellschaft der epidemiologischen Krebsregister in Deutschland e. V. (Ed.). (19.02.2008). *Krebs in Deutschland 2003-2004, Häufigkeiten und Trends*, 6. Auflage. Robert Koch Institute, ISBN 978-3-89606-182-9, Berlin

Robert Koch Institute (Ed.) und Gesellschaft der epidemiologischen Krebsregister in Deutschland e. V. (Ed.). (23.02.2010). *Krebs in Deutschland 2005/2006. Häufigkeiten und Trends*. 7 Ausgabe. Robert Koch Institute, ISBN 978-3-89606-207-9, Berlin

Ronellenfitsch, U.; Kyobutungi, C.; Becher, H. & Razum O. (2004). Large-scale. population-based epidemiological studies with record linkage can be done in Germany. *Eur J Epidemiol*, 19, 12, (April 2004), pp. 1073-4, ISSN 0393-2990

Ronellenfitsch, U.; Kyobutungi, C.; Ott, JJ.; Paltiel, A.; Razum, O.; Schwarzbach, M.; Winkler, V. & Becher, H. (2009). Stomach cancer mortality in two large cohorts of migrants from the Former Soviet Union to Israel and Germany: are there implications for prevention? *Eur J Gastroenterol Hepatol*, 21, 4, (April 2009), pp. 409-16, ISSN 1473-5687

Saarland cancer registry. (2008). *Interactive Database*, 19.04.2011, Availaible from: http://www krebsregister.saarland.de/datenbank/datenbank.html

Statistisches Bundesamt. (2007). *Deutschland Anzahl der Gestorbenen nach Kapiteln der International Statistical Classification of Diseases and Related Health Problems Version 2.24.0. 2007*, 22.04.2011, Availaible from: http://www.destatis.de

Thomas, DB. & Karagas, MR. (1987). Cancer in first and second generation Americans. *Cancer Res*, 47, 21, (November 1987), pp. 5771-6, ISSN 0008-5472

WHO. (2011). *European health for all database*, 02.05.2011, Availaible from: http://data.euro.who.int/hfadb/

WHO. (2011). *WHO Mortality Database*, 02.02.2011, Available from: http://www.who.int/healthinfo/morttables/en/index.html

Winkler, V.; Ott, JJ.; Holleczek, B.; Stegmaier, C. & Becher, H. (2009). Cancer profile of migrants from the Former Soviet Union in Germany: incidence and mortality. *Cancer Causes Control*, 20, 10, (December 2009), pp. 1873-9, ISSN 1573-7225

World Health Organization. (2004). Annex Table 2: Deaths by cause. sex and mortality stratum in WHO regions, In: *The world health report 2004 - changing history*, 11.10.2010, Available from: http://www.who.int/whr/2004/en/report04_en.pdf

Zeeb, H.; Razum, O.; Blettner, M. & Stegmaier, C. (2002). Transition in cancer patterns among Turks residing in Germany. *Eur J Cancer* 38, 5, (March 2003), pp. 705-11, ISSN 0959-8049

Ziegler, H.; Stabenow, R.; Holleczek B. & Stegmaier C. (21.08.2009). *Krebs im Saarland, Ministerium für Justiz*, 03.05.2010, Availaible from: http://www.krebsregister.saarland.de/krebsatlas/EKRS_Krebsatlas_21082009.pdf

Polymorphism Analysis of TRAIL Gene and Correlation TRAIL Expression in Prostate Cancer

Yuanyuan Mi[1,2], Lijie Zhu[2] and Ninghan Feng[1,*]
[1]Department of Urology, The First Affiliated Hospital
of Nanjing Medical University, Nanjing
[2]Department of Urology, Third Affiliated Hospital
of Nantong University, Wuxi
China

1. Introduction

Prostate cancer (PCa) is the most common male non-dermatological cancer in Europe and the United States of America (USA), and the sixth leading cause of cancer related-deaths, accounting for 14% (903,500) of total new diagnosed cancer cases and 6% (258,400) of whole cancer deaths in males in 2008 [1]. Because the increased use of screening techniques testing serum concentrations of prostate-specific antigen (PSA) has meant that PCa is more commonly diagnosed and can be detected at an earlier stage, the incidence rates recorded primarily in the developed countries, such as Oceania, Europe and North America, were hight. In contrast, males of African individuals in the Caribbean region have the highest PCa mortality rates in the world, which is thought to reflect partly difference in genetic susceptibility [2, 3].

Death rates for PCa have been decreasing in many developed countries, including Australia, Canada, USA, the United Kingdom, Italy and Norway in part due to the improved treatment with curative intent [4-6]. Recently, one European-based trial on the efficacy of PSA testing could reduce the rate of death from PCa by 20% [7]. In contrast to the trends of western countries, incidence and mortality rates are rising in several Asian and central/eastern-European countries, such as Japan, China and Poland, suggesting an increasingly westernized lifestyle in these regions [4, 5]. The underlying etiology of PCa remains poorly understood, with both genetic predisposition and environmental factors (diet, lifestyle, older age, race, family history and hormone) likely to play an important role [8-10]. Despite this strong evidence for a genetic component in PCa, little progress has been made to identify a major gene or genes [11].

Tumor necrosis factor-related apoptosis inducing ligand (TRAIL) is a novel member of the TNF super-family and was first identified by Wiley in 1995 [12]. TRAIL is mapped to the long arm of chromosome 3q26 in humans and is composed of five exons. It encodes 1.77 kb mRNA. Similar to FasL, TRAIL is also a type II membrane protein which induces apoptosis in a wide variety of cancer cells and spares normal cells [12]. TRAIL-induced apoptosis is a multi-step process: it binds to death receptor 4 (DR4) and DR5 cell surface receptors leading

* Corresponding author: Ninghan Feng, MD, PhD.

to the formation of the death inducing signaling complex (DISC) that recruits caspase-8 via the adaptor protein Fas-associated with death domain protein (FADD). The formation of DISC and recruitment of caspase-8 leads to proteolytic activation of caspase-3 and caspase-7 leading to DNA fragmentation and apoptosis [13-15] (Fig. 1).

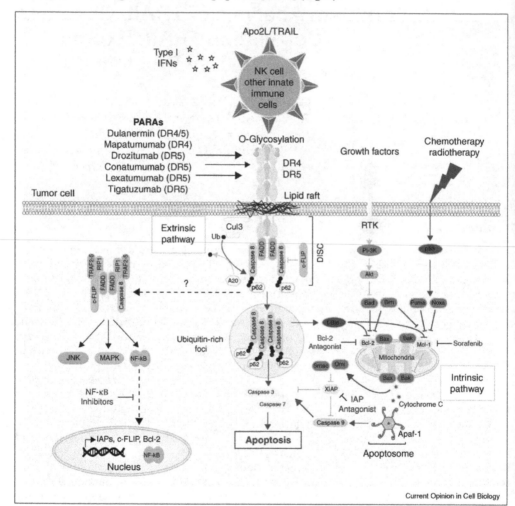

Fig. 1. TRAIL pathway for cancer therapy. DR4 and DR5 activation by PARAs (either trimeric rhApo2L/TRAIL or agonistic DR4 or DR5-specific antibodies) or Apo2L/TRAIL expressed by innate immune cells. FADD is recruited to DR4 or DR5 located within lipid raft containing regions of the membrane, which promotes receptor clustering and autocatalytic processing of the apoptosis initiating proteases caspase-8 or caspase-10 to form the active DISC. Caspase-8 can be polyubiquitylated at the DISC by a cullin-3/Rbx1-based E3 ubiquitin ligase, which facilitates caspase-8 activation. This process is negatively regulated by the de-ubiquitinating enzyme, A20. The signaling adaptor p62 can bind to ubiquitilated caspase-8 and translocate it to ubiquitin-rich foci, which may also enhance its activity. In many cancer cells, proapoptotic

signaling involves the mitochondrial pathway via caspase-8-mediated cleavage of Bid to t-Bid. Proapoptotic signaling through the intrinsic pathway is further regulated by pro apoptotic and anti apoptotic members of the Bcl-2 family. Receptor tyrosine kinase (RTK) signaling and chemotherapy or radiotherapy can further modulate the intrinsic proapoptotic pathway through targeting Bcl-2 family members. Under certain circumstances, DR4 or DR5 signaling can promote alternative signaling pathways such as JNK, MAPK or NF$_k$B, which may require recruitment of RIP1 and TRAF2 or TRAFs5 to form secondary signaling complexes. Depicted in blue are inhibitors that may enhance proapoptotic signaling by PARAs by targeting mechanisms of resistance in tumor cells. (This picture was cited from Yang et al. [50] Current Opinion in Cell Biology. 2010)

Several single nucleotide polymorphisms (SNPs) present along the TRAIL gene located in the 3q26 region have been found in both healthy and disease individuals, including four SNPs in the 5′ regulatory region [16], two SNPs within exons, and five SNPs in the 3′ untranslated regions[17-18]. TRAIL gene polymorphisms were also identified in patients with multiple sclerosis [19, 20] and fatty liver disease [21].
Recently, a SNP of -716A>G polymorphism (rs12488654) in the promoter region of TRAIL gene has been found to be associated with breast cancer with functional implications both in vitro and vivo studies [22]. To date, there have been no data about the association between this polymorphism and PCa, so we first explored the role of the TRAIL A>G polymorphism in PCa patients in southern Chinese Han descent. Moreover, we detected the serum levels of TRAIL expression with different genotypes in cases to characterize the functional consequences of TRAIL -716 A>G polymorphism.

2. Materials and methods

2.1 Study population
One hundred and eighty-seven PCa patients were newly diagnosed between November 2009 and May 2010 in the First Affiliated Hospital of Nanjing Medical University (Jiangsu Province Hospital) in Nanjing, China. All PCa cases were between 51 and 94 years of age and were diagnosed with the disease within the last one year; all controls were between 47 and 96 years of age. All cases were diagnosed with PCa through needle biopsy (ultrasoundguided transrectal needle biopsy of prostate, 13-fold biopsy) or operation (radical prostatectomy and transurethral resection of the prostate). All the patients were southern Chinese Han descent. The control group (n = 237) was age-matched and the subjects were healthy checkup examinees without cancer history and were collected in the same period. Controls were excluded if they ever had abnormal appearance of pathology, abnormal prostate-specific antigen test (i.e., ≥ 4 ng/ml), abnormal digital rectal examination, other previous cancer diagnosis, symptom of any prostate disease or abnormal appearance of other auxiliary examination including computed tomography urography (CTU), magnetic resonance urography (MRU), positron emission tomographic (PET), transrectal ultrasonography and so on.
After informed consent was obtained, 2 ml peripheral blood sample was collected and each subject was asked to finish a questionnaire including age, weight, height, race, tobacco use, alcohol use, family history of cancer and so on. In our present research, smoking more than five cigarettes per day for more than 5 years was defined as smoking; drinking habit was defined as drinking at least three times per week and lasting more than 10 years; family history of cancer was defined as cancer in first-degree relatives (parents, siblings, or

children); disease stage was determined by pathologic findings, pelvic computed tomography, magnetic resonance image and radio-nucleotide bone scans, the tumor stage was determined using tumor-node-metastasis (TNM) classification and graded according to WHO guidelines; pathologic grade was recorded as the Gleason score.

2.2 Genotyping

Polymorphisms were analyzed by polymorphism chain reaction and ligase detection reaction (PCR-LDR). Each PCR reaction was done in a total volume of 15 ul, which contains 1 ul genomic DNA, 2.5 pmol of each promer, 10× buffer 1.5 ul, $MgCl_2$ 1.5 ul, 0.3 ul of dNTP (MBI, Inc.), 0.25 ul of Taq DNA Polymerase (MBI, Inc.) and ddH_2O 9.95 ul. PCR was subjected to 35 thermal cycles at 94°C 15 sec, 56°C for 15 sec, and 72°C for 60 sec conducted on the ABI 9600 (ABI, Inc.). Primers were 5′-TGACGACTTCTTCCTCTTTGC-3′ (sense) 5′-GATAGTGACAGCGAGACATTG-3′ (antisense). The probes for LDR were: 5′-P-GTAGGAAGTAGTTGACACACTCAGATTT-FAM-3′ with common phosphorylated 5′-end and 6-carboxy X-uorescein (FAM) labeled 3′-end, the A-specific probe 5′ TTTTCATGCCTGTGTGTTAGGCTGCACAA-3′, the G-specific probe 5′-tttttTTCATGCCTGTGTGTTAGGCTGCACAG-3′. For each PCR product, the ligation reaction was performed in a final volume of 10 ul, which contains 3 ul PCR product, 10×Taq DNA ligase buffer 1 ul, 5 U of Taq DNA ligase (NEB, Inc.,), 0.1 pmol of each probe, and ddH_2O 5.575 ul. The LDR parameters were as follows: 25 thermal cycles at 94 °C for 30 sec and 60°C for 30 min. The LDR reaction products were analyzed on ABI 3730 DNA Sequencer (ABI, Inc.,). To confirm the accuracy of PCR-LDR genotyping method, direct DNA sequencing of randomly selected PCR products was performed. The proportion of the sequencing samples were about 5%, the results of the PCR-LDR genotyping showed 100% concordance to direct DNA sequencing of the randomly selected PCR products.

2.3 Enzyme-linked immunosorbent assay (ELISA)

Blood was collected in standard cubes without anticoagulant and was immediately centrifuged for 20 min, at 3,000 rpm. Serums were stored at -808°C until serum TRAIL levels were measured by ELISA kit (R&D Systems, Inc.). The optical density was determined by measuring the absorbance at 450 nm. The absorbance was correlated against a standard curve.

2.4 Statistical analysis

Hardy–Weinberg equilibrium (HWE) was tested among controls using the Pearson chi-square test. Differences in the distributions of demographic characteristics, selected variables and frequencies of genotypes of TRAIL -716 A>G polymorphism between the cases and controls were evaluated by using the student's t-test (for continuous variables) or chi-square (χ^2) test (for categorical variables). The odds ratios (OR) and 95% confidence internals (CI) were calculated by logistic regression analysis to quantify the association between TRAIL -716 A>G polymorphism and risk of PCa with the adjustment for potential covariates (age, BMI, cigarette smoking, alcohol drinking and family history of cancers). The correlation between the serum TRAIL levels and genotypes of TRAIL -716 A>G polymorphism were evaluated by one-way ANOVA. A P-value < 0.05 was considered statistically significant and all statistical tests were two sided. All statistical analyses were performed with Statistics Analysis System software (Version 9.1.3; SAS Institute, Inc., Cary, NC).

3. Results

3.1 Characteristics of the study population

One hundred and eighty-seven patients and 237 cancer-free controls were enrolled in our study. The distribution of relevant demographic and clinical characteristics is presented in Table 1. Baseline characteristics were similar between cases and controls, except that the frequency of relatives with cancer from the case group was higher, compared to non-relatives (27.27% vs. 15.61%, $P = 0.003$); there were more subjects who had larger body mass index (>23 kg/m^2) among the cases than among the controls (60.43% vs. 50.21%, $P = 0.036$), the frequency of ever alcohol drinking in cases was higher than in controls (34.22% vs. 20.68%, $P = 0.002$) and the mean ± SD PSA levels of PCa patients and control subjects were 80.45 ± 262.25 and 2.14 ± 1.42 ng/ml, respectively ($P < 0.001$).

Characteristics	Csaes (n=187)		Controls (n=237)		P-Value
	n	%	n	%	
Age (year)					0.687
≤70	55	29.41	74	31.22	
>70	132	70.59	163	68.78	
BMI (kg/m2)					0.036
≤23	74	39.57	118	49.79	
>23	113	60.43	119	50.21	
Cigarette smoking					0.839
Never	81	43.32	105	44.30	
Ever	106	56.68	132	55.70	
Alcohol drinking					0.002
Never	123	65.78	188	79.32	
Ever	64	34.22	49	20.68	
Family history of cancers					0.003
No	136	72.73	200	84.39	
Yes	51	27.27	37	15.61	
PSA(ng/ml)					
Mean ± SD	80.45	±262.25	2.14	±1.42	<0.001
Clinical stage					
Localized	86	46.00			
Advanced	101	54.00			
Gleason score					
<7	50	26.74			
= 7	70	37.43			
>7	67	35.82			

BMI: body mass index

Table 1. Demographic characteristic of PCa cases and controls

3.2 Genotype distributions of TRAIL -716 A>G polymorphism and risk of PCa

The distribution of TRAIL -716 A>G in the control group was 21.10% for AA homozygote, 51.48% for AG heterozygote, 27.42% for GG homozygote, and was in Hardy–Weinberg equilibrium ($\chi^2 = 0.268$, $P = 0.604$). As shown in Table 2, the TRAIL -716 A>G polymorphism was not associated with total PCa. After adjusting for potential covariates (age, BMI, cigarette smoking, alcohol drinking, family history of cancers), compared with AA homozygote, subjects carrying GG homozygote did not have any association between cases and controls (OR = 0.94, 95%CI = 0.69-1.27, P = 0.397). In addition, no association was also found between subjects carrying AG/GG genotypes and AA homozygote (OR = 0.87, 95%CI = 0.54-1.41, P = 0.577).

Genotype	PCa, No. (%)	Controls[a], No. (%)	P-value[b]	Adjusted OR(95%CI)[c]
Total	187	237		
AA	44(23.53)	50(21.10)		1.00(reference)
AG	98(52.41)	122(51.48)	0.712	0.89(0.54-1.47)
GG	45(24.06)	65(27.42)	0.397	0.94(0.69-1.27)
AA	44(23.53)	50(21.10)		1.00(reference)
AG+GG	143(76.47)	187(78.90)	0.577	0.87(0.54-1.41)

[a]The genotype frequencies among the control subjects were in agreement with the Hardy-Weinberg equilibrium ($\chi2$ = 0.268, P = 0.604).
[b]Two-sided $\chi2$ test for the distributions of genotypes frequencies between the cases and controls.
[c]Odd ratios (ORs) were obtained from a logistic regression model with adjusting for age, BMI, cigarette smoking, alcohol drinking, family history of cancers; 95%CI, 95% confidence interval.

Table 2. Genotypes in patients with PCa and controls

3.3 Stratified analysis
The association between genotypes and PCa risk stratified by disease stage (Localized: $T_{1-2}N_0M_0$; Advanced: $T_{3-4}N_XM_X$ or $T_XN_1M_X$ or $T_XN_XM_1$), pathologic grade (Gleason score < 7, = 7 and >7) and serum PSA level ($\leq$ 20 and >20) is shown in Table 3. These associations were in the same direction for advanced, higher grade disease and PSA level but were not statistically significant.

Variables	TRAIL-716A/G AA,No.(%)	TRAIL-716A/G AG/GG,No.(%)	P-value[a]	Adjusted OR (95% CI)[b]
Control	50(21.10)	187(78.90)		1.00(reference)
Clinical stage[c]				
Localized	15(17.65)	70(82.35)	0.644	1.17(0.60-2.27)
Advanced	29(28.43)	73(71.57)	0.158	0.67(0.38-1.17)
Gleason score				
<7	6(12.00)	44(88.00)	0.117	2.14(0.83-5.53)
= 7	19(27.14)	51(72.86)	0.226	0.68(0.36-1.27)
>7	19(28.36)	48(71.64)	0.117	0.59(0.31-1.14)
PSA				
$\leq$ 20	16(17.58)	75(82.42)	0.626	1.17(0.62-2.23)
>20	28(28.87)	69(71.13)	0.121	0.64(0.36-1.13)

[a]Two-sided $\chi2$ test for the distributions of genotypes frequencies between the cases and controls.
[b]Odd ratios (ORs) were obtained from a logistic regression model with adjusting for age, BMI, cigarette smoking, alcohol drinking, family history of cancers; 95%CI, 95% confidence interval.
[c]Localized: T1-2N0M0; Advanced: T3-4NXMX or TXN1MX or TXNXM1 [according to the international tumor-node-metastasis (TNM) staging system for PCa].

Table 3. TRAIL-716A/G and clinico-pathological characteristics in patients with PCa

In addition, as show in Table 4, the association between TRAIL -716 A>G polymorphism and PCa did not vary by cigarette smoking and alcohol drinking. However, the association appeared stronger in subgroups of BMI >23kg/m² (OR = 0.58, 95%CI = 0.31-0.89), age ≤70 years (OR = 0.32, 95%CI = 0.12-0.87) and no family history of cancers (OR = 0.86, 95%CI = 0.51-0.96).

Variables	N (case/control)	Genotypes(case/control)				P-value[a]	Adjusted OR(95%CI) [b]
		AA genotype		AG/GG genotype			
		n	%	n	%		
Total	187/237	44/50	23.53/ 21.10	143 /187	76.47/ 78.90	0.577	0.87 (0.54-1.41)
Age(years)							
≤ 70	55/74	13/9	23.64/ 12.16	42/65	76.36/ 87.84	0.026	0.32 (0.12-0.87)
>70	132/163	31/41	23.48/ 25.15	101/ 122	76.52/ 74.85	0.575	1.17 (0.67-2.04)
BMI (kg/m2)							
≤ 23	74/118	12/27	16.22/ 22.88	62/91	83.78/ 77.12	0.165	1.78 (0.79-3.99)
>23	113/119	32/23	28.32/ 19.33	81/96	71.68/ 80.67	0.042	0.58 (0.31-0.89)
Cigarette smoking							
Never	81/105	20/26	24.69/ 24.76	61/79	75.31/ 75.24	0.967	0.99 (0.49-1.97)
Ever	106/132	24/24	22.64/ 18.18	82/ 108	77.36/ 81.82	0.535	0.81 (0.41-1.58)
Alcohol drinking							
Never	123/188	29/39	23.58/ 20.74	94/ 149	76.42/ 79.26	0.513	0.83 (0.48-1.45)
Ever	64/49	15/11	23.44/ 22.45	49/38	76.56/ 77.55	0.944	0.97 (0.38-2.45)
Family history of cancers							
No	136/200	34/44	25.00/ 22.00	102/ 156	75.00/ 78.00	0.034	0.86 (0.51-0.96)
Yes	51/37	10/6	19.61/ 16.22	41/31	80.39/ 83.78	0.972	1.02 (0.31-3.32)

[a]Two-sided χ2 test for the distributions of genotypes frequencies between the cases and controls.
[b]Odd ratios (ORs) were obtained from a logistic regression model with adjusting for age, BMI, cigarette smoking, alcohol drinking, family history of cancers; 95%CI, 95% confidence interval. BMI: body mass index.

Table 4. Association and stratification between TRAIL-716A/G and PCa risk.

3.4 Association of TRAIL -716 A>G polymorphism with expression levels of TRAIL

We collected 83 tumor serum samples obtained from in present study with different genotypes of the TRAIL -716 A>G polymorphism, and the distribution of the AA, AG, and

GG genotypes was 27 (32.53%), 44 (53.01%) and 12 (14.46%), respectively. Moreover, serum TRAIL levels in PCa patients with AG/GG genotypes were significantly higher than those with AA genotypes (901.18 ± 189.58 µg/L vs. 819.13 ± 111.00 µg/L, $P = 0.041$; Fig. 2)

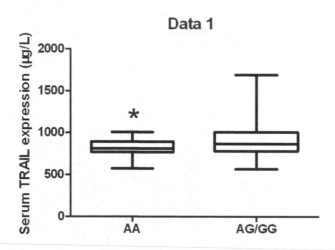

Fig. 2. Analysis of serum TRAIL levels in three groups of PCa cases with mean values (horizontal lines, mean values). * $P = 0.041$ compared with the AG/GG and AA genotypes.

4. Discussion

Recently, Kuribayashi et al. [23] indicated a direct regulation of TRAIL gene by p53 protein. Moreover, early growth response protein (EGR) [24], interferon regulatory factor 1 (IRF1) [25], NF-$_k$B [26], SP1 [27] and PU1 [28] have been implicated in the regulation of TRAIL. TRAIL is present in various tissues, particular in the prostate, spleen and lung.

TRAIL binds to two different types of receptors: death receptors and decoy receptors. TRAIL can also bind to osteoprotegerin (OPG) (a soluble inhibitor of receptor activator of NF-$_k$B ligand) at low affinity. To date, four human receptors specific for TRAIL have been recognized: the death receptors TRAIL-R1 (also know as DR4), TRAIL-R2 (also known as DR5), the putative decoy receptors TRAIL-R3 (DcR1) and TRAIL-R4 (DcR2). TRAIL-R1 (DR4) is expressed at very low levels in most human tissues including the spleen, thymus, liver, peripheral blood leukocytes, activated T cells, small intestine and some tumor cell lines. TRAIL-R2 (DR5) is ubiquitiously distributed both in normal and tumor cell lines but is more abundant in spleen, peripheral blood leukocytes, activated lymphocytes and hepatocyes [29-31].

TRAIL has attained the centre stage in anti-tumor drug discovery because of its efficacy in killing tumor cells without lethal toxicity in pre-clinical models apart from the inherent property to activate both the extrinsic and intrinsic apoptotic pathways [32-34].

Single nucleotide polymorphisms (SNPs) are the most abundant form of genetic variation in the human genome. By convention, a point mutation is referred to as a SNP when the frequency of the minor (rarer) allele exceeds 1% in at least one population. For example, a

SNP in a regulatory region may have an influence on gene transcription, a SNP located in a RNA splice site may affect RNA splicing, a SNP in the 3'-untranslated region of a gene may have an effect on mRNA stability, and a SNP in the coding region may result in an amino acid substitution in the encoded protein. It is thought that SNPs contribute to interindividual variability in susceptibility to common diseases such as cancer [35, 36].

So far, some published meta-analyses have confirmed that a number of SNPs are associated with increased or decreased PCa risk in different races, such as A49T in steroid-5-alpha-reductase, alpha polypeptide 2 (SRD5A2) gene [37], Gly388Arg in fibroblast growth factor receptor 4 (FGFR4) gene [38], -160C/A in E-cadherin (CDH1) gene [39], Val16Ala in manganese superoxide dismutase (MnSOD) gene [40], C677T in 5,10-methylenetetrahydrofolate reductase (MTHFR) gene [41].

Several studies have investigated the possible role of anti-tumor gene polymorphisms and the prevalence of PCa. This impairment of host factors might result in susceptibility or resistance to tumor progression. The transcription factor Sp3 (stimulatory protein 3) exhibits a similar DNA binding affinity for Sp1 consensus sequence [42-44] and represses the Sp1-mediated trans-activation of promoters with two or more Sp1 sites [45-47]. TRAIL has two Sp1 consensus sequences in the basal promoter [48, 49]. AA genotype at -716 in TRAIL promoter with additional Sp1 consensus sequence can decrease TRAIL expression due to the repression caused by binding of Sp3, whereas, GG genotype background at the same position can increase TRAIL expression because of the lower probability of Sp3 driven repression. To date, only one study [22] showed the association between TRAIL -716 A>G polymorphism and cancer risk: individuals with -716 GG genotype were at a greater risk of developing breast cancer, in addition, G allele resulted in a higher expression than the A allele to regulate the expression of TRAIL in four different cancer cell lines (HeLa, MCF-7, HepG2, HT1080).

To the best of our knowledge this is the first study investigating the genetic association of polymorphism of the -716 site in TRAIL gene with PCa and the expression of TRAIL with different genotypes in serum of cases in southern Chinese Han descent. No statistically significant association was observed between TRAIL -716 A>G polymorphism and PCa. Moreover, when stratifying the case group by clinical characteristics, the present study also did not find any association among PSA, Gleason and clinical stage. There must be some factors that would contribute to this discrepancy. First, TRAIL -716 A>G polymorphism might play a different role in different cancers. Second, multiple genes and environmental factors may lead to cancer formation. Third, race may be related to cancer. Either through common risk factors or other genes in linkage disequilibrium with TRAIL suggests that a possible role of ethnic differences is in genetic backgrounds and the environment they lived in.

Furthermore, we found that the decreased risk associated with the AG/GG genotypes was more pronounced in: subjects with age ≤70 years (OR = 0.32, 95%CI = 0.12-0.87) and no family history of cancers (OR = 0.86, 95%CI = 0.51-0.96). It confirmed the concept that younger age and no family history of cancers might be protective factors for PCa. In addition, we found that the OR for AG/GG genotypes was 0.58(95%CI = 0.31-0.89) among subjects with BMI >23kg/m². This finding may reflect that PCa formation may be subject to a variety of environmental and genetic factors. In these subgroups, other high level of genetic susceptibilities or other unknown risk factors may influence our results.

Except for above associated results, we detected the expression of TRAIL in the serums of the cases. We found that the protective genotypes AG/GG were associated with higher serum TRAIL expression when compared with the AA genotype. Previous one study [22] have reported that the G allele resulted in a higher expression than the A allele. Our work confirmed the findings of this study. Furthermore, since TRAIL can be measured in the blood and the serum level has been found significantly different in different genotypes in PCa cases, this may be a novel tumor marker and provide a future screening target. We need further investigations on the molecular mechanisms of how genetic variants might affect the TRAIL expression.

This study has several potential limitations. First of all, it is well known that sporadic and familial PCa have frequently quite different epidemiological and molecular peculiarities, clinical evolution and prognosis, so it is better to analysis these two kinds of PCa, respectively, however, we got together as a whole case group. Second, the numbers of cases/controls in our studies were not sufficiently large for a comprehensive analysis. Third, the control group in our study contained not only the healthy old matched man but also the benign prostatic hyperplasia (BPH), which was not the strict 'control'.

5. Conclusions

Our study suggested that a functional polymorphism -716 A>G in the TRAIL gene may play a role in the development of PCa in southern Chinese Han descent, and the protective genotypes AG/GG of -716 A>G were associated with increased TRAIL expression in serum, which makes it a potential role in early detection for PCa. Moreover, further investigations with larger sample size are needed to confirm this relationship and to elucidate the mechanism responsible for this association.

6. Acknowledgments

This study was supported by Natural Science Foundation of Jiangsu Province (No. BK2010577) and the foundation of medical key department of Jiangsu Province— Department of General Surgery of Jiangsu Province Hospital. We also thank professor Avi Ashkenazi (Genentech Inc., 1 DNA Way, South San Francisco, CA 94080, USA) with kindly help.

7. Conflict of interest

The authors declare that they have no conflict of interest related to the publication of this manuscript.

8. References

[1] Jemal A, Bray F, Center MM, Ferlay J, Ward E, Forman D. Global cancer statistics. CA Cancer J Clin. 2011;61:69-90.

[2] Bock CH, Schwartz AG, Ruterbusch JJ, Levin AM, Neslund-Dudas C, Land SJ, Wenzlaff AS, Reich D, McKeigue P, Chen W, Heath EI, Powell IJ, Kittles RA, Rybicki BA. Results from a prostate cancer admixture mapping study in African-American men. Hum Genet. 2009;126:637-642.

[3] Miller DC, Zheng SL, Dunn RL, Sarma AV, Montie JE, Lange EM, Meyers DA, Xu J, Cooney KA. Germ-line mutations of the macrophage scavenger receptor 1 gene:

association with prostate cancer risk in African-American men. Cancer Res. 2003;63:3486-3489.

[4] Baade PD, Youlden DR, Krnjacki LJ. International epidemiology of prostate cancer: geographical distribution and secular trends. Mol Nutr Food Res. 2009;53:171-184.

[5] Bray F, Lortet-Tieulent J, Ferlay J, Forman D, Auvinen A. Prostate cancer incidence and mortality trends in 37 European countries: an overview. Eur J Cancer. 2010;46:3040-3052.

[6] Kvåle R, Møller B, Angelsen A, Dahl O, Fosså SD, Halvorsen OJ, Hoem L, Solberg A, Wahlqvist R, Bray F. Regional trends in prostate cancer incidence, treatment with curative intent and mortality in Norway 1980-2007. Cancer Epidemiol. 2010;34:359-367.

[7] Schröder FH, Hugosson J, Roobol MJ, Tammela TL, Ciatto S, Nelen V, Kwiatkowski M, Lujan M, Lilja H, Zappa M, Denis LJ, Recker F, Berenguer A, Määttänen L, Bangma CH, Aus G, Villers A, Rebillard X, van der Kwast T, Blijenberg BG, Moss SM, de Koning HJ, Auvinen A; ERSPC Investigators. Screening and prostate-cancer mortality in a randomized European study. N Engl J Med. 2009;360:1320-1328.

[8] Johns LE, Houlston RS. A systematic review and meta-analysis of familial   prostate cancer risk. BJU Int. 2003;91:789-794.

[9] Bunker CH, Patrick AL, Konety BR, Dhir R, Brufsky AM, Vivas CA, Becich MJ, Trump DL, Kuller LH. High prevalence of screening-detected prostate cancer among Afro-Caribbeans: the Tobago Prostate Cancer Survey. Cancer Epidemiol Biomarkers Prev. 2002;11:726-729.

[10] Platz EA, Rimm EB, Willett WC, Kantoff PW, Giovannucci E. Racial variation in prostate cancer incidence and in hormonal system markers among male health professionals. J Natl Cancer Inst. 2000;92:2009-2017.

[11] Ostrander EA, Stanford JL. Genetics of prostate cancer: too many loci, too few genes. Am J Hum Genet. 2000;67: 1367-1375

[12] Wiley SR, Schooley K, Smolak PJ, Din WS, Huang CP, Nicholl JK, Sutherland GR, Smith TD, Rauch C, Smith CA, et al. Identification and characterization of a new member of the TNF family that induces apoptosis. Immunity. 1995;3:673-682.

[13] Tenniswood M, Lee EC. On the trail of cell death pathways in prostate cancer. Cancer Biol Ther. 2004;3:769-771.

[14] Srivastava RK. TRAIL/Apo-2L: mechanisms and clinical applications in cancer. Neoplasia. 2001;3:535-546.

[15] Suliman A, Lam A, Datta R, Srivastava RK. Intracellular mechanisms of TRAIL: apoptosis through mitochondrial-dependent and -independent pathways. Oncogene. 2001;20:2122-2133.

[16] Wang Q, Ji Y, Wang X, Evers BM. Isolation and molecular characterization of the 5'-upstream region of the human TRAIL gene. Biochem Biophys Res Commun. 2000;276:466-471.

[17] Unoki M, Furuta S, Onouchi Y, Watanabe O, Doi S, Fujiwara H, Miyatake A, Fujita K, Tamari M, Nakamura Y. Association studies of 33 single nucleotide polymorphisms (SNPs) in 29 candidate genes for bronchial asthma: positive

association a T924C polymorphism in the thromboxane A2 receptor gene. Hum Genet. 2000;106:440-446.

[18] Gray HL, Sorensen EL, Hunt JS, Ober C. Three polymorphisms in the 3' UTR of the TRAIL (TNF-related apoptosis-inducing ligand) gene. Genes Immun. 2001;2:469-470.

[19] Kikuchi S, Miyagishi R, Fukazawa T, Yabe I, Miyazaki Y, Sasaki H. TNF-related apoptosis inducing ligand (TRAIL) gene polymorphism in Japanese patients with multiple sclerosis. J Neuroimmunol. 2005;167:170-174.

[20] Weber A, Wandinger KP, Mueller W, Aktas O, Wengert O, Grundström E, Ehrlich S, Windemuth C, Kuhlmann T, Wienker T, Brück W, Zipp F. Identification and functional characterization of a highly polymorphic region in the human TRAIL promoter in multiple sclerosis. J Neuroimmunol. 2004;149:195-201.

[21] Yan X, Xu L, Qi J, Liang X, Ma C, Guo C, Zhang L, Sun W, Zhang J, Wei X, Gao L. sTRAIL levels and TRAIL gene polymorphisms in Chinese patients with fatty liver disease. Immunogenetics. 2009;61:551-556.

[22] Pal R, Gochhait S, Chattopadhyay S, Gupta P, Prakash N, Agarwal G, Chaturvedi A, Husain N, Husain SA, Bamezai RN. Functional implication of TRAIL -716 C/T promoter polymorphism on its in vitro and in vivo expression and the susceptibility to sporadic breast tumor. Breast Cancer Res Treat. 2011;126:333-343.

[23] Kuribayashi K, Krigsfeld G, Wang W, Xu J, Mayes PA, Dicker DT, Wu GS, El-Deiry WS. TNFSF10 (TRAIL), a p53 target gene that mediates p53-dependent cell death. Cancer Biol Ther. 2008 Dec;7(12):2034-8.

[24] Droin NM, Pinkoski MJ, Dejardin E, Green DR. Egr family members regulate nonlymphoid expression of Fas ligand, TRAIL, and tumor necrosis factor during immune responses. Mol Cell Biol. 2003 Nov;23(21):7638-47.

[25] Clarke N, Jimenez-Lara AM, Voltz E, Gronemeyer H. Tumor suppressor IRF-1 mediates retinoid and interferon anticancer signaling to death ligand TRAIL. EMBO J. 2004 Aug 4;23(15):3051-60.

[26] Ravi R, Bedi GC, Engstrom LW, Zeng Q, Mookerjee B, Gélinas C, Fuchs EJ, Bedi A. Regulation of death receptor expression and TRAIL/Apo2L-induced apoptosis by NF-kappaB. Nat Cell Biol. 2001 Apr;3(4):409-16.

[27] Xu J, Zhou JY, Wei WZ, Philipsen S, Wu GS. Sp1-mediated TRAIL induction in chemosensitization. Cancer Res. 2008 Aug 15;68(16):6718-26.

[28] Ueno S, Tatetsu H, Hata H, Iino T, Niiro H, Akashi K, Tenen DG, Mitsuya H, Okuno Y. PU.1 induces apoptosis in myeloma cells through direct transactivation of TRAIL. Oncogene. 2009 Nov 19;28(46):4116-25.

[29] Pan G, O'Rourke K, Chinnaiyan AM, Gentz R, Ebner R, Ni J, Dixit VM. The receptor for the cytotoxic ligand TRAIL. Science. 1997 Apr 4;276(5309):111-3.

[30] Pan G, Ni J, Wei YF, Yu G, Gentz R, Dixit VM. An antagonist decoy receptor and a death domain-containing receptor for TRAIL. Science. 1997 Aug 8;277(5327):815-8.

[31] Sheridan JP, Marsters SA, Pitti RM, Gurney A, Skubatch M, Baldwin D, Ramakrishnan L, Gray CL, Baker K, Wood WI, Goddard AD, Godowski P, Ashkenazi A. Control of TRAIL-induced apoptosis by a family of signaling and decoy receptors. Science. 1997 Aug 8;277(5327):818-21.

[32] Ashkenazi A. Directing cancer cells to self-destruct with pro-apoptotic receptor agonists. Nat Rev Drug Discov. 2008;7: 1001–1012.

[33] Smyth MJ, Takeda K, Hayakawa Y, Peschon JJ, van den Brink MR, Yagita H. Nature's TRAIL — on a path to cancer immunotherapy. Immunity. 2003;18:1–6.

[34] Yagita H, Takeda K, Hayakawa Y, Smyth MJ, Okumura K. TRAIL and its receptors as targets for cancer therapy. Cancer Sci. 2004;95:777–783.

[35] Matsumura S, Oue N, Nakayama H, Kitadai Y, Yoshida K, Yamaguchi Y, Imai K, Nakachi K, Matsusaki K, Chayama K, Yasui W. A single nucleotide polymorphism in the MMP-9 promoter affects tumor progression and invasive phenotype of gastric cancer. J Cancer Res Clin Oncol. 2005;131:19-25.

[36] Sugimoto M, Yoshida S, Kennedy S, Deguchi M, Ohara N, Maruo T. Matrix metalloproteinase-1 and -9 promoter polymorphisms and endometrial carcinoma risk in a Japanese population. J Soc Gynecol Investig. 2006;13:523-529.

[37] Li X, Huang Y, Fu X, Chen C, Zhang D, Yan L, Xie Y, Mao Y, Li Y. Meta-analysis of three polymorphisms in the steroid-5-alpha-reductase, alpha polypeptide 2 gene (SRD5A2) and risk of prostate cancer. Mutagenesis. 2011 May;26(3):371-83.

[38] Xu B, Tong N, Chen SQ, Hua LX, Wang ZJ, Zhang ZD, Chen M. FGFR4 Gly388Arg polymorphism contributes to prostate cancer development and progression: a meta-analysis of 2618 cases and 2305 controls. BMC Cancer. 2011 Feb 24;11:84.

[39] Qiu LX, Li RT, Zhang JB, Zhong WZ, Bai JL, Liu BR, Zheng MH, Qian XP. The E-cadherin (CDH1)--160 C/A polymorphism and prostate cancer risk: a meta-analysis. Eur J Hum Genet. 2009 Feb;17(2):244-9.

[40] Mao C, Qiu LX, Zhan P, Xue K, Ding H, Du FB, Li J, Chen Q. MnSOD Val16Ala polymorphism and prostate cancer susceptibility: a meta-analysis involving 8,962 subjects.

[41] Bai JL, Zheng MH, Xia X, Ter-Minassian M, Chen YP, Chen F. MTHFR C677T polymorphism contributes to prostate cancer risk among Caucasians: A meta-analysis of 3511 cases and 2762 controls. Eur J Cancer. 2009 May;45(8):1443-9.

[42] Yu B, Datta PK, Bagchi S. Stability of the Sp3-DNA complex is promoter-specific: Sp3 efficiently competes with Sp1 for binding to promoters containing multiple Sp-sites. Nucleic Acids Res. 2003;31:5368–5376.

[43] Kumar AP, Butler AP. Transcription factor Sp3 antagonizes activation of the ornithine decarboxylase promoter by Sp1. Nucleic Acids Res. 1997;25:2012–2019.

[44] Geltinger C, Hortnagel K, Polack A. TATA box and Sp1 sites mediate the activation of c-myc promoter P1 by immunoglobulin kappa enhancers. Gene Expr. 1996;6:113–127.

[45] Safe S, Abdelrahim M. Sp transcription factor family and its role in cancer. Eur J Cancer. 2005;41:2438–2448.

[46] Li L, He S, Sun JM, Davie JR. Gene regulation by Sp1 and Sp3. Biochem Cell Biol. 2004;82:460–471.

[47] Resendes KK, Rosmarin AG. Sp1 control of gene expression in myeloid cells. Crit Rev Eukaryot Gene Expr. 2004;14:171–181.

[48] Xu J, Zhou JY, Wu GS. Tumor necrosis factor-related apoptosis-inducing ligand is required for tumor necrosis factor alpha-mediated sensitization of human breast cancer cells to chemotherapy. Cancer Res. 2006;66:10092–10099.

[49] Wang Q, Ji Y, Wang X, Evers BM. Isolation and molecular characterization of the 50-upstream region of the human TRAIL gene. Biochem Biophys Res Commun. 2000;276:466–471.

[50] Yang A, Wilson NS, Ashkenazi A. Proapoptotic DR4 and DR5 signaling in cancer cells: toward clinical translation. Curr Opin Cell Biol. 2010;22:837-844.

3

NSAID Induction of p75^{NTR} in the Prostate: A Suppressor of Growth and Cell Migration Via the p38 MAPK Pathway

Daniel Djakiew
Georgetown University Medical School
USA

1. Introduction

Chronic consumption of Non-Steroidal Anti-Inflammatory Drugs (NSAIDs) has been associated with a reduced incidence of prostate cancer (Nelson & Harris, 2000). Pathologic inflammation can induce oxidative stress generating free radicals that can subsequently react with infectious agents and surrounding cells during induction of innate immunity. Different forms of reactive oxygen species can form DNA adducts by halogenation, nitration and oxygenation of bases (Kang & Sowers, 2008). DNA repair of reactive oxygen species damaged bases can seal in mutations that may eventually lead to transformation of cells and carcinogenesis (Burrows, 2009). NSAIDs inhibit inflammation (Masferrer et al., 1995, Tegeder et al., 2001) and therefore may reduce the incidence of carcinogenesis by preventing free radical transformation of cells. NSAID inhibition of the cyclo-oxygenases (COXs) reduces inflammation, however, the mechanism of action of NSAIDs associated with reduced risk of prostate cancer appears independent of COX inhibition (Quann et al., 2007a; Quann et al., 2007b). NSAIDs represent a diverse category of pharmacological compounds with the common biological activity to reduce inflammation, temperature and pain, but with diverse chemical structures that undoubtedly interact with multiple target molecules with multiple mechanisms of action. In the prostate, selected aryl propionic acid NSAIDS such as ibuprofen and r-flurbiprofen (profens) inhibit epithelial cell growth in a COX independent manner (Quann et al., 2007a; Quann et al., 2007b). A mechanism by which these profens inhibit prostate growth appears to be via re-induction of the p75 neurotrophin receptor (p75^{NTR}) which has been shown to exhibit both tumor suppressor and metastasis suppressor activity (Krygier & Djakiew, 2001a; Krygier & Djakiew, 2002). In pathologic human prostate cancer tissues, the p75^{NTR} protein exhibits focal loss of expression which is further lost with malignant progression of tissues (Perez et al., 1997). Significantly, treatment of prostate tumor cells with profen NSAIDs promotes re-expression of the p75^{NTR} protein that inhibits growth (Quann et al., 2007a; Quann et al., 2007b) consistent with p75^{NTR} dependent tumor and metastasis suppressor activity (Krygier & Djakiew, 2001;2002). The COX independent pathway by which profen NSAIDs induce p75^{NTR} re-expression involves rapid phosphorylation of p38 MAPK and down stream effectors leading to re-expression of p75^{NTR} protein and suppressor activity (Quann et al., 2007b). This review discusses the body of evidence for the inhibitory role of the p75^{NTR} in prostate growth; the pathologic loss of p75NTR expression during progression to prostate cancer, and the ability of profen NSAIDs to re-induce p75NTR protein expression through the p38 MAPK pathway with concomitant tumor and metastasis suppressor activity which provides a basis for NSAID associated reduced risk of prostate cancer.

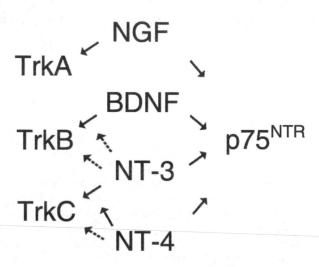

Fig. 1. Affinities of the neurotrophin ligands, nerve growth factor (NGF), brain derived neurotrophic factor (BDNF), neurotrophin-3 (NT-3) and neurotrophin-4 (NT-4) for the family of tropomyosin receptor kinases (Trks) and the p75 neurotrophin receptor (p75NTR). Solid arrows show primary affinities, while dotted arrows show secondary affinities.

2. Expression of neurotrophins and their receptors (p75^{NTR} and Trks) in the prostate

The progression of prostate cancer is accompanied by modifications in the expression of growth factors and their receptors (Bostwick et al, 2004). Amongst these are nerve growth factor (NGF) and its receptors, p75NTR and the Trk family (Djakiew, 2000). The neurotrophin family of ligands (Leibrock et al., 1989, Maisonpierre et al., 1990, Hallbook et al., 1991) consisting of nerve growth factor (NGF), brain derived neurotrophic factor (BDNF), neurotrophin-3 (NT-3) and neurotrophin-4 (NT-4) which is identical to NT-5, all of which can bind with similar affinity to the p75NTR (Bothwell, 1995) and with differential affinities to the Trk family (TrkA, TrkB, TrkC) of high affinity receptors (Figure 1). TrkA preferentially binds with NGF, but also binds BDNF. TrkB preferentially binds BDNF (Soppert et al., 1991), but also binds NT-3 and NT-4 (Berkemeier et al., 1991) and TrkC preferentially binds NT-3 (Lamballe et al., 1991), but also binds NT-4 (Figure 1). NGF immunoreactive protein has been localized to normal epithelium (MacGrogan, 1992; Paul et., 1992) and the stroma of normal, BPH (Djakiew et al., 1991) and cancer tissues of the human prostate (MacGrogan et al., 1992; Djakiew, 1991; Graham et al., 1992). Exogenous NGFβ has been shown to stimulate proliferation *in vitro* (Delsite & Djakiew, 1999; Angelsen et al., 1998; Pflug & Djakiew, 1998), and anchorage independent growth of several prostate tumor cell lines (Chung et al., 1992).

BDNF also is also expressed by human prostate stromal cells (Dalal & Djakiew, 1997). Hence, the two neurotrophins, NGF and BDNF appear to function as paracrine factors for prostate epithelial cell growth (Dalal & Djakiew, (1997).

The p75^NTR is expressed by normal human prostate epithelial cells (MacGrogan et al., 1992; Graham et al., 1992). Immunoblot (Pflug et al., 1992), immunofluorescence (Graham et al., 1992), and immunohistochemical (Pflug et al., 1992) studies have shown that p75^NTR protein expression progressively declines in human prostate cancer (Perez et al., 1997; Pflug et al., 1995; Djakiew et al., 1996). The p75^NTR is expressed in PIN tissue (Perez et al., 1997), and shows a gradual decline in the percentage of cells that retain expression with increasing Gleason score of pathologic prostate tissues (Perez et al., 1997). Hence, loss of p75^NTR expression appears to be correlated with cancer grade in organ-confined disease (Perez et al., 1997). The p75^NTR is also absent in three human cancer cell lines derived from metastases (Pflug et al., 1992). Loss of p75^NTR expression in prostate cancer may be related to its role in the induction of programmed cell death (Pflug & Djakiew, 1998; Djakiew et al., 1996). In this context, the p75 neurotrophin receptor (p75^NTR) is a 75 kD cell surface receptor glycoprotein that shares both structural and sequence homology with the tumor necrosis factor receptor super-family of proteins (Chao, 1994; Chapman, 1995). Some of these proteins (e.g. p75^NTR, p55^TNFR, Fas, DRs3-5) have similar sequence motifs of defined elongated structure (Chao, 1994) designated "death domains" based upon their apoptosis inducing function (Chao, 1994). Hence, re-expression of p75^NTR by stable and transient transfection showed that the p75^NTR inhibits growth of prostate epithelium *in vitro*, at least in part, by induction of programmed cell death (Pflug & Djakiew, 1998). Hence, loss of p75^NTR expression appears to eliminate a potential programmed cell death pathway in prostate cancer cells (Figure 2), thereby facilitating the growth of these cancer cells during carcinogenesis (Perez et al., 1997; Djakiew et al., 1996).

Since expression of the p75^NTR is lost during malignant progression and transformation of the prostate (Figure 2), NGF mediated growth of cancer cells has been shown to occur via the family of high affinity Trk receptors (Pflug & Djakiew, 1998; Dalal & Djakiew, 1997; Pflug et al., 1995). Differential expression of TrkA, TrkB and TrkC occurs in normal, organ confined and metastatic prostate cancer tissue (Chapman, 1995) and cell lines (Dalal & Djakiew, 1997) suggesting the presence of a neurotophin mediated proliferative stimulus via the Trk receptors (Figure 2). Expression of the TrkA receptor has been observed in normal prostate epithelial cells, organ confined prostate adenocarcinoma tissues (Djakiew et al., 1996; Pflug et al., 1995; Djakiew et al., 1996; Dionne et al., 1998), in prostate tumors that have metastasized to the bone (Dionne et al., 1998), as well as in several human prostate tumor cell lines derived from metastases (Djakiew et al., 1996). Interestingly, although normal prostate epithelial cells do the not express either TrkB or TrkC (Dionne et al., 1998), these receptors are expressed in metastatic prostate cancer of the bone (Dionne et al., 1998). Hence, it appears that normal prostate epithelial cells express TrkA, and that cancer cells continue to express TrkA within primary tumors and at metastatic foci, while TrkB and TrkC expression is subsequently up-regulated within metastatic prostate tumors (Dionne et al., 1998). Pharmacological inhibition of the Trk family of receptors has provided a basis for their role in mediating a proliferative stimulus is tumor cells. In this context, the indolocarbazole kinase inhibitors selectively antagonize Trk receptors at nanomolar concentrations (Berg et al., 1992) and inhibit NGF-stimulated Trk phosphorylation in cancer cell lines (Delsite & Djakiew, 1996). Concurrently, Trk selective indolocarbazoles inhibit growth of cancer cell lines *in vitro* (Delsite & Djakiew, 1996), and *in vivo* (Dionne et al., 1998).

Interestingly, Trk family mutations within the human prostate have not been identified (George et al., 1998). However, the absence of mutations in otherwise genetically unstable prostate tumor DNA suggests that intact Trk family signaling pathways may be important in prostate cancer development (George et al., 1998) consistent with a role as a proto-oncogene.

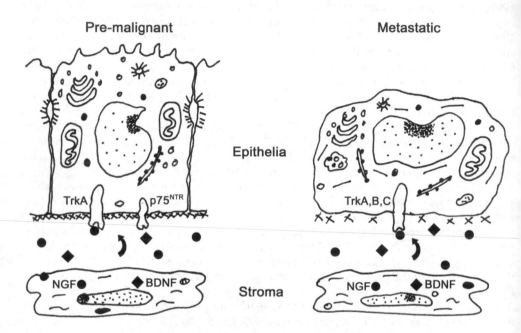

Fig. 2. Schematic diagram showing expression of NGF and BDNF in prostatic stroma for the paracrine regulation of epithelial cell growth. Pre-malignant epithelial cells express both TrkA and the p75NTR, whereas metastatic tumor cells have lost expression of the p75NTR and gained expression of both TrkB and TrkC.

3. Ectopic re-expression of p75^NTR induces tumor suppressor, metastasis suppressor and differentiation phenotypes in prostate tumor cells

Whereas the gene encoding p75NTR is intact in prostate cancer cells (Krygier & Djakiew, 2001b), expression of the p75NTR protein is suppressed (Perez et al., 1997; Pflug et al., 1992; Pflug et al., 1995). Moreover, transient transfection of two constructs of p75NTR into prostate cell lines that do not express the protein, one construct containing the full 2-kb 3' untranslated region and another that contains just a few hundred bases of the 3' untranslated region, showed that only the truncated construct allowed expression of the p75NTR protein (Krygier & Djakiew, 2001b). This lead to the conclusion that elements of the 3' untranslated region of p75NTR contribute to mRNA stability and p75NTR protein expression (Krygier & Djakiew, 2001b). Utilizing the truncated p75NTR expression vector that allows protein expression, a series of stable prostate cell lines were developed that express different levels of p75NTR protein (Pflug et al., 1992, Pflug et al., 1995). These cancer cells that ectopically expressed the p75^{NTR} protein exhibited a retardation of cell cycle progression characterized by accumulation of cells in G1 phase with a corresponding reduction of cells in the S phase of the cell cycle (Krygier & Djakiew, 2001a). In rank order, prostate cancer cells that expressed increased levels of p75^{NTR} protein exhibited increased rates of apoptosis and reduced rates of proliferation (Krygier & Djakiew, 2001a). When the same series of tumor cells were injected into the flanks of SCID mice the growth of prostate tumors was suppressed in proportion to increased p75^{NTR} expression levels (Krygier & Djakiew, 2001a) thereby functionally demonstrating that the p75^{NTR} exhibits tumor suppressor activity (Krygier & Djakiew, 2001a). Further evidence for the tumor suppressor function of p75^{NTR} was show utilizing a gene therapy strategy based upon intra-tumoral injection into xenografts of PC-3 prostate tumor cells of a lipoplex containing the p75^{NTR} gene. Administration of the p75^{NTR} gene into subcutaneous PC-3 xenografts suppressed in a dose-dependent manner the growth of tumors (Allen et al., 2004). Within the gene therapy treated tumors re-expression of the p75^{NTR} gene product was associated with increased apoptosis and reduced proliferation of tumor cells (Allen et al., 2004), the net effect of which was to reduce overall growth and tumor volume. Utilizing the same prostate tumor cells that exhibited a rank order (dose-dependent) increase in p75^{NTR} expression for growth of subcutaneous tumors in SCID mice (Krygier & Djakiew, 2001a), treatment of these tumors with NGF stimulated both proliferation as indicated by PCNA expression, and apoptosis as indicated by TUNEL assay, the net result of which was no change in the overall growth of the tumors (Krygier & Djakiew, 2002). However, NGF was found to increase the formation of smaller secondary satellite tumors, both contiguous and non-contiguous with respect to the primary tumor mass, indicating dose-dependent induction of metastasis (Krygier & Djakiew , 2002). Significantly, the formation of satellite tumors was suppressed by the expression of p75^{NTR} thus showing that p75^{NTR} is a tumor suppressor of growth and a metastasis suppressor of NGF stimulated migration (Djakiew et al, 1993) of human prostate tumor cells (Krygier & Djakiew, 2002). To better understand the molecular mechanism of p75^{NTR} on tumor and metastasis suppression a cDNA microarray composed of approximately 6,000 human cancer-related genes was used to determine the gene expression pattern altered by re-introduction of p75^{NTR} into PC-3 prostate tumor cells (Nalbandian et al., 2005). Comparison of the transcripts in the *neo* control and p75^{NTR}-transfected cells revealed 52 differentially expressed genes, of which 21 were up-regulated and 31 were down-regulated in the presence of p75^{NTR}. The known biological functions of these p75^{NTR} regulated genes suggested a role in the regulation of differentiation as well as cell adhesion, signal transduction, apoptosis, tumor cell invasion and metastasis (Nalbandian et al., 2005). Quantitative real-time polymerase chain reaction and immunoblot analysis confirmed increased CRABPI and IGFBP5 protein levels and decreased level of PLAUR protein with increasing p75^{NTR} protein expression. Indeed, CRABPI was elevated far more than any other genes (Nalbandian et al., 2005). In this context, the retinoids, ATRA and 9-*cis* RA, that bind CRABPI, promoted functional cell differentiation in p75^{NTR} PC-3 cells, but not in *neo* control PC-3 cells. Subsequent examination of the retinoic acid receptors expression levels demonstrated an absence of RAR-β in the *neo* control cells and re-expression in the p75^{NTR} expressing cells, consistent with previous findings where RAR-β is believed to play a critical role as a tumor suppressor gene which is lost during de-differentiation of prostate epithelial cells. Whereas the RAR-α and -γ protein levels remained unchanged, RXR-α and -β also exhibited increasing protein levels with re-expression of the p75^{NTR} protein (Nalbandian et al., 2005). Moreover, the ability of p75^{NTR} siRNA to knockdown levels of RAR-β, RXR-α, and

RXR-β support the specificity of the functional involvement of p75[NTR] in differentiation. Hence, re-expression of the p75[NTR] appears to partially reverse de-differentiation of prostate cancer cells by up-regulating expression of CRABPI for localized sequestration of retinoids that are available to newly up-regulated RAR-β, RXR-α, and RXR-β proteins (Nalbandian et al., 2005). Hence, the p75[NTR] has been shown to exhibit tumor suppressor (Krygier & Djakiew, 2001a), metastasis suppressor (Krygier & Djakiew, 2002) and differentiation (Nalbandian et al., 2005) functions all of which contribute to an anti-cancer phenotype in the prostate.

4. Effectors of signal transduction, cell cycle and apoptosis following constitutive p75[NTR] expression in the prostate

Ectopic re-expression of p75[NTR] down regulates the NFκB and JNK pathways leading to reduced survival of tumor cells (Allen et al., 2005). As a member of the TNF receptor super-family the p75[NTR] has been shown to mediate signal transduction through it's intracellular death domain. Expression of two adaptor proteins, TRAF2 and RIP are down-regulated following restoration of p75[NTR] protein by stable transfection of prostate tumor cells (Allen et al., 2005). Significantly, TRAF2 has previously been implicated as an upstream signaling molecule of both the NFκB and JNK pathways (MacEwan, 2002), both of which function as potent effectors of transcription. Similarly, RIP has also been shown to interact with death receptors that signal through both the NFκB and JNK pathways (Harper et al, 2003). Moreover, deletion constructs that lack much of the intracellular death domain were shown to rescue p75[NTR] down-regulation of RIP (Allen et al., 2005). This p75[NTR]-dependent reduction in RIP protein appeared to be a consequence of caspase-8 cleavage of RIP, since a caspase-8 inhibitor rescued the p75[NTR]-dependent reduction in the levels of RIP. This observation is consistent with previous reports where caspase-8 cleavage of RIP was shown to prevent activation of the NFκB pathway (Lin et al., 1999; Martinon et al., 2000) and suggests that caspase-8 cleavage of RIP is capable of preventing the previously reported RIP activation of the JNK pathway (Kelliher et al., 1998). Hence, both the NFκB and JNK pathways appear to be regulated by p75[NTR] expression (Allen et al., 2005). With regard to the NFκB signaling bifurcation, ectopic re-expression of p75[NTR] reduces levels of IKKs, with consequent reduced phosphorylation levels of IκBα, stabilized levels of unphosphorylated IκBα, and reduced levels of RelA (Allen et al., 2005). Moreover, the activity of the IKKs is regulated through the serine/threonine kinase activity of upstream full length RIP (Hur et al., 2003). Hence, the p75[NTR]-dependent reduction in the levels of RIP, via caspase-8 cleavage of RIP, leads to an overall reduction in signal transduction components required for activation of NFκB (Allen et al., 2005). Several of these p75[NTR] dependent changes in signaling components are rescued with dominant negative death domain deletion constructs, thereby further establishing a link between the NFκB pathway downstream of p75[NTR] (Allen et al., 2005). With regard to the JNK signaling bifurcation, ectopic restoration of p75[NTR] levels is associated with a reduction in the expression of the MKK4 kinase and a reduction in the phosphorylated (active) form of JNK. Since MKK4 phosphorylation of JNK has been shown to promote nuclear translocation (Cobb, 1999; Gonzalez et al., 2000) where activated JNK may function as an effector of transcription for growth (Gee et al., 2000; Herr & Debatin, 2001), p75[NTR] associated suppression of JNK phosphorylation and suppression of translocation is consistent with the suppression of the JNK signaling pathway. Moreover, deletion constructs that lack much of the intracellular death domain were shown to rescue p75^{NTR} down-regulation of MKK4 and phosphorylated JNK (Allen et al., 2005) thereby further establishing a link between the JNK pathway downstream of p75^{NTR} (Allen et al., 2005). At the functional level, ectopic re-expression of p75^{NTR} reduces cell survival (Allen et al., 2005), and dominant negative antagonism of IKKβ or MKK4 partially rescues survival (Allen et al., 2005). Hence, it appears that both the NFκB and JNK pathways promote cell survival and that p75^{NTR} down regulation of these pathways inhibits survival in prostate cancer cells, thereby providing a signal transduction pathway for the observed suppressor activities of the p75^{NTR} protein (Krygier and Djakiew, 2001a; Krygier and Djakiew, 2002). The observation that both signaling pathways bifurcate from the p75^{NTR} suggests a redundancy whereby robust down regulation of either pathway may function independently to promote suppressor activity.

Ectopic re-expression of p75^{NTR} alters the cell cycle kinetics of prostate tumor cells (Krygier & Djakiew, 2001a). Cell cycle initiation and progression is cooperatively regulated by several classes of cyclin-dependent kinases (cdks). The expression of cyclin D1-cdk6 (Boonstra, 2003; Sherr, & Roberts, 1995) complexed with PCNA has been shown to promote hyperphosphorylation of Rb during progression through early to mid-G1 (Satyanarayana & Rudolph, 2004). Conversely, p16^{INK4a} binds and induces an allosteric conformational change in cdk6 that inhibits the binding of ATP thereby disrupting the formation of the cdk6-cyclin D1 complex (Satyanarayana & Rudolph, 2004; Golsteyn, 2005). Prostate cancer cells that express rank-order (dose-dependent) increased levels of p75^{NTR} show suppression of cdk6, PCNA and hypophosphorylated Rb, and up-regulation of p16^{INK4a} levels indicates that p75^{NTR} selectively regulates specific components of the holoenzyme complex (Khwaja et al., 2006) associated with retarded progression through early to mid-G1 of the cell cycle (Meyer et al., 2002). The rescue of cdk6, PCNA and phosphorylated Rb levels, and conversely suppression of p16^{INK4a} levels, by both a death domain deleted dominant-negative antagonist of p75^{NTR} and by NGF ligand, show a p75^{NTR}-dependent regulation of early to mid-G1 in prostate tumor cells (Khwaja, et al., 2006). Beyond mid-G1, near the G1/S restriction point, the expression of cyclin E complexed with cdk2 has been shown to promote hyper-phosphorylation of Rb (Boonstra, 2003; Shintani et al., 2002).

A rank-order increase in p75^{NTR} suppression of cyclin E and cdk2 in prostate tumor cells (Khwaja et al., 2006) indicate that progression through the G1/S restriction point is regulated by p75^{NTR} protein expression. (Figure 3). Since the Rb protein is a major effector of cell proliferation through its ability to regulate entry into the S phase (Sellers & Kaelin, 1996; , Huang et al., 2002), and the cyclin E/cdk2 holoenzyme complex hyper-phosphorylates Rb during the G1/S transition, the observation that p75^{NTR} expression can stabilize hypo-phosphorylated Rb and diminish the phosphorylation of Rb is consistent with a mechanism by which p75^{NTR} retards progression through the G1/S restriction point of the cell cycle (Khwaja et al., 2006). Furthermore, hypophosphorylated Rb has been shown to bind the E2F1 transcription factor (Harbour & Dean, 2000), so that the Rb/E2F1 complex can no longer promote transcription of PCNA preventing progression into the S phase of the cell cycle. Hence, the observation that p75^{NTR} associated hypo-phosphorylation of Rb in conjunction with suppression of E2F1 and PCNA expression (Westwood et al., 2002) further supports a role of p75^{NTR} in G1/S restriction point cytostasis (Khwaja et al., 2006). Beyond the G1/S restriction point, expression of the cyclin A/cdk2 holoenzyme complex has been shown to maintain hyper-phosphorylation of Rb during the S phase of the cell cycle (Sherr, 1996). Hence, observations that p75NTR-potentiated suppression of cdk2 and cyclin A support a selective effect of p75NTR expression on maintaining hypo-phosphorylation of Rb (Khwaja et al., 2006), thereby retarding progression through the S phase of the cell cycle (Figure 3). Significantly, the rescue of cyclin E, cdk2, PCNA, phosphorylated Rb, E2F1 and PCNA by both a death domain deleted dominant–negative antagonist of p75NTR and also by NGF ligand (Khwaja et al., 2006) show a p75NTR-dependence of the regulation of progression through both the G1/S restriction point and the S phase in prostate tumor cells. Hence, it seems clear that p75NTR expression selectively alters specific cell cycle regulatory molecules that retard progression through early to mid-G1, the G1/S restriction point and the S phase of the cell cycle (Figure 3). Moreover, in the absence of ligand, the ability of p75NTR to retard cell cycle progression is dependent on the intracellular death domain, and that addition of NGF ligand attenuates inhibition of cell cycle progression at the level of the cyclin/cdk holoenzyme complex and related effects on Rb expression and tumor cell proliferation. Hence, p75NTR-dependent regulation of specific cyclin-dependent kinases and associated cell cycle effectors to retard progression of prostate tumors through the G1 phase and entry into S phase of the cell cycle (Figure 3) provides a biochemical basis upon which p75NTR inhibits prostate cell proliferation (Khwaja et al., 2006).

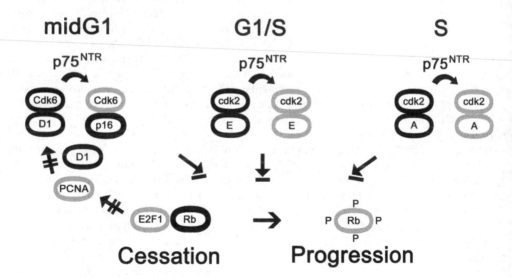

Fig. 3. Effects of p75NTR on regulation of the cell cycle. Re-expression of p75NTR induces midG1 suppression of cdk6 and up-regulation of p16Ink4a. During the G1/S transition re-expression of p75NTR induces suppression of cdk2 and cyclin E. Similarly, during S phase re-expression of p75NTR induces suppression of cdk2 and cyclin A. The net effect of these changes is to diminish phosphorylation of Rb thereby preventing progression of the cell cycle in favor of cessation.

In addition to cell cycle effects, ectopic re-expression of p75NTR has been shown to modify mitochondrial effector proteins that activate the caspase cascade leading to apoptosis (Khwaja, et al., 2006). Mitochondrial mediated apoptosis is facilitated by members of the Bcl-2 homology (Puthalakath & Strasser, 2002) family of proteins (O'Neill et al., 2004) that include both pro- and anti-apoptotic members (Puthalakath & Strasser, 2002). In this context, a rank-order increase in p75^NTR levels (Khwaja et al., 2006) was associated with a decrease in the mitochondrial pro-survival effector, Bcl-xL, and concomitantly, an increase in proapoptotic effectors (Smac, Bax, Bak, Bad). In the absence of NGF ligand the ability of a death domain deleted dominant–negative antagonist of p75^NTR to rescue p75^NTR-dependent changes in Smac and BH family proteins, and the addition of NGF having a comparable effect, suggest a ligand independent p75^NTR-potentiated apoptosis in prostate cells that occurs via a mitochondrial stress pathway (Khwaja et al., 2006). Release of Smac from the intermembranous space of the mitochondria into the cytosol (Shiozaki & Shi, 2004) also initiates apoptosis where it competes with caspases for binding to XIAP. Indeed, to protect against inadvertent activation of apoptosis, the IAP family of proteins (Shiozaki & Shi, 2004) have been shown to bind and prevent activation of caspases. Hence, p75^NTR-dependent down-regulation of XIAP in prostate cells allows for activation of the caspase cascade. Significantly, a rank-order increase in p75^NTR levels was shown to activate both caspase-9 and caspase-7 (Khwaja et al., 2006). In the intrinsic mitochondrial dependent pathway, the assembly of the apoptosome requires the recruitment of the initiator caspase-9 (Shiozaki & Shi, 2004) which subsequently activates the effector caspase-7. Interestingly, a specific peptide inhibitor of procaspase-9 cleavage was shown to prevent cleavage/activation of procaspase-7. Since the initiator procaspase-9 is a proximate component of the caspase cascade, it is clear that procaspase-7 is downstream from procaspase-9 during mitochondrial mediated p75^NTR potentiation of apoptosis (Shiozaki & Shi, 2004). Moreover, in p75^NTR expressing prostate cells the activation of caspase-7 appears to facilitate subsequent cleavage of PARP. PARP cleavage has been shown to be a key event in the execution phase of apoptosis leading to cellular demise (Lazebnik et al., 1994). Clearly, the ability of a death domain deleted dominant–negative antagonist of p75^NTR and NGF ligand to rescue p75^NTR potentiated changes in XIAP, caspase-9, caspase-7, PARP and apoptotic nuclear fragmentation show that mitochondrial mediated apoptosis is dependent, in part, on p75^NTR in the prostate. Moreover, the effect of p75^NTR-dependent down regulation of NFκB and JNK survival pathways, regulation of cell cycle regulatory molecules of the cyclin/cdk holoenzyme complex that produce stasis in G1 and/or inhibition of progression to S phase of the cell cycle and regulation of mitochondrial effector proteins that activate the caspase cascade leading to apoptosis, in combination, all inhibit growth of prostate cells as a function of it's tumor suppressor activity (Krygier & Djakiew, 2001a; Khwaja et al., 2006).

5. Constitutive p75^NTR expression regulates protease activity in the prostate

Ectopic re-expression of p75^NTR down regulates protease activities in prostate cancer cells (Nalbandian & Djakiew, 2006). The urokinase plasminogen activator (uPA) and its receptor (uPAR) are associated with tumor malignancy through an extracellular cascade of proteolysis (Andreasen et al., 2000; Reuning et al., 1998) including activation of the type IV collagen matrix metalloproteinases (MMP-2 and MMP-9) during invasion and tumor progression (Mazzier et al., 1997). Ectopic re-expression of p75^NTR reduces enzymatic protein levels and activity of uPA, MMP-2 and MMP-9 in prostate tumor cells (Nalbandian & Djakiew, 2006). Conversely, expression of an MMP-9 antagonist, tissue inhibitor of matrix metalloproteinase-1 (TIMP-1) exhibits an increase in protein levels with an increase in p75^NTR levels. Whereas, levels of TIMP-2 were not detectable (Nalbandian & Djakiew, 2006) transient transfection with an inducible death domain deleted dominant–negative antagonist of p75^NTR rescued uPA, MMP-

2, and MMP-9 protein levels and protease activities, and conversely suppressed TIMP-1 levels (Nalbandian & Djakiew, 2006). Since ectopic p75[NTR] signal transduction has been shown to suppress the NFκB and JNK pathways (Allen et al., 2005), antagonism of signaling intermediaries in these pathways, using dominant negative IKKβ or dominant negative MKK-4, respectively, was shown to further decrease expression of uPA, MMP-2, and MMP-9 protein and enzymatic activity levels, and conversely up-regulate levels of TIMP-1. Hence, expression of uPA, MMP-2, MMP-9, and TIMP-1 are directly regulated by expression of p75[NTR] and its downstream signal transduction cascade. This suggests that the metastasis suppressor activity of p75[NTR] (Krygier & Djakiew, 2002) is mediated, in part, by down-regulation of specific proteases (uPA, type IV collagenases) implicated in cell migration and metastasis (Nalbandian & Djakiew, 2006).

6. NSAIDS selectively induce pharmacological re-expression of the p75[NTR]

NSAIDs represent a diverse and often structurally unrelated group of compounds that exhibit a range of anti-inflammatory, anti-pyretic and analgesic activities. NSAIDs can be classified into three broad categories as carboxylic acids, enolic acids, and COX-2 inhibitors, or coxibs (Figure 4). The carboxylic acid group is further divided into salicylic acids and esters, acetic acids, and propionic acids. The enolic acids are divided into pyrazolones and oxicams. Many NSAIDs used to treat inflammation inhibit cyclooxygenase (COX) activity. Two well known isoforms of COX exist, COX-1 and COX-2. COX-1 is considered to be a house keeping gene, and is expressed constitutively and ubiquitously at low levels. COX-2 is highly inducible in response to cytokines, hormones, and growth factors. The COX enzymes catalyze the conversion of arachidonic acid to various prostaglandins, which play a role in biological processes including immune response, blood pressure regulation, angiogenesis, ovulation, pain and inflammatory responses. Nonselective NSAIDs inhibit both COX-1 and COX-2, and are frequently associated with gastrointestinal side effects. Whereas, NSAIDs that selectively inhibit COX-2 have significantly decreased gastrointestinal side effects, they often exhibit enhanced cardiovascular toxicity (Dubois et al., 2004). Overexpression of COX-2 is observed in several cancer types including colon, breast, pancreas, and lung (Sarkar et al., 2007; Mascaux et al., 2006). Increased COX-2 expression is believed to contribute to tumorigenesis through several mechanisms including stimulation of growth, promotion of angiogenesis, increased inflammation, increased invasion and migration, immune suppression, and inhibition of apoptosis (Liao et al., 2007). Hence, NSAID inhibition of COX-2 activity may suppress these mechanisms that contribute to tumorigenesis. Consistently, several reports have linked long term NSAID use to decreased cancer risk for colon (Thun et al., 1991), bladder (Castelao et al., 2000), and prostate (Nelson & Harris, 2000) and possibly other organ specific sites. Although it has been the subject of multiple reports, there is not a consensus concerning the expression and role of COX-2 in prostate cancer. Several studies show that COX-2 is overexpressed, while others found that it is low or absent in most prostate cancers (Madaan et al., 2000; Kirschenbaum et al., 2000; Yoshimura et al., 2000). In addition, expression of COX-2 is absent in the metastatic human prostate cancer cell lines LNCaP, DU145, and PC-3 (Yoshimura et al., 2000). Although reports of COX-2 expression in prostate cancer vary, long term NSAID use is associated with decreased prostate cancer risk (Nelson & Harris, 2000), and several COX inhibitors consistently induce apoptosis in prostate cancer cells regardless of COX-2 expression (Zha et al., 2001; Jacobs et al., 2007; Roberts et al., 2002; Hsu et al., 2000; Johnson et al., 2001). Indeed, NSAIDS that do not inhibit the cyclo-oxygenases (R-flurbiprofen) or NSAIDs that inhibit COX null tumor cells demonstrates an alternate COX independent mechanism of action for selected NSAID inhibition of some tumor cells. In this context, NSAIDs exhibit selective activity to induce p75^NTR-dependent cell death (Khwaja et al., 2004). The propionic acids, ibuprofen and r-flurbiprofen, as well as the indolacetic acid, indomethacin, exhibit greater pharmacological activity to induce p75^NTR-dependent cell death than the salicyclate, aspirin, or acetaminophen (Khwaja et al., 2004). Within the aryl propionic acid NSAIDs, r-flurbiprofen exhibits greater activity to induce p75^NTR in descending rank-order than ibuprofen, oxaprozin, fenoprofen, naproxen and least of all ketoprofen (Quann et al., 2007a). Significantly, this activity appears relatively selective for induction of p75^NTR (Quann et al., 2007a), since r-flurbiprofen and ibuprofen do not induce expression of Fas, p55^TNFR, DR3, DR4, DR5 or DR6 in prostate cancer cells (Quann et al., 2007a). Some other NSAIDs have also been reported to induce expression of certain TNF receptor super family members, particularly DR5.

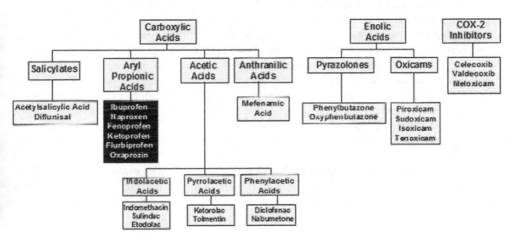

Fig. 4. Classification of the Non-Steroidal Anti-Inflammatory Drugs (NSAIDs) into three categories of carboxylic acids, enolic acids and COX-2 inhibitors. Sub-classifications of NSAIDs are further delineated with specific examples.

For instance, sulindac sulfide induces DR5 associated cell death in prostate cancer cells (Huang et al., 2001) and celocoxibs induce DR5 in both prostate and colon cancer cells (He et al., 2008). Moreover, aryl propionic acid induction of p75^NTR appears somewhat selective for urogenital cancer cell lines such as prostate, bladder, kidney, ovary, and colon (Khwaja et al., 2004), whereas cell lines derived from the lung, or breast do not exhibit induction of the p75^NTR protein (Khwaja et al., 2004). Hence, induction of p75^NTR appears to represent a COX independent mechanism for NSAID associated reduced risk of prostate cancer.

7. NSAID induced phosphorylation of p38 MAPK is necessary for induction of p75^{NTR} expression

NSAIDs exhibit a range of efficacy to inhibit survival of prostate cancer cells (Andrews et al., 2002). Induction of p75NTR dependent cell death by selected NSAIDs (R-flurbiprofen, ibuprofen) occurs through hyper-phosphorylation of p38 MAPK (Quann et al., 2007b). Although p75NTR is transcribed at a high level (Quann et al., 2007b; Krygier & Djakiew, 2001b), prostate cancer cells have very little p75NTR mRNA or protein due to increased mRNA instability mediated through the 3'UTR (Krygier & Djakiew, 2001b). Since, increased 3'UTR length provides increased potential for post-transcriptional regulation through the 3'UTR (Mazumder et al., 2003) R-flurbiprofen and ibuprofen appear to modulate mRNA stability as a determinant in regulating the expression level of p75NTR protein (Quann et al., 2007b). Significantly, activity of the p38 MAPK pathway is an important regulator of mRNA stability (Zarubin & Han, 2005; Kennedy et al., 2007; Gaestel, 2006). Pretreatment of prostate cancer cells with a p38 MAPK selective pharmacological inhibitor or siRNA knockdown of p38 MAPK prior to R-flurbiprofen and ibuprofen treatment prevents induction of p75NTR protein. In addition, the phytoestrogens biochanin A and to a lesser extent genestein, inhibit ibuprofen induced phosphorylation of p38 MAPK which in turn suppresses p75NTR expression and increases cell survival (El Touny et al., 2010). R-flurbiprofen and ibuprofen cause increased p38 MAPK phosphorylation within 5 minutes of treatment (Quann et al., 2007b). Whereas, p38 MAPK can be phosphorylated by MKK6 and MKK3, R-flurbiprofen and ibuprofen induce hyperphosphorylation of only MKK6 but not MKK3 within 30 seconds of treatment (Figure 5) indicating that the target molecule of these NSAIDs is immediately proximal to MKK6. Significantly, several oxidative stress pathways converge upstream of MKK6, thereby providing a basis by which NSAID inhibition of inflammation (Masferrer et al., 1995; Tegeder et al., 2001) may regulate p38 MAPK dependent expression of the p75NTR tumor suppressor to reduce the incidence of prostate cancer. Downstream of p38 MAPK R-flurbiprofen and ibuprofen induced activation of the kinase MK2 (Quann et al., 2007b). MK2 and the closely related MK3 are known to be responsible for mediating the mRNA stabilizing effects of the p38 MAPK pathway (Ronkina et al., 2007). Moreover, siRNA knockdown of both MK2 and MK3 together prevents induction of p75NTR by R-flurbiprofen or ibuprofen to a greater extent than knockdown of either MK2 or MK3 separately, indicating that p38 MAPK is able to induce p75NTR by acting through both MK2 and MK3 (Quann et al., 2007b).

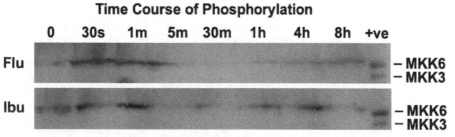

Fig. 5. Western blot showing the time course in seconds (s), minutes (m) and hours (h) of the phosphorylation forms of MKK6, but not MKK3, in PC-3 prostate cancer cells treated with r-flurbiprofen (Flu), or ibuprofen (Ibu). The positive controls for the phosphorylated forms of both MKK6 and MKK3 are shown to the right.

The mRNA stabilizing effects of the p38 MAPK pathway (Ronkina et al., 2007) also involves the RNA binding protein HuR (Tran et al., 2003; Lin et al., 2006; Jin et al., 2007; Song et al., 2005). Its ability to stabilize target mRNAs is linked to its subcellular localization, and activation of p38 MAPK and MK2 have been shown to cause translocation of HuR from the nucleus to the cytoplasm, resulting in increased mRNA stability of a number of p38 MAPK regulated genes (Tran et al., 2003; Lin et al., 2006; Jin et al., 2007; Song et al., 2005). HuR has repeatedly been shown to stabilize transcripts containing the AUUUA sequence (Tran et al., 2003; Song et al., 2005). The human p75^{NTR} transcript contains AUUUA sites located in the 3'UTR at positions 2946 and 3124, suggesting they may be involved in regulating p75^{NTR} expression. Significantly, treatment with R-flurbiprofen or ibuprofen results in an increase in the cytoplasmic level of HuR and binding to the p75^{NTR} transcript (Quann et al., 2007b) although this is not the sole mechanism responsible for increased p75^{NTR} expression. Indeed, eIF4E is also phosphorylated by kinases downstream of p38 MAPK (Scheper & Proud, 2002). eIF4E has also been shown to control the nuclear export as well as translation of a subset of transcripts (Culjkovic et al., 2007). eIF4E has been linked to the control of mRNA stability by removal of the 5'-cap during mRNA degradation (von der Haar et al., 2004). R-flurbiprofen or ibuprofen treatment increases the level of phosphorylated eIF4E (Quann et al., 2007b) involved in translation initiation and this appears to occur at least partially through the p38 MAPK pathway since the increase in phosphorylation is substantially inhibited in the presence of p38 MAPK siRNA. Therefore, modulation of eIF4E activity is another mechanism by which the p38 MAPK pathway may control post-transcriptional events in response to R-flurbiprofen or ibuprofen treatment (Figure 6). R-flurbiprofen or ibuprofen stabilization of the p75^{NTR} transcript allows levels of the p75^{NTR} protein to accumulate (Quann et al., 1997a, Quann et al., 197b) that then exhibit biological activity to inhibit prostate cancer cell survival and induce apoptosis (Quann et al., 1997a) consistent with its tumor suppressor activity (Krygier & Djakiew, 2001a). Significantly, NSAID induction of p38 MAPK dependent p75^{NTR} expression and tumor suppressor activity may represent a new pathway to medicinal drug design. Rather that inhibit kinase dependent proliferation pathways, pharmacological induction of the p75^{NTR} tumor suppressor, as shown with NSAIDs (Figure 6), may represent an alternate approach to the targeting of cancer cell survival pathways. Presumably, target molecules that activate this pathway appear to occur immediately proximal to MKK6 and the p38 MAPK (Figure 5).

8. NSAIDs induce expression of NAG-1 down stream of p75^{NTR} via the p38 MAPK pathway

R-flurbiprofen and ibuprofen treatment of prostate cancer cells induces expression of the NSAID activated gene-1 (Nag-1) protein, a divergent member of the transforming growth factor beta (TGF-β) family (Wynne & Djakiew, 2010). Moreover, a selective pharmacological inhibitor of p38 MAPK and p38 MAPK specific siRNA, both reduce Nag-1 induction following NSAID treatment. Hence, NSAID induced Nag-1 expression is regulated by the p38 MAPK pathway (Figure 6). Interestingly, p75^{NTR} specific siRNA pretreatment abrogates Nag-1 induction by NSAIDs (Wynne & Djakiew, 2010) thereby demonstrating that Nag-1 is downstream of p75^{NTR} induction (Figure 6). Functionally, decreased survival of NSAID treated cells is rescued by p75^{NTR} specific siRNA (Quann et al., 2007a; Wynne & Djakiew, 2010) but not by Nag-1 siRNA. Transwell chamber and *in vitro* wound healing assays demonstrate decreased cell migration upon NSAID treatment (Wynne & Djakiew, 2010). Pre-treatment of prostate cancer cells with p75^{NTR} and Nag-1 specific siRNA shows that

NSAID inhibition of cell migration is mediated by Nag-1 and p75NTR (Wynne & Djakiew, 2010). Additionally, prostate cancer cells stably expressing Nag-1 exhibit decreased migration relative to the parental cell line (Wynne & Djakiew, 2010), thereby independently confirming a role for this protein in reduced prostate cancer cell migration. Hence, it appears that NSAID induction of Nag-1 functions in the inhibition of cell migration, but not survival (Figure 6). Interestingly, NSAIDs have been linked to metastasis suppression in a variety of cancers including prostate cancer (Lloyd et al., 2003; Jin et al., 2010; Kamei et al., 2009). Hence, NSAID induction of Nag-1 via the p38 MAPK pathway may contribute to the metastasis suppressor activity of p75NTR (Krygier & Djakiew, 2002).

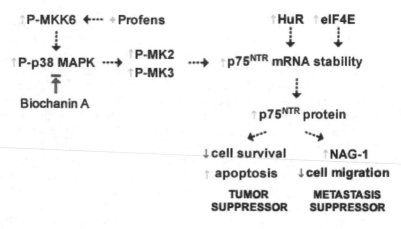

Fig. 6. Schematic diagram showing the biochemical pathway by which profen NSAIDs positively stimulate and the phytoestrogen, biochanin A, negatively inhibits phosphorylation of the p38 MAPK pathway leading to p75NTR expression with consequent tumor suppressor and metastasis suppressor activity.

9. Summary and conclusions

Paracrine regulated growth of the prostate is mediated, in part, by neurotrophin dependent interactions with the Trk family of receptors and the p75NTR (Djakiew, 2000). In the normal prostate neurotrophins stimulate proliferation via the Trk family of receptors and abrogate p75NTR apoptotic activity. However, p75NTR protein expression progressively declines in human prostate cancer (Perez et al., 1997; Pflug et al., 1995; Djakiew et al., 1996). Hence, in the absence of p75NTR inhibition of growth, prostate tumor cells respond to neurotrophins with a stiochiometry that favors Trk family dependent proliferation. Even though the p75NTR protein is no longer expressed in many prostate cancer cells the gene has remained intact (Krygier & Djakiew, 2001b). Indeed, reduced p75NTR protein in cancer cells occurs via loss of mRNA stability (Krygier & Djakiew, 2001b). Ectopic re-expression of p75NTR in cancer cells induces tumor suppressor (Krygier & Djakiew, 2001a), metastasis suppressor (Krygier & Djakiew, 2002) and differentiation phenotypes (Nalbandian et al., 2005). The tumor suppressor activity of p75NTR is manifest as a suppression of the NFκB and JNK pathways, modification of cyclin-dependent holoenzyme complexes resulting in accumulations of cells in G1 and restriction of entry into the S1 phase of the cell cycle, and modification of mitochondrial effector proteins that activate the caspase cascade leading to apoptosis. The metastasis suppressor activity of p75^{NTR} is manifest as down-regulation of urokinase plasminogen activator and type IV collagenases (MMP-2, MMP-9) as well as increased expression of the tissue inhibitor of matrix metalloproteinase-1 (Nalbandian & Djakiew, 2006). The differentiation activity of p75^{NTR} is manifest as up-regulated expression of CRABPI for localized sequestration of retinoids that are available to newly up-regulated RAR-β, RXR-α, and RXR-β proteins (Nalbandian et al., 2005). Moreover, certain aryl propionic acid type NSAIDs (profens) restore p75^{NTR} protein levels that inhibit growth via a COX independent mechanism of action. Indeed, these profens induce hyperphosphorylation of p38 MAPK that initiates a signal transduction cascade leading to mRNA stability of the p75^{NTR} transcript and increased protein levels (Quann et al., 2007a; Quann et al., 2007b). Profen NSAIDs also induce Nag-1 expression downstream of p75^{NTR} (Wynne & Djakiew, 2010). Functionally, profen dependent induction of p75^{NTR} inhibits growth and downstream Nag-1 inhibition of cell migration consistent with the tumor suppressor (Krygier & Djakiew, 2001a) and metastasis suppressor (Krygier & Djakiew, 2002) activities of p75^{NTR} expression, respectively. Hence, these profen NSAIDs induce multiple activities of the p75^{NTR} and downstream Nag-1 consistent with observations that chronic consumption of NSAIDs is associated with a reduced incidence of prostate cancer (Nelson & Harris, 2000).

10. Acknowledgements

The author thanks his former graduate students (Drs. Robert Delsite, Beth Pflug, Scott Krygier, Jeff Allen, Angele Nalbandian, Emily Quann, Shehla Wynne) and research associates (Drs. Rhaki Dalal, Ashia Tabassum, Fatima Khwaja, Lara El Touny) for their dedication and tireless efforts that contributed to much of this work. A significant amount of this research was supported by the National Institutes of Health (DK52626). Research support was also provided by the Department of Defense (PC060409) to graduate students (EQ, SW).

11. References

Allen, J., Khwaja, F., Byers, S. & Djakiew, D. (2005). The p75^{NTR} Mediates a Bifurcated Signal Transduction Cascade through the NFκB and JNK Pathways to Inhibit Cell Survival. *Experimental Cell Research,* Vol.304, No.1, (March 2005), pp69-80, PMID 15707575

Allen, J., Khwaja, F. & Djakiew, D. (2004). Gene therapy of prostate xenograft tumors with a p75^{NTR} lipoplex. *Anticancer Research,* Vol.24, No.5A, (September-October 2004), pp2997-3003, PMID 15517907

Andreasen, P., Egelund, R. & Petersen, H. (2000). The plasminogen activation system in tumor growth, invasion, and metastasis. *Cellular and Molecular Life Sciences,* Vol.57, No.1, (January 2000), pp 25-40, PMID 10949579

Andrews, J., Djakiew, D., Krygier, S. & Andrews, P. (2002). Superior effectiveness of ibuprofen compared with other NSAIDs for reducing the survival of human prostate cancer cells. Cancer Chemotherapy and Pharmacology, Vol. 50, No.4, (October 2002), pp 277-284, PMID 12357301

Angelsen, A., Sandvik, A., Syversen, U., Stridsberg, M. & Waldum, H. (1998). NGF-beta, NE-cells and prostatic cancer cell lines. A study of neuroendocrine expression in the human prostatic cancer cell lines DU-145, PC-3, LNCaP, and TSU-pr1 following stimulation of the nerve growth factor-beta. *Scandinavian Journal of Urology and Nephrology,* Vol.32, No.1 (February 1998), pp 7-13, PMID 9561567

Berkemeier, L., Winslow, J., Kaplan, D., Nikolics, K., Goeddel, D. & Rosenthal, A. (1991). Neurotrophin-5: a novel neurotrophic factor that activates trk and trkB. *Neuron*, Vol.7, No.5, (November 1991), pp 857-866, PMID 1742028

Berg M.M., Sternberg D.W., Parada L.F. & Chao M.V. (1992). K-252a inhibits nerve growth factor-induced trk proto-oncogene tyrosine phosphorylation and kinase activity. *Journal of Biological Chemistry*, Vol.267, No.1 (January 1992), pp13-16, PMID 1730579

Boonstra, J. (2003). Progression through the G1-phase of the on-going cell cycle. *Journal of Cellular Biochemistry*, Vol.90, No.2, (October 2003), pp 244-252, PMID 14505341

Bothwell, M. (1995). Functional interactions of neurotrophins and neurotrophin receptors. *Annual Reviews of Neuroscience*, Vol.18, (March 1995), pp 223-253, PMID 7605062

Bostwick, D., Burke, H., Djakiew, D., Euling, S., Ho, S., Landolph, J., Morrison, H., Sonawane, B., Shifflett, T., Waters, D., Timms, B. (2004). Human prostate cancer risk factors. *Cancer*, Vol.101, Supplement 10, (November 2004), pp 2371-490, PMID 15495199

Burrows, C. (2009). Surviving an Oxygen Atmosphere: DNA Damage and Repair. *ACS symposium Series American Chemical Society* (December 2009); pp.147–156, PMID 20458355

Castelao, J., Yuan, M., Gago-Dominguez, M., Yu, M. & Ross, R. (2000). Non-steroidal anti-inflammatory drugs and bladder cancer prevention. *The British Journal of Cancer*, Vol.82, No.7, (April 2000), pp 1364-1369, PMID 10755416

Chao, M. (1994). The p75 neurotrophin receptor. Journal of Neurobiology, Vol.25, No.11 (November 1994), pp1373-1385, PMID 7852992

Chapman, B. (1995). A region of the 75kD neurotrophin receptor homologous to the death domains of TNFR-1 and Fas. *Federation of Experimental Biology Society Letters* Vol.374, No. (October 1995), pp 216-220, PMID 7589538

Chung, L., Li, W., Gleave, M., Hsieh, J., Wu, H., Sikes, R., Zhau, H., Bandyk, M., Logothetis, J., Rubin, J. & von Eschenbach, A. (1992). Human prostate cancer model: roles of growth factors and extracellular matrices. *Journal of Cellular Biochemistry*, Supplement 16H (1992), pp 99-105, PMID 1289680

Cobb, M. (1999). MAP kinase pathways. *Progress in Biophysics and Molecular Biology*, Vol.71, No.3-4, (April 1999), pp 479-500, PMID 10354710

Culjkovic, B., Topisirovic, I. & Borden, K. (2007). Controlling gene expression through RNA regulons: the role of the eukaryotic translation initiation factor eIF4E. *Cell Cycle*, Vol.6, No.1, (January 2007), pp 65-69, PMID 17245113

Dalal, R. & Djakiew, D. (1997). Molecular characterization of neurotrophin expression and the corresponding tropomyosin receptor kinases (trks) in epithelial and stromal cells of the human prostate. *Molecular and Cellular Endocrinology*, Vol.134, No.1 (October 1997), pp 15-22, PMID 9406845

Delsite R. & Djakiew D. (1996). Anti-proliferative effect of the kinase inhibitor K252a on human prostatic carcinoma cell lines. *Journal of Andrology*, Vol.17, No.5 (September-October 1996), pp481-490, PMID 8957691

Delsite R. & Djakiew D. (1999). Characterization of nerve growth factor precursor protein expression by human prostate stromal cells: a role in selective neurotrophin stimulation of prostate epithelial cell growth. *Prostate*, Vol.41, No.1 (September 1999), pp 39-48, PMID 10440874

Dionne, C., Camoratto, A., Jani, J., Emerson, E., Neff, N., Vaught, J., Murakata, C., Djakiew, D., Lamb, J., Bova, S., George, D. & Isaacs, J. (1998). *Clinical Cancer Research, Vol.4*, No.8 (August 1998), pp1887-1898, PMID 9717816

Djakiew, D. (2000). Neurotrophins, p75^{NTR} and TRK in Prostate Cancer, In: *Neurobiology of the Neurotrophins,* I. Mocchetti, (Ed.), 525-539, F. P. Graham Publishing Co., Johnson City, Tennessee, USA, ISBN 1-929675-01-1

Djakiew, D., Delsite, R., Pflug, B., Wrathall, J., Lynch, J. & Onoda M. (1991). Regulation of growth by a nerve growth factor-like protein which modulates paracrine interactions between a neoplastic epithelial cell line and stromal cells of the human prostate. *Cancer Research,* Vol.51, No.12, (June 1991), pp 3304-3310, PMID 1710170

Djakiew, D., Delsite, R., Dalal, R. & Pflug, B. (1996). Role of the low-affinity nerve growth factor receptor and the high-affinity Trk nerve growth factor receptor in human prostate carcinogenesis. *Radiation Oncology Investigations,* Vol.3, (1996), 333-339.

Djakiew, D., & Pflug, B., Delsite, R., Onoda, M., Lynch, J., Arand, G. & Thompson, G. (1993). Chemotaxis and chemokinesis of human prostate tumor cell lines in response to human prostate stromal cell secretory proteins containing a nerve growth factor-like protein. *Cancer Research,* Vol.53, No.6, (March 1993), pp 1416-20, PMID 8443820

Dubois, R., Melmed, G., Henning, J. & Laine, L. (2004). Guidelines for the appropriate use of non-steroidal anti-inflammatory drugs, cyclo-oxygenase-2-specific inhibitors and proton pump inhibitors in patients requiring chronic anti-inflammatory therapy. *Alimentary Pharmacology and Therapeutics,* Vol.19, No.2, (January 2004), pp 197-208, PMID 14723611

El Touny, L., Henderson, F. & Djakiew, D. (2010). Biochanin A Reduces Drug-Induced p75^{NTR} expression and Enhances Cell Survival: a New *in Vitro* Assay for Screening Inhibitors of p75^{NTR} Expression. *Rejuvenation Research,* Vol.13, No.5, (October 2010), pp 527-537, PMID 20818983

Gaestel, M. (2006). MAPKAP kinases - MKs - two's company, three's a crowd. *Nature Reviews Molecular Cell Biology,* Vol.7, (February 2007), pp 120-130, PMID 16421520

Gee, J., Barroso, A., Ellis, I., Robertson, J. & Nicholson, R. (2000). Biological and clinical associations of c-jun activation in human breast cancer. *International Journal of Cancer,* Vol.89, No.2, (March 2000), pp 177-186, PMID 10754497

George, D., Suzuki, H., Bova, G. & Isaacs, J. (1998). Mutational analysis of the TrkA gene in prostate cancer. *Prostate,* Vol.36, No.3 (August 1998), pp172-180, PMID 9687989

Golsteyn, R. (2005). Cdk1 and Cdk2 complexes (cyclin dependent kinases) in apoptosis: a role beyond the cell cycle *Cancer Letters,* Vol.217, No.2, (January 2005), pp. 129-138, PMID 15617830

Gonzalez, M., Jimenez, B., Berciano, M., Gonzalez-Sancho, J., Caelles, C., Lafarga, M. & Munoz, A. (2000). Glucocorticoids antagonize AP-1 by inhibiting the Activation/phosphorylation of JNK without affecting its subcellular distribution. *Journal of Cell Biology,* Vol.150, No.5, (September 2000), pp 1199-1208, PMID 10974006

Graham, C., Lynch, J. & Djakiew, D. (1992). Distribution of nerve growth factor-like protein and nerve growth factor receptor in human benign prostatic hyperplasia and prostatic adenocarcinoma. *Journal of Urology,* Vol.147, No.5, (May 1992), pp. 1444-1447, PMID 1373782

Hallböök, F., Ibáñez, C. & Persson, H. (1991). Evolutionary studies of the nerve growth factor family reveal a novel member abundantly expressed in Xenopus ovary. *Neuron,* Vol.6, No.5, (May 1991), pp 845-858, PMID 2025430

Harbour, J. & Dean, D. (2000). The Rb/E2F pathway: expanding roles and emerging paradigms. *Genes and Development,* Vol.14, No.19, (October 2000), pp2393-2409, PMID 11018009

Harper, N., Hughes, M. MacFarlane, M. & Cohen, G. (2003). Fas-associated death domain protein and caspase-8 are not recruited to the tumor necrosis factor receptor 1 signaling complex during tumor necrosis factor-induced apoptosis. *Journal of Biological Chemistry*, Vol.278, No.28, (July 2003), pp 25534-25541, PMID 12721308

He, Q., Luo, X., Jin, W., Huang, Y., Reddy, M., Reddy, E. & Sheikh, M. (2008). Celecoxib and a novel COX-2 inhibitor ON09310 upregulate death receptor 5 expression via GADD153/CHOP. *Oncogene*, Vol.27, No.18 (April 2008), 2656-60, PMID 17968315

Herr, I. & Debatin, K. (2001). Cellular stress response and apoptosis in cancer therapy. *Blood*, Vol.98, No.9, (November 2001), pp 2603-2614, PMID 11675328

Hsu, A., Ching, T., Wang, D., Song, X., Rangnekar, V. & Chen, C. (2000). The cyclooxygenase-2 inhibitor celecoxib induces apoptosis by blocking Akt activation in human prostate cancer cells independently of Bcl-2. *Journal of Biological Chemistry*, Vol.275, No.15, (April 2000), pp 11397-11403, PMID 10753955

Huang, Y., He, Q., Hillman, M., Rong, R. & Sheikh, M. (2001). Sulindac sulfide-induced apoptosis involves death receptor 5 and the caspase 8-dependent pathway in human colon and prostate cancer cells. *Cancer Research*, Vol.61, No.18, (September 2001), pp 6918-6924, PMID 11559570

Huang, Z., Tang, X. & Cambi, F. (2002). Down-regulation of the retinoblastoma protein (rb) is associated with rat oligodendrocyte differentiation. *Molecular and Cellular Neuroscience*, Vol.19, No.2, (February 2002), pp250-262, PMID 11860277

Hur, G., Lewis, J., Yang, Q., Lin, Y., Nakano, H., Nedospasov, S. & Liu, Z. (2003). The death domain kinase RIP has an essential role in DNA damage-induced NF-kappa B activation. *Genes and Development*, Vol.17, No.7, (April 2003), pp 873-882, PMID 12654725

Jacobs, E., Thun, M., Bain, E., Rodríguez, C., Henley, S. & Calle, E. (2007). A large cohort study of long-term daily use of adult-strength aspirin and cancer incidence. *Journal of the National Cancer Institute*, Vol.99, No.8, (April 2007), pp 608-15, PMID 17440162

Jin, S., Kim, T., Yang, K. & Kim, W. (2007). Thalidomide destabilizes cyclooxygenase-2 mRNA by inhibiting p38 mitogen-activated protein kinase and cytoplasmic shuttling of HuR. *European Journal of Pharmacology*, Vol.558, No.1-3, (March 2007), pp 14-20, PMID 17208222

Jin, H., Wang, Z., Liu, L., Gao, L., Sun, L., Li, X., Zhao, H., Pan, Y., Shi, H., Liu, N., Hong, L., Liang, J., Wu, Q., Yang Z., Wu, K. & Fan, D. (2010). R-flurbiprofen reverses multidrug resistance, proliferation and metastasis in gastric cancer cells by p75(NTR) induction. *Molecular Pharmacology*, Vol.7, No.1, (February 2010), pp 156-168, PMID 19916560

Johnson, A., Song, X. Hsu, A. & Chen, C. (2001). Apoptosis signaling pathways mediated by cyclooxygenase-2 inhibitors in prostate cancer cells. *Advances in Enzyme Regulation*, Vol.41, pp 221-235, PMID 11384747

Kamei, S., Sakayama, K., Tamashiro, S., Aizawa, J., Miyawaki, J., Miyazaki, T., Yamamoto, H., Norimatsu, Y., Masuno, H. (2009). Ketoprofen in topical formulation decreases the matrix metalloproteinase-2 expression and pulmonary metastatic incidence in nude mice with osteosarcoma. *Journal of Orthopaedic Research*, Vol.27, No.7, (July 2009), 909-915.

Kang, J. & Sowers, L. (2008). Examination of hypochlorous acid-induced damage to cytosine residues in a CpG dinucleotide in DNA. *Chemical Research in Toxicology*, Vol.21, No.6, (June 2008), pp 1211-1218, PMID 18826175

Kelliher, M., Grimm, S., Ishida, Y., Kuo, F., Stanger, B. & Leder, P. (1998). The death domain kinase RIP mediates the TNF-induced NF-kappaB signal. *Immunity*, Vol.8, No.3, (March 1998), pp 297-303, PMID 9529147

Kennedy, N., Cellurale, C. & Davis, R. (2007). A radical role for p38 MAPK in tumor initiation. *Cancer Cell*, Vol.11, No.2, (February 2007), p101-103, PMID 17292820

Khwaja, F., Allen, J., Lynch, J., Andrews, P. & Djakiew D. (2004). Ibuprofen inhibits survival of bladder cancer cells by induced expression of the p75^{NTR} tumor suppressor protein. *Cancer Research*, Vol.64, No.17, (September 2004), pp 6207-6213, PMID 15342406

Khwaja, F., Tabassum, A., Allen, J. & Djakiew D. (2006). The p75^{NTR} tumor suppressor induces cell cycle arrest facilitating caspase mediated apoptosis in prostate tumor cells. *Biochemical and Biophysical Research Communications*, Vol.341, No.4, (March 2006), pp 1184-1192, PMID 16460673

Kirschenbaum, A., Klausner, A., Lee, R., Unger, P., Yao, S., Liu, X., & Levine, A. (2000). Expression of cyclooxygenase-1 and cyclooxygenase-2 in the human prostate. *Urology*, Vol.56, No.4, (October 2000), pp 671-676, PMID 11018637

Krygier, S. & Djakiew, D. (2001a). The Neurotrophin Receptor p75^{NTR} is a tumor suppressor in the human prostate. *Anticancer Research* Vol.21, No.6A, (November-December 2001) pp. 3749-3756, PMID 11911243

Krygier, S. & Djakiew, D. (2001b). Molecular characterization of p75^{NTR} loss of the expression in human prostate tumor cells. *Molecular Carcinogenesis*, Vol.31, No.1, (May 2001), pp46-55, PMID 11398197

Krygier, S. & Djakiew, D. (2002). Neurotrophin Receptor p75^{NTR} suppresses growth and nerve growth factor-mediated metastasis of human prostate cancer cells. *International Journal of Cancer*, Vol.98, No.1, (March 2002) pp. 1-7, PMID 11857376

Lamballe, F., Klein, R. & Barbacid, M. (1991). trkC, a new member of the trk family of tyrosine protein kinases, is a receptor for neurotrophin-3. *Cell*, Vol.66, No.5, (September 1991), pp967-979, PMID 1653651

Lazebnik, Y., Kaufmann, S., Desnoyers, S., Poirier, G. & Earnshaw, W. (1994). Cleavage of poly(ADP-ribose) polymerase by a proteinase with properties like ICE. *Nature*, Vol.371, No.6495, (September 1994), pp. 346-347, PMID 8090205

Leibrock, J., Lottspeich, F., Hohn, A., Hofer, M., Hengerer, B., Masiakowski, P., Thoenen, H. & Barde, Y. (1989). Molecular cloning and expression of brain-derived neurotrophic factor. *Nature*, Vol.341, No.6238, (September 1989), pp 149-152, PMID 2779653

Liao, Z., Mason, K. & Milas, L. (2007). Cyclo-oxygenase-2 and its inhibition in cancer: is there a role? *Drugs*, Vol.67, No.6, pp 821-45, PMID 17428102

Lin, F., Chen, Y., Lin, Y, Tsai, J., Chen, J., Wang, H., Chen, Y., Li, C. & Lin S.. (2006). The role of human antigen R, an RNA-binding protein, in mediating the stabilization of toll-like receptor 4 mRNA induced by endotoxin: a novel mechanism involved in vascular inflammation. *Arteriosclerosis, Thrombosis, and Vascular Biology*, Vol.26, No.12, (December 2006), pp 2622-2629, PMID 16990552

Lin, Y., Devin, A., Rodriguez, Y. & Liu, Z. (1999). Cleavage of the death domain kinase RIP by caspase-8 prompts TNF-induced apoptosis. *Genes and Development*, Vol.13, No.19, (October 1999), pp 2514-2526, PMID 10521396

Lloyd, F., Slivova, V., Valachovicova, T. & Sliva, D. (2003). Aspirin inhibits highly invasive prostate cancer cells. *International Journal of Oncology*, Vol.23, No.5, (November 2003), pp 1277-1283, PMID 14532966

MacEwan, D. (2002). TNF receptor subtype signaling: differences and cellular consequences. *Cell Signalling*, Vol.14, No.6, (June 2002), pp 477-492, PMID 11897488

MacGrogan, D., Saint-Andre J. & Dicou E. (1992). Expression of nerve growth factor and nerve growth factor receptor genes in human tissues and in prostatic adenocarcinoma cell lines. *Journal of Neurochemistry*, Vol.59, No.4, (October 1992), pp 1381-1391, PMID 1383421

Madaan, S., Abel, P. Chaudhary, K., Hewitt, R., Stott, M., Stamp, G. & Lalani, E. (2000). Cytoplasmic induction and over-expression of cyclooxygenase-2 in human prostate cancer: implications for prevention and treatment. *British Journal of Urology International*, Vol.86, No.6, (October 2000), pp 736-41, PMID 11069387

Maisonpierre, P., Belluscio, L., Squinto, S., Ip, N., Furth, M., Lindsay, R. & Yancopoulos, G. (1990). Neurotrophin-3: a neurotrophic factor related to NGF and BDNF. *Science*, (March 1990) Vol.247, No. 4949, pp 1446-1451, PMID 2321006

Martinon, F., Holler, N., Richard, C. & Tschopp, J. (2000). Activation of a pro-apoptotic amplification loop through inhibition of NF-kappaB-dependent survival signals by caspase-mediated inactivation of RIP. *Federation of Experimental Biology Society Letters*, Vol.468, No.2-3, (February 2000), pp 134-136, PMID 10692573

Mascaux, C., Martin, B., Paesmans, M. Berghmans, T., Dusart, M., Haller, A., Lothaire, P., Meert, A., Lafitte, J. & Sculier, J. (2006). Has Cox-2 a prognostic role in non-small-cell lung cancer? A systematic review of the literature with meta-analysis of the survival results. *British Journal of Cancer*, Vol.95, No.2, (July 2006), pp 139-45, PMID 16786043

Masferrer, J., Zweifel, B.S., Colburn, S.M., Ornberg, R.L., Salvemini, D., Isakson, P. & Seibert, K. (1995). The Role of Cyclooxygenase-2 in Inflammation. *American Journal of Therapeutics*, Vol.2, No.9, (September 1995) pp. 607-610, PMID11854834

Mazumder, B., Seshadri, V. & Fox, P. (2003). Translational control by the 3'-UTR: the ends specify the means. *Trends in Biochemical Sciences*, 2003;Vol.28, No.2, (February 2003), pp 91-98, PMID 12575997

Mazzieri, R., Masiero, L., Zanetta, L., Monea, S., Onisto, M., Garbisa, S. & Mignatti, P. (1997). Control of type IV collagenase activity by components of the urokinase-plasmin system: a regulatory mechanism with cell-bound reactants. *The EMBO Journal*, Vol.16, No.9, (May 1997), pp 2319-32, PMID 9171346

Meyer, C., Jacobs, H. & Lehner, C. (2002). Cyclin d-cdk4 is not a master regulator of cell multiplication in Drosophila embryos. *Current Biology*, Vol.12, No.8, (April 2002), pp 661-666, PMID 11967154

Nalbandian A. & Djakiew, D. (2006). The p75[NTR] metastasis suppressor inhibits urokinase plasminogen activator, matrix metalloproteinase-2 and matrix metalloproteinase-9 in PC-3 prostate cancer cells. *Clinical and Experimental Metastasis*, Vol.23, No.2, (August 2006), pp. 107-116, PMID 16912916

Nalbandian, A., Pang, A., Rennert, O., Chan, W., Ravindranath, N. & Djakiew, D. (2005). A novel function of differentiation revealed by cDNA microarray profiling of p75[NTR]-regulated gene expression. *Differentiation*, Vol.73, No.8 (October 2005), pp385-396, PMID 16316409

Nelson, J. & Harris, R. (2000). Inverse association of prostate cancer and non-steroidal anti-inflammatory drugs (NSAIDs): results of a case-control study. *Oncology Reports*, Vol.7, No.1, (January-February 2000), pp. 69-70, PMID 10601612

O'Neill, J., Manion, M., Schwartz, P. & Hockenbery, D. (2004). Promises and challenges of targeting Bcl-2 anti-apoptotic proteins for cancer therapy *Biochimica Biophysica Acta*, Vol.1705, No.1, (December 2004), pp 43-51, PMID 15585172

Paul, A., Grant, E. & Habib, F. (1992). The expression and localisation of beta-nerve growth factor (beta-NGF) in benign and malignant human prostate tissue: relationship to neuroendocrine differentiation. *British Journal of Cancer*, Vol.74, No.12, (December 1992), pp 1990-1996, PMID 8980402

Perez, M., Regan, T., Pflug, B., Lynch, J. & Djakiew, D. (1997). Loss of low-affinity nerve growth factor receptor during malignant transformation of the human prostate. *Prostate*, Vol.30, No.4, (March 1997), pp. 274-279, PMID 9111606

Pflug, B., Dionne, C., Kaplan, D., Lynch, J. & Djakiew, D. (1995). Expression of a Trk high affinity nerve growth factor receptor in the human prostate. *Endocrinology*, Vol.136, No.1 (January 1995), pp. 262-268, PMID 7828539

Pflug, B. & Djakiew, D. (1998). Expression of p75^NTR in a human prostate epithelial tumor cell line reduces nerve growth factor-induced cell growth by activation of programmed cell death. *Molecular Carcinogenesis* Vol.23, No.2 (October 1998), pp 106-114, PMID 9808164

Pflug, B., Onoda, M., Lynch, J. & Djakiew, D. (1992). Reduced expression of the low affinity nerve growth factor receptor in benign and malignant human prostate tissue and loss of expression in four human metastatic prostate tumor cell lines. *Cancer Research*, Vol.52, No.19 (October 1992), pp. 5403-5406, PMID 1382843

Puthalakath, H. & Strasser, A. (2002). Keeping killers on a tight leash: transcriptional and post-translational control of the pro-apoptotic activity of BH3-only proteins *Cell Death and Differentiation*, Vol.9, No.5, (May 2002), pp505-512, PMID 11973609

Quann, E., Khwaja, F., & Djakiew, D. (2007b). The p38 MAPK Pathway Mediates Aryl Propionic Acid-Induced messenger RNA Stability of p75^NTR in Prostate Cancer Cells. *Cancer Research*, Vol.67, No.23, (December 2007) pp. 11402-11410, PMID 18056468

Quann, E., Khwaja, F., Zavitz, K. & Djakiew, D. (2007a). The Aryl Propionic Acid R-Flurbiprofen Selectively Induces p75^NTR-Dependent Decreased Survival of Prostate Tumor Cells. *Cancer Research* Vol.67, No.7, (April 2007) pp 3254-3262, PMID 17409433

Reuning, U., Magdolen, V., Wilhelm, O., Fischer, K., Lutz, V., Graeff, H. & Schmitt, M. (1998). Multifunctional potential of the plasminogen activation system in tumor invasion and metastasis (review). *International Journal of Oncology*, Vol.13, No.5, (November 1998), pp. 893-906, PMID 9772277

Roberts, R., Jacobson, D., Girman, C., Rhodes, T., Lieber, M. & Jacobsen, S. (2002). A population-based study of daily nonsteroidal anti-inflammatory drug use and prostate cancer. *Mayo Clinic Proceedings*, Vol.77, No.3 (March 2002), pp 219-25, PMID 11888024

Ronkina, N., Kotlyarov, A., Dittrich-Breiholz, O., Kracht, M., Hitti, E., Milarski, K., Askew, R., Marusic, S., Lin, L., Gaestel, M. & Telliez, J. (2007). The mitogen-activated protein kinase (MAPK)-activated protein kinases MK2 and MK3 cooperate in stimulation of tumor necrosis factor biosynthesis and stabilization of p38 MAPK. *Molecular and Cellular Biology*, Vol.27, No.1, (January 2007), pp 170-181, PMID 17030606

Satyanarayana, A. & Rudolph, K. (2004). p16 and ARF: activation of teenage proteins in old age. *Journal of Clinical Investigation*, Vol.114, No.9, (November 2004), pp 1237-1240, PMID 15520854

Sarkar, F, Adsule, S., Li, Y. & Padhye, S. (2007). Back to the future: COX-2 inhibitors for chemoprevention and cancer therapy. *Mini Reviews in Medicinal Chemistry*, Vol.7, No.6, (June 2007), pp 599-608.

Scheper, G., & Proud, C. (2002). Does phosphorylation of the cap-binding protein eIF4E play a role in translation initiation? *European Journal of Biochemistry*, Vol.269, No.22, (November 2002), pp 5350-5359, PMID 12423333

Sellers, W. & Kaelin W. (1996). RB [corrected] as a modulator of transcription. *Biochimica Biophysica Acta*, Vol.1288, No.3, (August 1996), Pp M1-5, PMID 8764839

Sherr, C. (1996). Cancer cell cycles. *Science,* Vol. 274, No. 5293 (December 1996), pp1672-1677, PMID 8939849

Sherr, C. & Roberts, J. (1995). Inhibitors of mammalian G1 cyclin-dependent kinases. *Genes and Development,* Vol.9, No.10, (May 1995), pp 1149-1163, PMID 7758941

Shintani, S., Mihara, M., Nakahara, Y., Kiyota, A., Ueyama, Y., Matsumura, T. & Wong, D. Expression of cell cycle control proteins in normal epithelium, premalignant and malignant lesions of oral cavity. *Oral Oncology,* Vol.38, No.3, (April 2002), pp235-243, PMID 11978545

Shiozaki, E. Y. Shi (2004). Caspases, IAPs and Smac/DIABLO: mechanisms from structural biology. *Trends in Biochemical Sciences,* Vol.29, No.9, (September 2004), pp. 486-494, PMID 15337122

Song, I., Tatebe, S., Dai, W. & Kuo, M. (2005). Delayed mechanism for induction of gamma-glutamylcysteine synthetase heavy subunit mRNA stability by oxidative stress involving p38 mitogen-activated protein kinase signaling. Journal of Biological Chemistry, Vol.280, No.13, (August 2005), pp 28230-28240, PMID 15946948

Soppet, D., Escandon, E., Maragos, J., Middlemas, D., Reid, S., Blair, J., Burton, L., Stanton, B., Kaplan, D., Hunter, T., Nikolics, K. & Parada, L. (1991). The neurotrophic factors brain-derived neurotrophic factor and neurotrophin-3 are ligands for the trkB tyrosine kinase receptor. *Cell,* Vol.65, No.5, (May 1991), pp 895-903, PMID 1645620

Tegeder, I., Pfeilschifter, J., & Geisslinger, G. (2001). Cyclooxygenase-independent actions of cyclooxygenase inhibitors. *Federation of American Society of Experimental Biology Journal,* Vol.15, No.12, (October 2001) pp. 2057-2072, PMID 11641233

Thun, M., Namboodiri, M. & Heath, C. (1991). Aspirin use and reduced risk of fatal colon cancer. *The New England Journal of Medicine,* Vol.325, No.23, (December 1991), pp 1593-6, PMID 1669840

Tran, H., Maurer, F. & Nagamine, Y. (2003). Stabilization of urokinase and urokinase receptor mRNAs by HuR is linked to its cytoplasmic accumulation induced by activated mitogen-activated protein kinase-activated protein kinase 2. *Molecular and Cellular Biology,* Vol.23, No.20, (October 2003), pp 7177-7188, PMID 14517288

von der Haar, T., Gross, J., Wagner, G. & McCarthy, J. (2004). The mRNA cap-binding protein eIF4E in post-transcriptional gene expression. *Nature Structure and Molecular Biology,* Vol.11, No.6, (June 2004), pp 503-511, PMID 15164008

Westwood, G., Dibling, B., Cuthbert-Heavens, D. & Burchill, S. (2002). Basic fibroblast growth factor (bFGF)-induced cell death is mediated through a caspase-dependent and p53-independent cell death receptor pathway. *Oncogene,* Vol.21, No.5, (January 2002), pp 809-824, PMID 11850809

Wynne, S. & Djakiew, D. (2010). NSAID-inhibition of prostate cancer cell migration is mediated by Nag-1 induction via the p38 MAPK-p75[NTR] pathway. *Molecular Cancer Research,* Vol.8, No.12, (December 2010), pp 1656-1664, PMID 21097678

Yoshimura, R., Sano, H., Masuda, C., Kawamura, M., Tsubouchi, Y., Chargui, J., Yoshimura, N., Hla, T. & Wada, S. (2000). Expression of cyclooxygenase-2 in prostate carcinoma. *Cancer,* Vol.89, No.3, (August 2000), pp 589-596, PMID 10931458

Zarubin, T. & Han, J. (2005). Activation and signaling of the p38 MAP kinase pathway. *Cell Research,* Vol.15, No.1, (January 2005), p11-18, PMID 15686620

Zha, S., Gage, W., Sauvageot, J., Saria, E., Putzi, M., Ewing, C., Faith, D., Nelson, W., De Marzo, A. & Isaacs, W. (2001). Cyclooxygenase-2 is up-regulated in proliferative inflammatory atrophy of the prostate, but not in prostate carcinoma. *Cancer Research,* Vol.61, No.24, (December 2001), pp 8617-8623, PMID 11751373

4

Development of Miniature ^{125}I - Seeds for the Treatment of Prostate Cancer

Sanjay Kumar Saxena and Ashutosh Dash
Radiopharmaceuticals Division, Bhabha Atomic Research Centre, Trombay, Mumbai
India

1. Introduction

Cancer of prostate is one of the very common diseases of ageing men with incidence rises up 40% over the age of 75-80 years. It has also been noticed recently, that incidences of prostate cancers are on increase specially in many developing countries mainly because of long survival time due to better health care facilities available now-a-days and also due to changes in lifestyles of population of these countries. As compared with white men, black men have a 40% higher risk of the disease and twice the rate of death. The mortality due to prostate cancer has steadily declined for a decade, and it decreased by 4% per year between 1999 and 2003. This decrease may be attributable to several factors, including earlier detection of cancer and improved local and possibly systemic treatment [1]. Thanks to the recent advancements in diagnostic tools, more and more patients are being diagnosed with potentially curable localized prostate cancer at a time where radical local treatment is deemed to be appropriate. For disease that is likely confined to the prostate and the immediate surrounding area, surgery, external beam radiation (EBRT) and seed implantation are the primary treatment options. In recent years, seed implantation has become more popular as a treatment option as it is simpler, less traumatic and the duration of relief is comparable. It has been estimated that up to 50% of patients with early stage prostate cancer are now receiving ultra sound guided seed implantation [2].

2. Historical background

Seed implantation for prostate cancer began in 1911. Louis Pasteur suggested that surgical insertion of radium seed into the prostate may eradicate this malignancy [3]. A number of techniques were subsequently used with limited success. In the 1960s, Drs. Scardino and Carlton at Baylor College of Medicine, Houston, reintroduced permanent prostate brachytherapy using ^{198}Au interstitial implantation in combination with external beam radiation therapy (EBRT)[4].

At about the same time, Dr. Whitmore and colleagues at Memorial Sloan Kettering Cancer Center (MSKCC) also began to insert ^{125}I seeds through an open incision as a sole treatment [5]. Unfortunately, these early techniques did not allow for clear visualization of the seeds as they were being inserted into the prostate and, as a result, there was often poor dose coverage of the prostate gland. However, some important information was obtained from these early seed implantation approaches. Local control was better in patients who received high-quality implants and who had low-grade and early-stage cancer. The subsequent development of the transperineal, ultrasound guided approach provided a means to more accurately place seeds and thereby improve dose coverage. In the 1980s, several investigators were exploring new brachytherapy approaches to the treatment of prostate cancer. Drs. Syed and Puthawala pioneered a temporary seed technique of placing the needles while visualizing them through an open laparotomy [6]. In 1983, Dr. Holm introduced the use of transrectal ultrasound to visualize the permanent placement of 125I seeds via needles inserted through the perineum directly into the prostate[7]. Drs Blasko and Ragde [8] began the first transperineal ultrasound-guided approach in the United States. The transperineal ultrasound-guided, approach resulted in increased accuracy of seed placement and relatively even distribution of seeds throughout the prostate. This marked a major advance in prostate brachytherapy in that it allowed more precise planning of the implant prior to the procedure. These advances also significantly increased the accuracy of seed placement and insured that the prostate would receive the proper number, strength, and positioning of radioactive sources.

The first transrectal ultrasound-guided, template-guided 125I implant procedure was carried out at the Seattle Prostate Institute in late 1985 and is now being practiced around the world. The original Seattle approach has been modified and improved several times since the original implants. As this procedure has become more popular, many technical improvements have been added to improve the consistency and quality of the procedure. The availability of better imaging techniques such as transrectal ultrasound, fluoroscopy, high quality CT scan, etc. have now made permanent prostate implants much more refined. Today, the implant is planned prior to the procedure either on the day of or several weeks prior to the implant. Typically, the implant is completed in a 45-90 minute outpatient procedure under spinal anesthesia or light general anesthesia [8].

In addition to the availability of loose sealed radioactive sources, seeds incorporating radionuclides such as 125I ,103Pd and 131Cs are now available in continuous strand form, increasing the likelihood that the seeds will remain in place after implantation. About 60-140 radioactive seeds encompassing the entire prostate gland are used to eradicate the tumor. While slight differences in technique are expected to grow as more and more physicians perform this procedure and as more technical advances are made, the basic approach is quite similar and it remains to be determined whether any single technique will prove superior in controlling the cancer.

3. Selection of radionuclide

Beginning in 1967, 125I became the first radioisotope sealed within a titanium capsule popularly known as seed. While its use continues to this day, many patients and doctors in recent years have chosen shorter half-life isotopes other than 125I such as 103Pd and 131Cs.

Radionuclides used in the prostate radiotherapy are 125I, 103Pd or 131Cs. The radiation characteristics of these three isotopes are given in Table 1. The high energy (10-50 MeV) cyclotron produced 103Pd is not yet available in India. The reactor production of 131Cs is difficult due to low percentage abundance of 130Ba (~1%) in natural targets and the logistics and cost considerations of this isotope do not permit its use at present. On the other hand, 125I with its relatively longer half-life and suitable gamma energy coupled with ease of production is a cost effective isotope and can be easily produced by (n,γ) reaction of natural 124Xe gas in a special set up provided in the research reactors (DHRUVA) of BARC, Mumbai, India. The production and processing procedures for ^{125}I have been developed and regular production of this isotope has been commenced by Radiopharmaceuticals Division, BARC, Mumbai.

The Indian pursuit of developing technology for ^{125}I brachytherapy sources was driven mainly by three considerations, namely, (a) well-established and ease of reliable production of ^{125}I in several GBq quantities in the research reactors in BARC, (b) need to provide ^{125}I-brachytherapy sources at an affordable cost to meet the domestic needs, (c) help to ease reliance on import and to promote the beneficial use of ^{125}I- brachytherapy sources in the country.

Isotope	$T_{1/2}$	Specific Activity (TBq/g)	Mode of Decay	Average Energy (keV)	Dose Delivery	Total Dose	Production methods
^{125}I	60d	650	EC (100%)	28.5	90% in 204 days	145 Gy	^{124}Xe$(n,\gamma)^{125}$Xe$\rightarrow^{125}$I Nuclear Reactor
^{103}Pd	17d	2763	EC (100%)	21	90% in 58 days	125 Gy	^{103}Rh$(p,n)^{103}$Pd Cyclotron
^{131}Cs	9 d	3808	EC (100%)	30.4	90% in 33 days	115 Gy	^{130}Ba$(n,\gamma)^{131}$Ba$\rightarrow^{131}$Cs Nuclear Reactor

Table 1. Radiation Characteristics of radionuclides used in prostate seed implantation

4. Source requirements

The encapsulated source's outer dimensions are ~ 4.75 mm length and 0.8mmdia. The active core is situated within the shell of the capsules, often of 50 micron thickness. Iodine belongs to the halogen group of elements which is highly reactive. Although several stable compounds of iodides are reported in the literature, most of them have a definite solubility in water/saline. The main challenge, therefore, is to develop a non-leachable source core containing ^{125}I incorporated in a solid substrate at very high specific activity. Production of the source core in a highly reproducible manner within acceptable dimensional tolerances is yet another challenge. An innovative strategy has to be devised to develop the necessary technology for fabrication of ^{125}I source core, capsules and encapsulation technique. Preparation of ^{125}I-brachytherapy sources addresses the following main issues:
a. Immobilization of ^{125}I in a suitable solid matrix.
b. Quality evaluation of the sources.
c. Fabrication of titanium capsules of suitable dimensions.
d. Hermetic Sealing of the capsules by Laser welding.
e. Quality assurance of the encapsulated sources.

5. Preparation of ^{125}I minature source cores

Two types of source core are used for the preparation of ^{125}I seed; namely
- Rod/wire type sources
- Spherical type sources

Silver is chosen as the basic matrix for immobilization of iodine which functions both as the active support and as the x-ray marker. Iodine-125 can be used directly in its elemental form, or as iodide, iodate, hypoiodate, or other ionic forms, or in the form of compounds such as aliphatic or aromatic iodo labeled compounds. The choice of anion(s) depend on the methodology intended to use. Owing to volatile nature of elemental iodine, iodide ions are used for source preparation. Iodine-125 as iodide may be physically trapped in or on the substrate, by adsorption, or may be chemically attached to it in some way. The radioactive source core should be of an overall size and dimensions to fit inside a conventional seed container suitable for encapsulation. The range of desired activity is about 0.3 to 4.0 mCi per seed.

5.1 Preparation of rod/wire type source cores

Silver wires of guranted purity of 3 mm length & 0.5mm dia are used to incorporate Iodine-125. The following methodologies were explored for preparing [125I]-silver rod source core.
1.   Electrodeposition
2.   Physical & physico-chemical adsorption

5.1.1 Electro deposition

Anodic electro deposition of radio iodine ([125I]) was carried out in a quartz bath size [1.2 cm (dia.), 2.5 cm (ht)] with platinum cathode (1mm). The wires were arranged in the cell as shown in Fig.1. Various experimental parameters such as the current used, radioiodine concentration in the cell and time for deposition were optimized to obtain maximum activity on the silver wire. By this method, more than 85% of the initial radioactivity could be firmly deposited on the source at 20 µA current for 25-30 min duration on the silver wires. These sources with extremely good reproducibility and consistency with respect to activity content, could by this method [9].

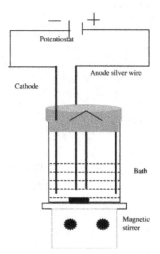

Fig. 1. Schematic diagram of the electro-deposition set-up.

Cieszykowska et al.[10] have also developed an electrochemical method of depositing [125I] form an electrolyte containing 0.01 M NaOH. In brief, 10 ml of solution containing appropriate amount of I-125 was taken in a platinum crucible which served as cathode. The cathode consists of a single silver bar of 3 mm long and 0.5 mm in diameter. The volume of the electrolyte used was 10 mL and the distance between the electrodes was about 20 mm.

The potential of the cell was kept at 233 mV. The electrodeposition was carried out under ultra violet radiation.

5.1.2 Iodination of the silver rod

Zhang et al. [11] have described a method of depositing ^{125}I using chlorinated silver rod. In brief, the procedure involved coating a layer of AgCl on the silver rod of 3 mm long and 0.5 mm in diameter. The activated silver rods were put into 4 mol/l nitric acid and heated for 5 minutes. They were then put into a mixed solution of sodium hypochlorite and hydrochloric acid. The chlorinated silver rods were put in Na^{125}I solution at pH > 6.5 to deposit required amount of ^{125}I.

5.1.3 Absorption of ^{125}I on a ceramic matrix

Han et al. [12] have described a method of depositing ^{125}I using a ceramic rods. The ceramic rods of 3 mm long and 0.5 mm sizes were immersed in conc. HF solution for 4 hours, scratched with a specially made pin along the length at regular intervals to made miniature horizontal cavities of ~ 0.1 mm depth. they were then immersed aqueous AgNO$_3$ solution to absorb the solution. Impregnation of ^{125}I on to the treated rod was carried out by the controlled addition of Na^{125}I solution at pH > 9 to deposit required amount of ^{125}I. Extending this theme, Park et al.[13] have investigated the possibility of adsorption of ^{125}I on a Ag + Al$_2$O$_3$ rod as a carrier body. The adsorption capacity was more than 95% after 4 hours at a volume of 50 μl containing about 5 mCi of ^{125}I.

5.1.4 Physico-chemical adsorption

Our group have used a novel method to adsorb radioiodine(^{125}I) on silver wires, by precoating the wires with palladium[14-15]. The experimental conditions such as amount of radioactivity, carrier concentration, reaction time, reaction temperature, reaction volume, pH of the reaction mixture, etc. were systematically optimized to achieve best results. More than 80% of the initial radioactivity could be firmly deposited on the source core. The sources with extremely good reproducibility and consistency with respect to activity content and other quality parameters could be produced.

The microstructures of plain silver wire and palladium coated silver wires are shown in Fig. 2 (a) and (b) respectively, indicating the presence of huge sites for sorption of iodine on palladium cated silver wires.

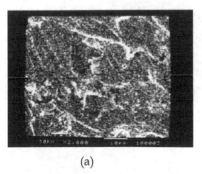 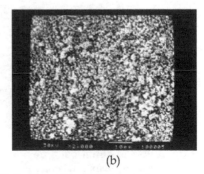

      (a)   (b)

Fig. 2. (a) SEM of Plain Silver wire Fig. 2 (b) SEM of Palladium Coated Silver wire

5.1.5 Comparison of techniques

The electrodeposition method of preparing ^{125}I source core is a straight forward procedure and used by many commercial manufacturers of these sources. Quantitative firm and uniform deposition could be obtained by the optimized parameters, with low leaching of activity. However this method is labour intensive, require high skill and would be exposing personnel to long time to radiation. The electro deposition method is attractive only if automated system where radioactive iodine is electrodeposited on a long piece of silver wire of the required diameter and subsequently precision cut in to the required dimensions by remotely operated electro mechanical cutting devices, is available.

The inherent drawbacks of absorption of 125I on a ceramic matrix and iodination of the silver rod, include a tedious time-consuming matrix preparation procedure, need for strict adherence to the operational protocol, and the requirement for well-trained, skilled operator.

Chemisorption of ^{125}I activity on the $PdCl_2$ treated silver wire as more suitable for adsorption of ^{125}I than plain silver wires in terms of quantitative adsorption and non-leachability of ^{125}I activity. The procedure is straightforward and easily performed. The workload to use this protocol is small. The incidence of serious error may be low. The mild experimental conditions of adsorption at neutral to alkaline pH facilitates the safe handling of high amounts of radioactivity for the preparation of therapeutic sources without the release of air activity. The stability of ^{125}I on Pd coated silver wire is due to the formation of insoluble palladous iodide on the surface of the wire and accounts for low leachability. This procedure is routinely used by Radiopharmaceuticals Division, BARC, Mumbai. Fig. 3 depicts the laboratory used for the regular production of ^{125}I source core.

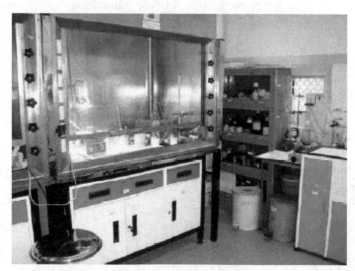

Fig. 3. Laboratory for the production of ^{125}I source core

5.2 Preparation of spherical type source cores

A linear assembly of six alumina microspheres or six palladium coated silver spheres of 0.5 mm(ϕ) were used for making spherical seed sources.

5.2.1 Alumina microspheres

A mixture of pre-cooled (5°C) solution of hexamethylenetetraamine and urea (3 M) with aluminum nitrate solution was dispersed as droplets into hot oil to bring about the formation of aluminium hydroxide in to solid gel sphere form. The spheres were dried in an air oven at 100°C and heat treated at 700°C for 5 h in a furnace to obtain alumina spheres. Spheres of uniform sizes were selected by passing through a 600 μm mesh. The experimental conditions such as amount of radioactivity, carrier concentration, reaction time, reaction temperature, reaction volume etc. were systematically optimised. By this method, more than 95% of the initial radioactivity could be firmly deposited on the source core and 0.6-0.8 mCi of radioiodine could be adsorbed on the alumina microsphere [9].

5.2.2 Metallic microspheres

Silver beads of dimension of 0.5 mm(ϕ) were pre-coated with palladium for the incorporation of radioiodine (^{125}I). The experimental conditions such as amount of radioactivity, carrier concentration, reaction time, reaction temperature, reaction volume, pH of the reaction mixture, etc. were systematically optimized [16]. By this method, more than 83 % of the initial radioactivity could be irreversibly adsorbed on the palladium coated on the source core and radioactive sources in the range of 20-251 MBq (0.5-0.6 mCi) can be prepared. The sources with extremely good reproducibility and consistency w.r.t. activity content and other quality parameters could be produced. All the sources were measured with calibrated ionization chambers and seed strength was quoted with an overall uncertainty of ± 10%.

5.2.3 Comparison of techniques

The physicochemical adsorption of radioiodine on alumina microspheres is easy and also less expensive. Quantitative adsorption of activity on the spheres is possible by using radioactive iodine in iodate (IO^-_3) form. However, it was found that the percentage leachability of radioactivity from the spheres was more than desirable. Further developments are needed to assess the potential of this approach on a reliable and continuous basis.

The physicochemical adsorption of Pd-silver microspheres is easy and ^{125}I-beads could be prepared in a nonleachable form. The radioactive sources upto ~111MBq (3 mCi) activity can be prepared by arranging six individual beads in a well-arranged geometry.

6. Fabrication of titanium capsules

The capsule matrix should have chemical compatibility with the source core which will be encapsulated inside. The capsule material need to be of low atomic weight so that it would attenuate radiation to a minimum extent. Titanium's unique combination of attributes such as light weight, high strength to weight ratio, corrosion resistance, amenability for easy welding, biocompatibility, and durability in extreme environments make it an excellent material for capsule fabrication. Titanium is used extensively for medical and dental implants because it is biocompatible with the human body. It is completely inert and immune to corrosion by all fluids and tissues of the body, making it ideal for encapsulation. The wall thickness of the capsule should be adequate to provide requisite mechanical strength to retain the source core, in order to reduce the risk of radioactive contamination in the event of source rupture during handling. At the same time it should not be too thick to attenuate the radiation emanating from the source. The wall thickness of the capsule is configured to provide adequate mechanical strength as well as required radiation output. About 0.05 mm thick titanium tubes is sufficient to allow gamma rays and low energy X-rays to pass through for providing therapeutic effect. It is preferred that the capsule have an open end and a closed end. The capsule is preferably sealed with a suitable end cap using techniques such as laser/electron beam welding.

The titanium Capsules of the required dimensions 4.75mm(l) x 0.8 mm(ϕ) x 0.05mm(t) along with suitable caps(lids) of 0.8mm(ϕ) are generally used. Fig.4 shows the cross-sectional view of titanium encapsulated wire source and microspheres.

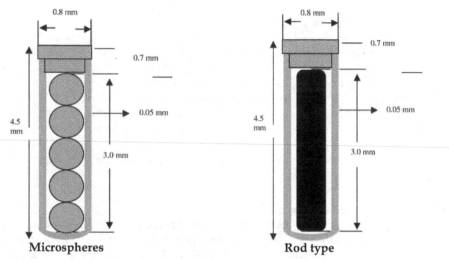

Fig. 4. Cross sectional view of encapsulated ^{125}I- sources.

7. Laser welding of titanium capsules

The welding of capsules containing radioactive sources requires that the following conditions are met:

- The welding has to be carried out in a well ventilated shielded enclosure
- The process of welding should be feasible in a remotely operated system.
- The welding should not change the geometry of the capsules.
- Loss of activity during the welding should be minimum(minimum heat input to the active source)
- Efficiency of welding should be such that there should not be leakage of activity after welding.(Welding should cause less porosity)

The activities of the ^{125}I rods/spheres were measured and the sources with activity within ± 5 % of the targeted activity (generally 111 MBq/source) were segregated and used for encapsulation. The rods were inserted individually into the titanium capsule followed by placement of a cap over it with the aid of magnifying glass. The source loading procedure adapted in radiopharmaceuticals Division of Bhabha Atomic Research Center is depicted in Fig.5.

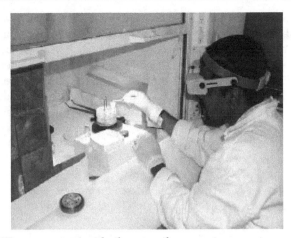

Fig. 5. Loading of ^{125}I source core inside the capsules

Although the tungsten inert gas (TIG) process is the most common method for welding SS capsules, this is not suited to our type of application.TIG welding cause molten titanium to flow down and the weld was observed to be porous. The most likely cause of porosity is the trapping of gas bubbles between dendrites during solidification and presence of hydrogen from moisture in the arc environment. This resulted in the leakage of radioactivity from the welded capsules significantly higher than the prescribed limit. Hence an alternative method of welding is to be adopted.

In order to circumvent these problems, a pulsed laser welding system was used for the encapsulation of capsules. This system consists of a laser head, power supply unit, chiller unit and welding system. As the welding is carried out in pulses, the heat input to the ^{125}I source is reduced. The Nd:YAG laser installed inside the fume-hood in our laboratory is shown in the Fig.6. The output of the laser is taken through the ports and it is connected to the welding head using optical fiber.

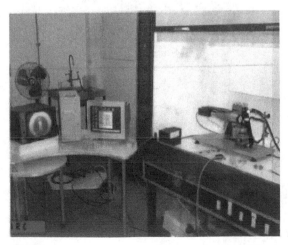

Fig. 6. Laser Welding System

Major advantages of laser beam welding are low welding stresses, low risk of distortion, creation of minimal heat affected zone with minimal ^{125}I contamination and capability of welding of varying mass that allows hermetic sealing of Ti capsules. Nd:YAG pulsed lasers have the ability to weld hard materials like Ti and produce an aesthetic weld with high depth/width ratio free from any weld buildup that eliminates many secondary operations such as grinding or honing. It has also high welding speed, good reproducibility, flexibility and the process can be easily be remotized and automated. Due to the extreme reactivity of titanium metal, it is essential to shield the molten pool and the hot metal from contact with air. Argon is used as inert gas protection.

Prior to welding, the welding parameters such as energy of laser pulse, frequency, pulse duration and rotational speed of sample are systematically optimized to obtain quality welds with negligible leakage. The laser-welding operations were carried out remotely using PC-based controlled system. Fig. 7 depicts a typical welded ^{125}I- seed.

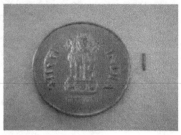

Fig. 7. Encapsulated ^{125}I- brachytherapy sources

The metallography test of welded capsules was carried out by optical metallography (The metallograph of a welded source is shown in Fig. 8.

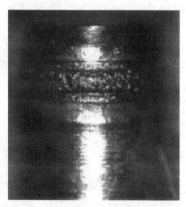

Fig. 8. Optical micrograph (50 times magnified) of a welded capsule.

The penetration depth in the samples was evaluated by Scanning Electron Microscopy(SEM). The SEM micrograph is depicted in Fig. 9. The penetration depth was found to be ~ 2-3 times the wall thickness of the capsules. The welded samples showed high integrity and superior metallurgical quality.

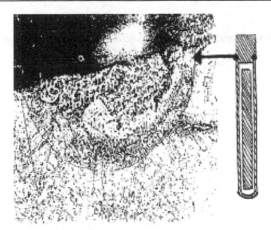

Fig. 9. SEM of welded capsule

8. Quality control of sealed sources

Quality is "the degree to which a set of inherent characteristics fulfils requirements." Control is "the need or expectation that is stated, generally implied or obligatory." Iodine-125 sources produced are subjected to numerous checks obligatory by regulatory authorities. The emphasis given is on the physical and chemical aspects. The schematic diagrm of an assembly of laser welded ^{125}I seed is shown in Fig. 10.

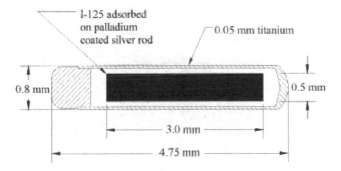

Fig. 10. Assembly of laser welded ^{125}I seed

8.1 Source strength measurement

The estimation of source activity/ strength for the seed was carried out by using a calibrated well-type ionization chambers. The charge collected per unit time by keeping the source at the position of peak response in the well chamber was multiplied by the calibration factor to estimate the activity content of source. The factor recommended by AAPM for converting the strength of ^{125}I-seeds from apparent activity (mCi) to source strength (i.e. air kerma strength) is 1.27 mGy/h-m^2 per mCi (irrespective of internal construction of the source) and the same was used as a reference for the studies carried out at our end. A source calibration accuracy of ~ 3% relative to existing air kerma standards seems reasonable. The radiation equipment should not be used whenever the level is exceeded.

8.2 Leachability

Source cores (Un-encapsulated) were immersed in 100 mL of still distilled water at ambient temperature for 48 hours. At the end of 48 hours, the total leached out radioactivity was assayed to determine the leachability of bare sources should be less than 0.01% of the total seed activity. The physico-chemical adsorption method [14] adapted by us was found to achieve this limit and thus complied with regulatory norms.

8.3 Swipe test

The sealed sources are tested for surface contamination or presence of any loose activity by swiping the sources using alcohol immersed cotton wool and checking the radioactive content in a NaI(Tl) scintillation counter. When the activities detected in the swipe is less than 185 Bq, the sealed source capsule is considered to be contamination free.

8.4 Uniformity of activity

Uniformity of deposition of ^{125}I activity was examined by autoradiography using a specially designed gadget (Fig. 11.) A circular disc [4.4 cm (ϕ), 1.4cm thick] made of brass with a central hole of 3mm diameter and 8 mm depth was taken and eight equidistant tunnels (45° angle between each successive tunnels) of uniform aperture were drilled through the central hole. One source was placed at a time in the central hole and autoradiographed simultaneously by wrapping a strip of photographic film all along the side of brass disc.

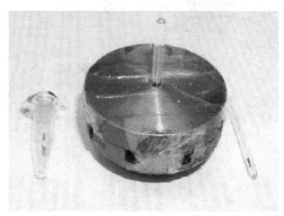

Fig. 11. Gadget for Auto-radiography

The film gets exposed from eight equidistant directions through the holes. The Optical density distribution of the exposed film at different angles was measured by B/W transmission densitometer. The variation in OD values at different positions should be ±10 %. Sources prepared by the physico-chemical adsorption methodology [14] in our laboratory has variation within ± 5% (Fig.12).

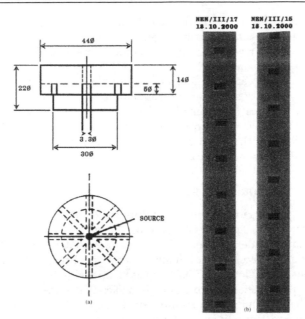

Fig. 12. (a) Specially designed autoradiography gadget; b) developed autoradiography film of the sources.

8.5 Leakage test

It was mandatory to check all the sealed sources to ascertain leak tightness of the sealing. The following tests are performed on all the sources.

Bubble test

The fabricated sealed sources are placed in nearly boiling water kept in a glass beaker for about 2 minutes. Appearance of bubbles from the sealed sources indicates improper sealing and such sources are discarded.

Pressure test

The fabricated sealed sources are immersed in a closed glass container containing ethylene glycol and the pressure inside the chamber is reduced to 100 mm of Hg. Any leak from the sources is shown by a string of bubbles, and such sources are rejected.

8.6 Immersion test

One sealed source is immersed in 20 mL of water taken in a glass beaker and heated to 50°C for 5 hours. The source is removed, the water concentrated to 1mL and the activity released is estimated in a well type NaI(Tl) counter. Activity measuring 185 Bq /source is considered to be the limit for acceptance of leak tightness. When the activities detected in the immersion test of the sealed source is less than 185 Bq, the sealed source capsule is considered to be leak tight.

The following steps should be taken during Quality Control of 125I seeds.

i.   The surface of each source must be checked regularly for visible damage. Sources with damaged surface must not be touched for wipe test.

ii.   All quality control results must be documented.

iii.   For each type of test separate instrument should be used.

iv.   Ion chamber used for measuring activity should be used solely for that purpose only and should be kept separately.

v.   Swipe test should be carried out using a dedicated surface contamination detector which can easily show even the smallest amount of radioactive material. The table used for keeping the surface contamination detector must be separated from the source preparation laboratory. The instruments may get contaminated and must be decontaminated regularly. The verification of the absence of radiation in the surface contamination detector should be a routine task.

9. Classification performance testing

For use of radioactive seeds in interstitial applications, where sources of higher radioactive strength of the order of 30 GBq to 370 GBq and comprising of radiologically more hazardous and longer lived radionuclides such as ^{137}Cs, ^{192}Ir etc. are used, the integrity of sources upto a temperature of 600°C is necessarily evaluated. In case of ^{125}I-seeds, the strength of a typical implant of 100 seeds is very low (1.85-3.7 GBq) as compared to the strength of ^{137}Cs or ^{192}Ir sources. However, the volatile nature of iodine makes the source vulnerable to air borne release of radioactivity at higher temperature exposure conditions. In view of the low levels of radioactivity, low radiotoxicity and less risk of accidents or hazards associated with ^{125}I - seeds, the exemption for test at 600°C seeds was sought from Atomic Energy Regulatory Board, India. ^{125}I -seeds were tested upto 400°C, a temperature that was experimentally found to release the radioactivity within the permissible levels of 185 Bq. Release of radioactivity from sources after subjecting them to various classification performance evaluation tests was found to be well within the permissible level of 185 Bq and the source design was approved by Atomic Energy Regulatory Board, India under class C-43211. Classification performance testing of indigenous ^{125}I-seeds was carried out for ensuring their safety in brachytheray applications [17] and following tests were performed.

9.1 Temperature and thermal shock tests

Sealed sources were tested for their integrity under extreme temperature as well as quick changes in temperature. Two sources are heated to of 400 °C in a controlled manner and kept at this temperature for one hour. Two other sources are heated to 400 °C for 15 minutes and then quenched to 20°C. Two other sources are cooled to - 40 °C and kept at this temperature for 20 minutes. All these sources are subjected to tests for leakage in hot water and surface contamination as described above. When the activities detected are less than 185 Bq, the sealed source pass this test.

9.2 Pressure test

In order to assess the strength of the sources to withstand extreme pressures, two sealed sources are subjected to a pressure of 2 MPa. In a separate set-up, two sources are subjected to a vacuum of 25 kPa. After repeating two cycles of both these tests for 5 minutes, tests for leakage in hot water and surface contamination are carried out. When the activities detected in the swipe as well as in water are less than 185 Bq, the sealed sources were consider withstanding extreme pressures.

9.3 Impact test

In order to evaluate the ability of the sealed source to withstand high impacts, a steel billet of 50 grams weight is dropped over the sealed sources from a height of one meter. The integrity the sealed source is then examined by visual examination as well as conducting leakage tests and surface contamination tests. If a wipe test or leakage tests detects less than 185Bq (0.005 µCi) of removable radioactive material, the sealed sources are consider withstanding high impacts.

10. Radiological safety

In view of radioactive nature of ^{125}I, safe and appropriate radioactive procedures should be adopted during the whole preparation process. Although gamma/X-ray emanating from ^{125}I have little penetrating power, they are hazardous if ^{125}I is ingested or inhaled. For this reason, it is recommended to wear protective clothing and safety glasses when working with ^{125}I. Radiation monitoring of personnel should be accomplished with TLD dosimeters worn while working. The room or area used for the preparation of ^{125}I sources must be posted with a sign having the words "Caution - Radioactive Materials". Ventilation of the source preparation laboratory should be sufficient to quickly reduce the presence of gaseous radioactive products. It is useful to locate a surveillance monitor in the source preparation laboratory which can give a warning signal if there is significant increase in the radiation level resulting from radioactive contamination on the work place. The sensitivity of the monitor should be easily adjustable. The ALARA principle should be observed with regard to the radiation exposure of the operating staff. Reduction of the dose during the preparation of ^{25}I-brachytherapy sources can be achieved by a combination of the following principles:

i.   Reduce the time of exposure during handling of activity, as the total dose is proportional with time. Materials and equipment used for source preparation must be set ready. Procedures must be practiced with non-active, dummy material to gain experience.

ii.   Keep the distance as large as possible. Radioactive materials should not be touched by hand. It is recommended to use long forceps or tweezers to handle the source cores. The inverse square law is the most effective method of dose reduction.

iii. Reduce the amount of radioactive materials handling as far as possible. Measures must be taken to reduce the exposure from the radioactive materials not used for source preparation. Each source must be subjected quality control separately, while any other source is stored in a shielded container and set aside at some distance.

iv.   Use the shielding material that is available. Examples are the shields at the preparation hood or movable shields besides the ion chamber.

Radioactive sources cannot be left in the laboratory hood. All fabricated sources must be registered. The register must contain information on the activity on a given date and eventually the batch number and the results of the QC checks. The sources have to be locked away safely in a storage container. The radiation level at 1 m from the container surface should be less than 1 mSv. h^{-1} and at the surface less than 2 mSv.h^{-1}. Storage containers must be fire resistant and carefully locked when in use to prevent access by unauthorized persons. The radiation symbols should be clearly visible on each container. A logbook must show the date of dispatch and the destination of the sources such as user's address.

11. Conclusion

The technique of permanent seed implantation in management of prostate carcinoma is historically proven and is being widely used in many advanced countries. Modern transrectal ultrasound-guided, interstitial permanent brachytherapy is a single outpatient treatment for the majority of men with early-stage prostate cancer. It has documented five- and ten-year biochemical, overall, and disease-specific relapse-free survival rates that equal the best that radical prostatectomy has thus far achieved. These favorable findings have established permanent prostate brachytherapy as a primary treatment option for early stage prostate cancer.

The potential utility of various methods for the preparation of ^{125}I-brachytherapy sources for prostate cancer have been documented. Quality control of ^{125}I-brachytherapy sources after preparation is an important part. Many publications give recommendations on frequencies of quality control procedures without describing the procedures. It is, however, of extreme importance for the general process of quality assurance that these procedures are well defined and understood by the source manufactures. The quality control procedure depicted in this manuscript can be applied universally irrespective of the source preparation method adapted. The procedures presented here are a set of minimum requirements and can serve as guidelines for developing a QC protocol. It should be noted, however, that if any national set of requirements exists, these should be followed. It is envisaged that any one of the source preparation strategy would serve for ensuring easy availability ^{125}I-brachytherapy sources particularly in Institution with Radiochemistry Laboratory facility where commercial sources are too expensive. Availability ^{125}I-brachytherapy sources at local level would promote the beneficial use of permanent seed implantation technique.

12. Acknowledgements

The authors express their gratitude to all who have contributed in the preparation of this chapter. The authors are highly grateful to Prof. M. R. A. Pillai, Head, Radiopharmaceuticals Division for his keen interest, guidance, encouragement, valuable scientific discussions and support. The authors also wish to thank Dr. Meera Venkatesh, former Head, Radiopharmaceuticals Division for her encouragement and administrative support. The authors wish to thank Prof. V. Venugopal, Director, Radiochemistry and Isotope Group and Prof. K.L. Ramkumar, Associate Director, Radiochemistry and Isotope Group for their administrative support. The authors are indebted to their ex-colleagues Mr. S.A.Balakrishnan, Dr. M.A. Majali, Mr. C. Mathew who have started the work and brought to the this shape. The authors also thanks Mr. P. Sreeramakrishnan and Mr. A.S.Tapase of Isotope Applications Division, BARC for their contribution in the autoradiography analysis, Mr. K.C. Sahoo and Mr. E.Ramadasan of Post Irradiation Examination Division, BARC for the metallography analysis of welded capsules,Dr. K.T. Pillai, Fuel Chemistry Division for his contribution in making the alumina microspheres, Dr. C.G.S.Pillai, Chemistry Division, BARC for his contribution in the SEM analysis. The authors are grateful to Dr. (Mrs.) A. Shanta and Dr. S.D.Sharma of Radiological Physics & Advisory Division of our Institute for establishing clinical dosimetric parameters. The authors are grateful to the Engineers of Centre for Design and Manufacture for undertaking the fabrication of titanium capsules.

13. References

[1] Localized Prostate Cancer-Patrick C. Walsh, Theodore L. DeWeese, and Mario A. Eisenberger- N Engl J Med 2007;357:2696-705.

[2] Prostate Canvcer Brachytherapy: Clinical and Financial Imperatives for Permanent Implantation, in Oncology Roundtable Annual Meeting. Washington, D.C., The Advisory Board Co., 2000, p 15

[3] Porter AT, Blasko JC, Grimm PD, Reddy SM, Ragde H: Brachytherapy for prostate cancer . CA Cancer J Clin 1995; 45:165-78

[4] Scardino P, Carlton C: Combined interstitial and external irradiation for prostatic cancer, in Principles and Management of Urologic Cancer. Edited by Javadpour N. Baltimore, Williams & Wilkins, 1983, pp 392-408.

[5] Whitmore WF, Jr., Hilaris B, Grabstald H: Retropubic implantation to iodine 125 in the treatment of prostatic cancer. J Urol 1972; 108:918-20 19. Blasko JC, Grimm PD, Ragde H: Brachytherapy and organ preservation in the management of carcinoma of the prostate. Semin. Radiat. Oncol. 1993; 3:240-249

[6] Puthawala A, Syed A, Tansey L: Temporary iridium implant in the management of carcinoma of the prostate. Endocurie Hyper Oncol 1985; 1:25-33

[7] Holm HH, Juul N, Pedersen JF, Hansen H, Stroyer I: Transperineal I-125odine seed implantation in prostatic cancer guided by transrectal ultrasonography. J Urol 1983; 130:283-286

[8] Blasko JC, Radge H, Schumacher D: Transperineal Percutaneous Iodine-125 Implantation For Prostatic Carcinoma Using Transrectal Ultrasound and Template Guidance. Endocurietherapy Hyperthermia Oncol 1987; 3:131-139

[9] R. B. Manolkar, S. U. Sane, K. T Pillai, M. A. Majali, Comparison of methods for preparation of 125I brachytherapy source cores for the treatment of eye cancer, Applied Radiation and Isotopes, Volume 59, Issues 2-3, August-September 2003, Pages 145-150

[10] Izabela Cieszykowska, Andrzej Piasecki, Mieczysław Mielcarski, An approach to the preparation of iodine-125 seed-type sources, NUKLEONIKA 2005;50(1):17 22

[11] Chunfu Zhang, Yongxian Wang, Haibin Tian, Duan Zhiyin Preparation of iodine-125 seed,Part I: Iodination of the silver rod, Journal of Radioanalytical and Nuclear Chemistry, Vol. 252, No. 1 (2002) 161–163

[12] H. S. Han, U. J. Park, A. Dash, The absorption of iodine-131 on a ceramic matrix, Journal of Radioanalytical and Nuclear Chemistry, Vol. 262, No. 3 (2004) 703.705.

[13] U. J. Park, J. S. Lee, K. J. Son, H. S. Han and S. S. Nam, The adsorption of 125I on a Ag+Al2O3 rod as a carrier body for a brachytherapy source, Journal of Radioanalytical and Nuclear Chemistry, Vol. 277, No. 7 (2008) 429-432.

[14] Saxena SK, Shanta A., Rajurkar Nilima S, Majali MA, Studies on the production and quality assurance of miniature 125 I radioactive sources suitable for treatment of ocular and prostate cancers. Appl. Radiat. Isot. 2006; 64: 441-447.

[15] Mathew C., Majali MA, Balakrishnan SA., A novel approach for the adsorption of 125I on silver wire as matrix for brachytherapy for the treatment of eye and prostate cancer. Appl. Radiat. Isot. 2002; 57:359-367.

[16] Sanjay Kumar Saxena, S.D.Sharma, Ashutosh Dash, Meera Venkatesh, Development of a new design 125I-brachytherapy seed for its application in the treatment of eye and prostate cancer Applied Radiation and Isotopes, 67 (2009) 1421–1425

[17] Saxena S.K.,Yogendra Kumar, Manoj Kumar, Ashutosh Dash and Meera Venkatesh (2008),Quality Assurance and Classification Performance Testing of 125I-brachytherapy Seeds, Proceedings of International Conference on Medical Physics (ICMP-2008) ,49-50

[18] Regulations for the Safe transport of Radioactive material, 2005 Edition, International Atomic Energy Agency (IAEA) No. TS-R-1

[19] International Standard ISO 2919:1999, Radiation protection- Sealed radioactive sources-General requirements and classification

[20] International Standard ISO 9978:1992, Radiation protection-Sealed radioactive sources-Leakage test methods

5

LNCaP Prostate Cancer Growth *In Vivo*: Oncostatic Effects of Melatonin as Compared to Hypoxia and Reoxygenation

L. Terraneo*, E. Finati*, E. Virgili, G. Demartini,
L. De Angelis, R. Dall'Aglio, F. Fraschini,
M. Samaja and R. Paroni
University of Milan, Milan
Italy

1. Introduction

Oxygen (O_2) is often thought of as a double-edged sword: all forms of life actually need O_2 for survival as the terminal acceptor of electrons in oxidative phosphorylation, but excess O_2 might increase formation of reactive O_2 species (ROS). Whereas on one hand ROS trigger uncontrolled burst of free radicals that lead to potentially lethal injury, on the other hand they act as messengers that elicit cell protection and improve survival through a variety of mechanisms. Although one can easily expect a link of O_2 with tumor growth and metastatic potential, there is no univocal role for O_2 in cancer.

1.1 Hypoxia in cancer

Lack of O_2, or hypoxia, has been extensively studied in cancer because the growth of solid tumors requires a local vascular network that supplies O_2 and nutrients to tumor cells. In the classical view, when cell proliferation exceeds angiogenesis, the vasculature might become unable to sustain the O_2 needs of tumor cells, which therefore have to cope with an environment chronically deficient in O_2 as a result of diffusion-limited O_2 supply (Vaupel, 2004). This triggers various mechanisms, most of which are mediated by over-expression of the hypoxia-inducible factor-1 (HIF-1α). HIF-1α stimulates a variety of mechanisms aimed at survival of hypoxic tissue, for example the angiogenic switch, which provides growth factors for the development of circulation to feed the growing tumor, as well as anti-apoptotic and cell cycle factors. Therefore, tumor hypoxia emerges as a major contributor to the malignant phenotype (Hockel *et al.*, 2001) and a cause of resistance to radiation therapy (Brown *et al.*, 1998).

There are several instances whereby the O_2 supply to tissues is altered. The term "hypoxia" is sometimes improperly attributed to any of them, but there are important differences with dramatically different phenotypes, as explained in Table 1.

---

* These Authors contributed equally to the work

Name	Relative experimental situation	Correlated pathologies
Chronic hypoxia	Prolonged O_2 supply/demand unbalance without interruption, typical of decreased tissue perfusion for altered geometry of O_2 diffusion from capillary to cell	Chronic obstructive pulmonary disease, congenital heart disease, cancer-derived anemia, blood O_2 carrying failure, CO poisoning, high altitude
CH with repeated reoxygenation	Animals housed in hypoxic chambers that are opened for cleaning and animal feeding	Some cases of immature capillary network with pulsing perfusion changes
Intermittent hypoxia	Repetitive hypoxic events, typical of immature capillary network with pulsing perfusion changes	Obstructive sleep apnea, sickle cell anemia crises, asthma, immature capillary network with pulsing perfusion changes

Table 1. Different types of hypoxia and examples of correlated pathologies.

1.2 Prostate cancer

Prostate cancer is the most common neoplasia and the second most frequent cause of male cancer death in the developed world and in many Western countries (Hsing et al., 2000). A malignant tumor derived from the interaction of genetic and environmental factors, potentially curative treatment options are available for management of early localized disease, whereas palliative hormonal therapy in the form of medical or surgical castration is the mainstay of treatment for patients with advanced prostate cancer. Approximately 80% of castrated patients will suffer from a relapse of the disease within 2 years, with progression of the tumor from a hormone-dependent to a hormone-independent stage (Wilding, 1995), which is associated with unfavorable prognosis.

In addition, prostate cancer may also represent an useful workbench to investigate the relationship between hypoxia and cancer, because HIF-1α is over-expressed compared with normal prostate epithelium (Zhong et al., 1999) and its up-regulation is recognized as an early event in carcinogenesis (Zhong et al., 2004). Furthermore, androgens and androgen receptors modulate HIF-1α levels (Kimbro et al., 2006), and hypoxia increases androgen receptor activity in LNCaP cells in vitro via HIF-1α (Park et al., 2006).

1.3 Melatonin and prostate cancer

Melatonin (N-acetyl-5-methoxytryptamine, **Figure 1**), a neurohormone synthesized during night time in the pineal gland, mediates many physiological, endocrinological and behavioral processes, including the well-known biorhythmic regulation of organism physiology, through its action on the biological clock at the hypothalamic suprachiasmatic nucleus (Tamarkin et al., 1985). Melatonin increases sleepiness, decreases core temperature, and increases peripheral temperature in humans (Brzezinski, 1997; Burgess et al., 2001; Lewy et al., 1996). The melatonin's regulatory roles are mediated through high affinity G protein–coupled receptors that reside primarily in the eye, kidney, gastrointestinal tract, blood vessels, and brain (Beyer *et al.*, 1998). This suggests some significant actions of melatonin on the cell biology of these target tissues outside the central nervous system as well (Cardinali *et al.*, 1997; Pang *et al.*, 1993). In addition, melatonin is known to exhibit antioxidant properties against the deleterious effects of reactive oxygen and nitrogen species (ROS and RNS, respectively) that are independent of its many receptor-mediated effects (Korkmaz *et al.*, 2009; Ochoa *et al.*, 2011). Melatonin has been reported to scavenge hydrogen peroxide (H_2O_2), hydroxyl radical (HO•), nitric oxide (NO•), peroxynitrite anion (ONOO-), hypochlorous acid (HOCl), singlet molecular oxygen [$O_2(^1\Delta_g)$] and superoxide anion (O_2•-) (Allegra *et al.*, 2003; Reiter, 1998; Reiter *et al.*, 2001; Tan *et al.*, 2000). Melatonin has also been shown to possess genomic actions, through regulation of the expression of several genes including glutathione peroxidase, superoxide dismutase, and catalase, both under physiological conditions and under conditions of elevated oxidative stress (Allegra *et al.*, 2003; Kotler *et al.*, 1998).

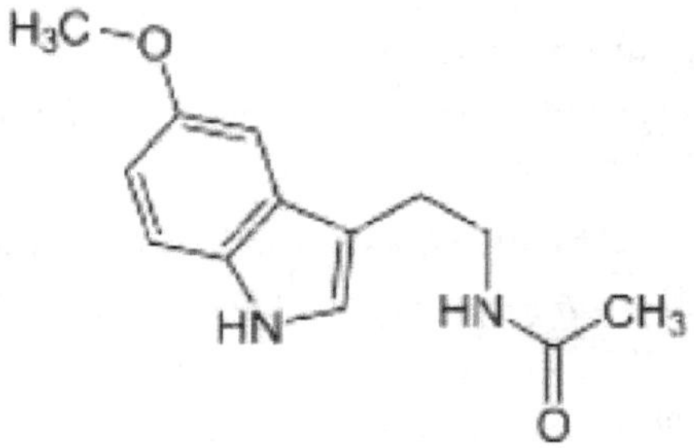

Fig. 1. Structure of melatonin, MW 232.2 Da.

A multitude of literature reports have documented a direct modulatory effect of melatonin on benign and malignant cell proliferation and an anti-tumor effect was reported both in vitro and in vivo in human tumors of the reproductive tissues (Cos *et al.*, 1998; Shiu *et al.*, 1999). Among these, a significant role of melatonin, by itself and by interaction with sex steroids, has been found in the pathobiology of prostate cancer and benign prostatic hyperplasia (Laudon *et al.*, 1996; Lupowitz *et al.*, 1999). Of the various experimental prostate cancer models, hormone (androgen)-sensitive and hormone (androgen)-insensitive metastatic human prostate cancer cell lines are widely used for the experimental evaluation of pharmacological agents with therapeutic potential for the disease (Cho *et al.*, 2011). In particular, the growth of the androgen-independent but androgen-sensitive (responsive) human LNCaP prostate cancer cells has been demonstrated to be inhibited by the pineal gland indoleamine hormone both in vitro and in vivo in a nude mice xenograft model (Siu *et al.*, 2002; Xi *et al.*, 2000). The antiproliferative action of melatonin seems to be mediated in part by means of MT1 receptor activation and partly by means of attenuation of dihydrotestosterone-induced calcium influx model (Xi *et al.*, 2000).

1.4 Solid lipid nanoparticles and cryopass laser therapy

Cytostatic and antitumoral drugs activity is often impaired by low plasma solubility, poor systemic absorbance, rapid metabolism, non-specific tissue distribution and toxic effects. The search for advanced methods to deliver these molecules to target tissues and to overcome the failure shown even with very active drugs is therefore mandatory.

Solid-lipid nanoparticles (SLN) is a technology able to produce sub-micrometric lipidic particles characterized by an average diameter <500 nm, with a narrow size distribution and a spherical shape. The several advantages of this technology are listed in Table 2 (Mehnert *et al.*, 2001). SLN formulation of antitumor drugs is predicted to be advantageous with respect to other formulations because it allows greater uptake into the malignant cell, with consequent intracellular accumulation and higher efficacy, still keeping the level of free circulating drug as low as possible, thereby preventing non-specific unwanted side effects.

Main advantages of SLN formulation for drugs delivery.
To control and direct the release of the drug against a specific target organ
To modify favorably drugs pharmacokinetics
To target directly to lymph bypassing the entero-hepatic circulation following oral administration
To obtain a stealth formulation that avoids recognition by the reticuloendothelial system
To allow oral administration of drugs poorly soluble and not easily adsorbed in the gastrointestinal tract
To overcome the blood-brain barrier
To permit administration routes as transdermal or eye topical

Table 2. Main advantages to administer drugs as solid-lipid nanoparticles (SLN).

Criopass therapy, is a procedure used to actively deliver drugs across the dermal barrier. It is based on topical application of a frozen drug emulsion in 1.5% hydroxymethylcellulose by means of a laser source that gives energy to penetrate the dermal barrier and deliver the active principle to the target area. The low energy photon flux generated by a laser beam hit the drug molecules frozen in the crystal lattice, exciting the electrons in the outer orbital. The drug molecules, when melt at the ice-skin interface, release the accumulated potential energy transforming into kinetic energy, which speeds up the passage of the drug across the skin membrane and allows to reach the target area. The last step consists in a laser scan on the area of drug application to optimize the adsorption through the skin and facilitate the drug to reach the desired site of activity. This treatment is particularly advantageous for treatment of bones cartilage, producing significant drug accumulation in a tissue difficult to be reached by traditional administration techniques. The main advantages of this non-invasive and painless treatment are speed of absorption (15-20 s), high capacity of penetration (6 cm depth), suitability for polar and non-polar molecules delivery, improved drug bioavailability and high specificity.

1.5 Aims

Solid tumors contain underperfused regions where hypoxia might induce adaptation and cell proliferation. Often, this response is mediated by HIF-1α over-expression in hypoxic cells. We demonstrated that systemic chronic *in vivo* hypoxia promotes prostate cancer growth regardless of HIF-1α expression level and neovascularization. We have also assessed that altering HIF-1α expression by use of non-pharmacological agents (intermittent hypoxia with reoxygenation) alter the phenotype of tumor growth. These observations suggest an important role for hypoxia dependent pathways that do not involve HIF-1α, and for the pharmacological treatments able to modulate these pathways.

Pharmacologic concentrations of melatonin inhibit *in vitro* expression of HIF-1α protein under both normoxic and hypoxic conditions in DU145, PC-3, and LNCaP prostate cancer cells (Park *et al.*, 2009). This effect, perhaps a result of the antioxidant activity of melatonin against ROS induced by hypoxia, and the subsequent suppression of HIF-1α transcriptional activity decreases VEGF expression in HCT116 human colon cancer cell line (Park *et al.*, 2010). Therefore, the main aim of this preliminary study was to focus into the role of melatonin as a therapeutic/adjuvant agent that reduces tumor growth in vivo as a proof-of-concept for further studies assessing melatonin interference with the hypoxia signaling paths. To this purpose, we used the *in-vivo* model of nude mice xenograft with human LNCaP prostate cancer cells under a variety of conditions spanning from chronic hypoxia with/out reoxygenation, and compared different routes of melatonin administration.

2. Methods

Cells. LNCaP cells (80-90% confluence) were maintained in RPMI-1640 medium containing 10% (v/v) heat-inactivated fetal bovine serum and L-glutamine, and cultured in 5% CO_2. To ensure that LNCaP cells were not injured when passing through G26 needles during xenografts, we verified that their vitality did not decreased by more 2 3% per each passage. To obtain positive controls for HIF-1α immunostaining, LNCaP cells were incubated for 24 h in the presence of 100 µM $CoCl_2$, washed, fixed in formalin and stained as described below.

Mice. Seven-week old Foxn1$^{nu/nu}$ mice (Harlan, n=46), weighing 25-30 g at the entry into the study, were cared in accordance to the Guide for the Care and Use of Laboratory Animals published by the National Institutes of Health (NIH Publication No. 85-23, revised 1996). Water and bedding were heat-sterilized, whereas food was sterilized by ^{60}Co γ-irradiation. Mice had free access to water and conventional laboratory diet until 24 h before sacrifice. A 12/12 h light/dark cycle was maintained.

Xenografts. LNCaP cells were resuspended in ice-cold Matrigel (1:1) at a final concentration of $3 \cdot 10^6/0.1$ ml. Mice were inoculated in each flank with 0.1 ml of cells using a 26G insulin syringe. The next day, mice were transferred into the gas chamber, where they were treated accordingly.

In vivo measurements of tumor growth. Body weight and tumor volume were measured three times a week during the various treatments. The tumor volume was calculated as length•width•height•0.5236, as measured by a caliper. Data are expressed as the ratio (tumor volume)/(body weight) to compensate different rates of growth in the various experimental situations (**Figure 2**).

Sacrifice. At the end of the observation period, mice were anesthetized by i.p. Na-thiopental (10 mg/100 g body weight) plus heparin (500 units), then they were thoracotomized to withdraw a blood sample into a heparinized syringe from the left ventricle, and tumors were quickly excised from surrounding skin.

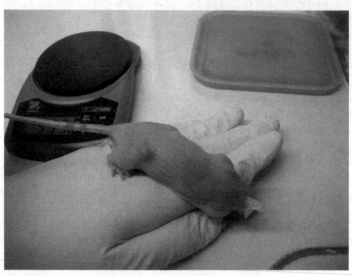

Fig. 2. Picture of a mouse at the end of the observation window. The tumors are clearly visible on both flanks.

Hemoglobin. Hemoglobin (Hb) concentration was measured in blood, by diluting 10 µl of well-stirred blood in 1 ml of Drabkin reagent, followed by incubation for 30 min at room temperature and absorbance reading at λ=540 nm. The concentration was calculated assuming λ=11.05 cm^{-1} mM^{-1}.

Effects of melatonin i.p.. For this set of experiments, mice xenografted with LNCaP cells as described above were treated with melatonin i.p. (30 µg, 1 mg/Kg), given either dissolved in in 100 µL isotonic saline (n=7) or encapsulated in 100 µL SLN (n=7). Mice treated with 100 µL saline acted as control. Whereas melatonin-saline was prepared fresh, melatonin-SLN was obtained from Nanovector S.r.L., Torino, Italy (Gasco *et al.*, 2007). Timing of treatments is given in *Figure 3*.

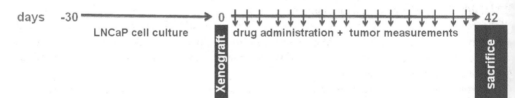

Fig. 3. Timing of melatonin treatments.

Effects of melatonin-laser. For this set of experiments, mice xenografted with LNCaP cells as described above were exposed to laser treatment with (n=11) or without (n=11) melatonin. Melatonin was prepared fresh every week by emulsifying 0.048 mg melatonin/mL of 1.5 % hydroxymethylcellulose for 7 min with a Ultraturrex at the maximum speed in ice and dark.

Then, 15 mL of the suspension or 0.72 mg melatonin was transferred in suitable devices and frozen at -20°C overnight. Each frozen stick (*Figure 4A*) was used to treat 6 mice. The final dose administered topically was about ~0.120 mg melatonin/mouse/treatment, i.e. 4 mg/Kg. For the administration, the stick containing frozen melatonin (or saline for the control group) was delivered topically for 2.4 min in the correspondence of the xenografts with the frozen stick connected to the laser beam. The duration of the treatment was kept within 2.4 min, because topical application of the frozen stick in small-size animals causes hypothermia (when necessary, mice were kept on a heating plate at 37°C during the treatment, not shown). The concentration of melatonin was selected in order to deliver the wanted amount in 2.4 min. After this first phase, mice were placed in a home-made device, immobilized and exposed for 15 min to the laser scan (the wide of the laser beam scan was set to the minimum value, so to cover only the small tumor area exposed on the mice back) (*Figure 4B*). We used an instrument LASERICE Med C.I.R.C.E. S.r.L., Magnago, Milano (230 V, 50 Hz, 150 mA) constituted by a device for freezing the drug emulsion and by a scanner connected to photodiode laser bean with λ= 635 nm, maximum power <5 mW, collimation lens <20 mV. For our experiments, we selected the software designed for veterinary use in small animals. The software automatically selects the most suitable laser power and frequency to target the drug at the right depth into the tissues.

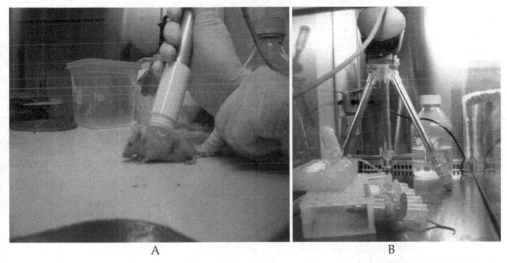

A   B

Fig. 4. (A) Topical administration of melatonin by a frozen stick connected to a low energy laser beam. (B) Experimental setup showing exposure of immobilized mice to high-energy laser scan.

Effects of hypoxia with/out reoxygenation. Data relative to this set of experiments have been published in (Terraneo *et al.*, 2010) and are here reported to enable comparing with the groups with melatonin. Briefly, mice xenografted with LNCaP cells as described above were exposed to either chronic hypoxia (10% O_2) or hypoxia with reoxygenation (3 times/week for 1 h), with normoxia as control (n=17, 19 and 20, respectively). Hypoxia was induced by using the hypoxic chambers described elsewhere that prevent any unwanted contact of the animal with room air during cleaning operations and sacrifice (Milano *et al.*, 2002).

Statistics. Data are expressed as mean±SEM. Significance level was P=0.05 (two-tailed). To detect differences among the groups, we performed one-way ANOVA. If this test resulted significant, the differences between selected pairs of data were tested using the Bonferroni procedure (Instat 3, GraphPad software).

3. Results

Table 3 shows the main characteristics of the mice considered in this study. No significant differences were detected among the various melatonin groups as far as the changes in body weight and Hb concentration are concerned. By contrast, hypoxia depressed the gain in body weight and increased the blood Hb concentration, as expected. The marked decrease in body weight in the mice exposed to hypoxia forced us to shorten the 42-day observation window to 28 days.

	n Surviving/total	*Body weight at entry, g*	*Final body weight, g (42 days of treatment)*	*Blood [Hb], g/L*
Effects of melatonin i.p.				
Saline	6/6	26.63±0.20	26.77±0.80	120±3
Melatonin-saline	7/7	27.71±0.32	32.17±0.46*#	119±6
Melatonin-SLN	7/7	27.96±0.25	31.94±0.90*#	119±3
Effects of melatonin laser				
Laser	11/11	27.24±0.31	29.70±0.91*	126±11
Laser+melatonin	11/11	27.40±0.30	30.58±0.74*	119±6
Effects of hypoxia (28 days of treatment)				
Normoxia	19/20	26.83±0.39	31.17±0.61*	134±3
Chronic hypoxia	16/17	28±0.46	27.38±0.52#	197±3#
Hypoxia with reoxygenation	9/9	27.55±0.37	23.92±0.28*#	205±5#

Table 3. Main characteristics of the mice considered in this study. Data from the hypoxia groups are published in (Terraneo *et al.*, 2010). *, $P<0.05$ with respect to body weight at entry (unpaired two-tailed Student's t-test); #, $P<0.05$ with respect to the relative control (ANOVA and Bonferroni post-test).

3.1 Effect of melatonin i.p.

This set of experiments aims at assessing whether the traditional way to administer melatonin results into an oncostatic situation, and whether administration of the same amount of melatonin is oncostatic as well. The xenograft rate of success was in the range 55-90%. Whereas **Figure 5A** reports the time course of the successful xenografts, **Figure 5B** reports the time after the xenograft necessary for the xenografted tumors to be palpable. Data confirm that i.p. treatment with melatonin in saline has important oncostatic potential. Of interest, melatonin does not delay appreciably the time of appearance of the tumors after the xenograft, but rather it decreases the growth rate. Melatonin in SLN has less oncostatic potential than melatonin in saline when given in the same amount, probably as the result of less delivery efficiency than in the melatonin-saline group.

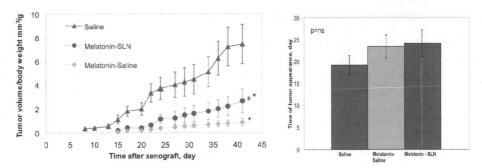

Fig. 5. Time course (A) and time necessary for the tumors to be palpable (B) in mice treated i.p. with either melatonin in saline or melatonin in SLN (0.51 mg melatonin/mouse in 17 administrations over a 42 day period), whereas saline-treated mice represent the control group. Data are expressed as mean ±SEM from 12, 10 and 8 tumors, respectively. *, P<0.05 from untreated; #, P<0.05 from melatonin SLN (ANOVA and Bonferroni post-test).

3.2 Effect of melatonin laser

This set of experiments aims at assessing whether administering melatonin topically by treatment with laser results into an oncostatic situation as that described above for i.p. melatonin. The xenograft rate of success was in the range 75-95%. Whereas **Figure 6A** reports the time course of the successful xenografts, **Figure 6B** reports the time after the xenograft necessary for the xenografted tumors to be palpable. Whereas laser+melatonin results into a oncostatic situation (compare with the saline-treated as reported in Figure 4), it is difficult to discern an effect due to melatonin in comparison with that driven by laser+melatonin.

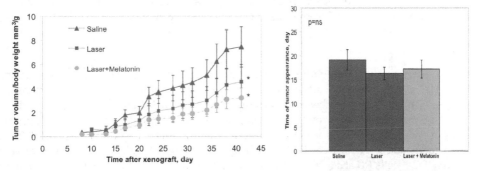

Fig. 6. Time course (A) and time necessary for the xenografted tumors to be palpable (B) in mice exposed to either laser only or laser+melatonin (2.04 mg melatonin/mouse in 17 administrations over a 42-day period). Data are expressed as mean±SEM from 12, 13 and 12 tumors, respectively. No significant difference between the two treatments was observed, but both laser groups are different from Saline control (*, P<0.05).

3.3 Effect of hypoxia

This set of experiments aims at assessing whether inducing local hypoxia increases the growth of prostate tumors as published elsewhere (Terraneo *et al.*, 2010). By decreasing arterial PO_2 from 85 to 34 mmHg, the selected hypoxia severity (10% O_2, equivalent to an altitude of about 5000 m) decreases the total O_2 arterial content by 35%, despite the increased blood Hb concentration. The xenograft success rate was 56-83% without any significant effect of hypoxia nor its way of administration. **Figure 7A** reports the time course of the successful xenografts, and **Figure 7B** reports the time after the xenograft necessary for the tumors to be palpable. Chronic hypoxia resulted into significant increase of the tumor growth rate. Interestingly, an operation aimed at increasing the cytosolic abundance of HIF-1α by approximately 10 times, e.g., exposing mice to repeated reoxygenation events during hypoxia, did not affected appreciably the tumor growth rate. This suggests that mechanisms other than those mediated by HIF-1α might have determined the increased tumor growth rate in hypoxic mice.

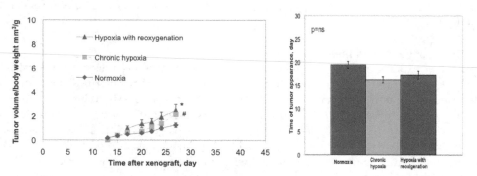

Fig. 7. Time course (A) and time necessary for the xenografted tumors to be palpable (B) in mice exposed to either laser only or laser+melatonin (n g melatonin/mouse in n administrations over a 42 day period). Data are expressed as mean±SEM from n, n and n tumors, respectively. *, P<0.05 from normoxia (ANOVA and Bonferroni post-test).

4. Discussion

Melatonin. After the first observation that in MCF-7 cells *in vitro*, 1 nM melatonin reduces tumor cells invasiveness in Falcon invasion chambers (Cos *et al.*, 1998), the oncostatic properties of melatonin have been thoroughly investigated. Melatonin acts synergistically with castration in inhibiting growth of androgen-sensitive LNCaP tumor through opposite changes in cyclin D1 levels induced by activated MT1 and EGF receptors (Siu *et al.*, 2002). As MT1 receptors are clearly involved in androgen-sensitive LNCaP, but not in androgen-insensitive PC-3 cells (Xi *et al.*, 2001), it is likely that the antiproliferative action of melatonin in LNCaP tumor growth is associated with MT1 receptor protein expression. Furthermore, the clear relationship found in MCF-7 xenografts between melatonin and telomerase activity, responsible of telomere elongation that activated in most human cancers (Leon-Blanco *et al.*, 2003), suggests that melatonin also influences telomerase decreasing its activity in the tumors. Although melatonin at physiologic concentration has no impact on VEGF expression in three human cancer cell lines (PANC-1, HeLa and A549), at high pharmacological concentrations it markedly reduces expression of VEGF and HIF-1α induced by $CoCl_2$ in cultured cancer cells (Dai *et al.*, 2008). A breakthrough in understanding the mechanisms underlying the oncostatic properties of melatonin came along with unraveling the relationship between melatonin and the hypoxia signaling path. Melatonin indeed inhibits HIF-1α protein expression in normoxic and hypoxic DU145, PC-3 and LNCaP prostate cancer cells without affecting HIF-1α mRNA levels (Park *et al.*, 2009). In HCT116 human colon cancer cells, melatonin destabilizes HIF-1α, suppresses its transcriptional activity, thereby decreasing VEGF expression (Park *et al.*, 2010). In turn, these features block in vitro tube formation and invasion and migration of human umbilical vein endothelial cells induced by hypoxia media, indicating that melatonin plays a pivotal role in tumor suppression via inhibition of HIF-1α-mediated angiogenesis. Our observation that melatonin inhibits LNCaP prostate cancer growth as opposite to enhanced growth in hypoxia agrees with the described findings.

Chronic hypoxia. Despite the acknowledged role of hypoxia in cancer biology, mainly acquired through *in vitro* and clinical studies, accurate analysis of existing literature revealed that the effects of *chronic* hypoxia *in vivo* had not been investigated experimentally as well. To mimic chronic hypoxia, we recently developed an experimental model whereby prostate tumor-bearing mice are exposed to various forms of hypoxia *in vivo*, while continuously monitoring tumor growth and finally assessing the molecular and cellular phenotypes (Terraneo *et al.*, 2010). We found that, although hypoxia *in vivo* promotes prostate cancer growth, this could not be entirely ascribed to HIF-1α, in the favor of other molecular pathways, such as those involving phosphatidyl inositol-3-phosphate/protein kinase B (Akt) pathway. This finding bears important implications especially when designing effective therapies: as a matter of facts, on clinical ground therapies targeting HIF-1α do not appear particularly successful (Fox *et al.*, 2011). Comparing the effects led by chronic hypoxia with/out reoxygenation contributed to univocally assess the latter issue.

Chronic hypoxia with reoxygenation. Reoxygenating the tumors during hypoxia increased HIF-1α cytosolic level >10-fold more than in chronic hypoxia, yet tumor growth was essentially similar to that of chronic hypoxia (Terraneo *et al.*, 2010). Higher HIF-1α in reoxygenated tumors with respect to chronic hypoxia could be a consequence of shorter normalization time since the last exposure to hypoxia (2-3 days), or of reoxygenation-induced HIF-1α stabilization or enhanced synthesis. As the reoxygenation of hypoxic tissues causes considerable oxidative stress (Milano *et al.*, 2004), the associated enhanced generation of mitochondrial ROS may stabilize HIF-1α (Chandel *et al.*, 2000). It has also been proposed that the persistent oxidative stress promoted by ROS during the reoxygenation further amplifies HIF-1α activation in a feed-forward mechanism through a mechanism involving mTOR (Semenza *et al.*, 2007). Therefore, although this finding was key to suppose non-centrality of HIF-1α in cancer growth, the effect of HIF-1α on metastatic potential is still to be investigated.

Therapeutic potential and future perspectives. The role of melatonin as anti-proliferative factor in the management of prostate cancer is currently under study by several research groups. However, its signaling mechanism and its crosstalk with other positive or negative growth regulator factors as HIF-1α, sex steroids, epidermal growth factor (EGF), vascular endothelial growth factor (VEGF) and others is still under debate and deserves to be thoroughly investigated. Moreover, to elucidate the biological effects of melatonin under physiological and pathological conditions, its putative antioxidant action is to be studied. Finally, the effect of melatonin on sarcosine (N-methyl derivative of the amino acid glycine), a potentially important metabolic intermediary of cancer cell invasion and aggressivity (Sreekumar et al., 2009) merits future attention.

5. Conclusion

In vivo systemic hypoxia promotes prostate cancer growth regardless of HIF-1α expression level and neovascularization, suggesting an important role for hypoxia-dependent pathways that do not involve HIF-1α, as the phosphatidyl inositol-3-phosphate signaling cascade. Melatonin experiments may not only provide a useful probe to assess the effects of HIF-1α on tumor growth, but may also represent the basis for the future introduction of this natural molecule as adjuvant active component in novel therapeutic strategies for the treatment of malignant prostate cancer in humans, for the prevention of cancer relapses, or simply for the amelioration of the quality of life of the oncologic patient.

6. Acknowledgments

We thanks to Dr. Enrico Bonizzoni and Dr. Emilio Bonizzoni C.I.R.CE. S.r.L., Magnago, Milano, who kindly borrowed the Laser equipment.

7. References

Allegra, M., Reiter, R.J., Tan, D.X., Gentile, C., Tesoriere, L.& Livrea, M.A. (2003) The chemistry of melatonin's interaction with reactive species. *J Pineal Res* 34(1): 1-10.

Beyer, C.E., Steketee, J.D.& Saphier, D. (1998) Antioxidant properties of melatonin--an emerging mystery. *Biochem Pharmacol* 56(10): 1265-1272.

Brown, J.M.& Giaccia, A.J. (1998) The unique physiology of solid tumors: opportunities (and problems) for cancer therapy. *Cancer Res* 58(7): 1408-1416.

Brzezinski, A. (1997) Melatonin in humans. *N Engl J Med* 336(3): 186-195.

Burgess, H.J., Sletten, T., Savic, N., Gilbert, S.S.& Dawson, D. (2001) Effects of bright light and melatonin on sleep propensity, temperature, and cardiac activity at night. *J Appl Physiol* 91(3): 1214-1222.

Cardinali, D.P., Golombek, D.A., Rosenstein, R.E., Cutrera, R.A.& Esquifino, A.I. (1997) Melatonin site and mechanism of action: single or multiple? *J Pineal Res* 23(1): 32-39.

Chandel, N., McClintock, D., Feliciano, C., Wood, T., Melendez, J., Rodriguez, A.& Schumacker, P. (2000) Reative oxygen species generated at mitochondria complex III stabilize HIF-1-alpha during hypoxia: a mechanism of oxygen sensing. *J Biol Chem* 275: 25130-25138.

Cho, S.Y., Lee, H.J., Jeong, S.J., Kim, H.S., Chen, C.Y., Lee, E.O.& Kim, S.H. (2011) Sphingosine kinase 1 pathway is involved in melatonin-induced HIF-1alpha inactivation in hypoxic PC-3 prostate cancer cells. *J Pineal Res.*

Cos, S., Fernandez, R., Guezmes, A.& Sanchez-Barcelo, E.J. (1998) Influence of melatonin on invasive and metastatic properties of MCF-7 human breast cancer cells. *Cancer Res* 58(19): 4383-4390.

Dai, M., Cui, P., Yu, M., Han, J., Li, H.& Xiu, R. (2008) Melatonin modulates the expression of VEGF and HIF-1 alpha induced by CoCl2 in cultured cancer cells. *J Pineal Res* 44(2): 121-126.

Fox, S.B., Generali, D., Berruti, A., Brizzi, M.P., Campo, L., Bonardi, S., Bersiga, A., Allevi,
    G., Milani, M., Aguggini, S., Mele, T., Dogliotti, L., Bottini, A.& Harris, A.L. (2011)
    The prolyl hydroxylase enzymes are positively associated with hypoxia-inducible
    factor-1alpha and vascular endothelial growth factor in human breast cancer and
    alter in response to primary systemic treatment with epirubicin and tamoxifen.
    Breast Cancer Res 13(1): R16.
Gasco, M.R.& Gasco, P. (2007) Nanovector. *Nanomedicine (Lond)* 2(6): 955-960.
Hockel, M.& Vaupel, P. (2001) Biological consequences of tumor hypoxia. *Semin Oncol* 28:
    36-41.
Hsing, A.W., Tsao, L.& Devesa, S.S. (2000) International trends and patterns of prostate
    cancer incidence and mortality. *Int J Cancer* 85(1): 60-67.
Kimbro, K.S.& Simons, J.W. (2006) Hypoxia-inducible factor-1 in human breast and prostate
    cancer. *Endocr Relat Cancer* 13(3): 739-749.
Korkmaz, A., Reiter, R.J., Topal, T., Manchester, L.C., Oter, S.& Tan, D.X. (2009) Melatonin:
    an established antioxidant worthy of use in clinical trials. *Mol Med* 15(1-2): 43-50.
Kotler, M., Rodriguez, C., Sainz, R.M., Antolin, I.& Menendez-Pelaez, A. (1998) Melatonin
    increases gene expression for antioxidant enzymes in rat brain cortex. *J Pineal Res*
    24(2): 83-89.
Laudon, M., Gilad, E., Matzkin, H., Braf, Z.& Zisapel, N. (1996) Putative melatonin receptors
    in benign human prostate tissue. *J Clin Endocrinol Metab* 81(4): 1336-1342.
Leon-Blanco, M.M., Guerrero, J.M., Reiter, R.J., Calvo, J.R.& Pozo, D. (2003) Melatonin
    inhibits telomerase activity in the MCF-7 tumor cell line both in vivo and in vitro. *J
    Pineal Res* 35(3): 204-211.
Lewy, A.J.& Sack, R.L. (1996) The role of melatonin and light in the human circadian system.
    Prog Brain Res 111: 205-216.
Lupowitz, Z.& Zisapel, N. (1999) Hormonal interactions in human prostate tumor LNCaP
    cells. *J Steroid Biochem Mol Biol* 68(1-2): 83-88.
Mehnert, W.& Mader, K. (2001) Solid lipid nanoparticles: production, characterization and
    applications. *Adv Drug Deliv Rev* 47(2-3): 165-196.
Milano, G., Bianciardi, P., Corno, A.F., Raddatz, E., Morel, S., von Segesser, L.K.& Samaja,
    M. (2004) Myocardial Impairment in Chronic Hypoxia Is Abolished by Short
    Aeration Episodes: Involvement of K+ATP Channels. *Exp Biol Med (Maywood)*
    229(11): 1196-1205.
Milano, G., Corno, A.F., Lippa, S., Von Segesser, L.K.& Samaja, M. (2002) Chronic and
    intermittent hypoxia induce different degrees of myocardial tolerance to hypoxia-
    induced dysfunction. *Exp Biol Med (Maywood)* 227(6): 389-397.
Ochoa, J.J., Diaz-Castro, J., Kajarabille, N., Garcia, C., Guisado, I.M., De Teresa, C.&
    Guisado, R. (2011) Melatonin supplementation ameliorates oxidative stress and
    inflammatory signaling induced by strenuous exercise in adult human males. *J
    Pineal Res.*
Pang, S.F., Dubocovich, M.L.& Brown, G.M. (1993) Melatonin receptors in peripheral tissues:
    a new area of melatonin research. *Biol Signals* 2(4): 177-180.
Park, J.W., Hwang, M.S., Suh, S.I.& Baek, W.K. (2009) Melatonin down-regulates HIF-1
    alpha expression through inhibition of protein translation in prostate cancer cells. *J
    Pineal Res* 46(4): 415-421.
Park, S.Y., Jang, W.J., Yi, E.Y., Jang, J.Y., Jung, Y., Jeong, J.W.& Kim, Y.J. (2010) Melatonin
    suppresses tumor angiogenesis by inhibiting HIF-1alpha stabilization under
    hypoxia. *J Pineal Res* 48(2): 178-184.

Park, S.Y., Kim, Y.J., Gao, A.C., Mohler, J.L., Onate, S.A., Hidalgo, A.A., Ip, C., Park, E.M., Yoon, S.Y.& Park, Y.M. (2006) Hypoxia increases androgen receptor activity in prostate cancer cells. *Cancer Res* 66(10): 5121-5129.

Reiter, R.J. (1998) Cytoprotective properties of melatonin: presumed association with oxidative damage and aging. *Nutrition* 14(9): 691-696.

Reiter, R.J., Tan, D.X., Manchester, L.C.& Qi, W. (2001) Biochemical reactivity of melatonin with reactive oxygen and nitrogen species: a review of the evidence. *Cell Biochem Biophys* 34(2): 237-256.

Semenza, G.L.& Prabhakar, N.R. (2007) HIF-1-dependent respiratory, cardiovascular, and redox responses to chronic intermittent hypoxia. *Antioxid Redox Signal* 9(9): 1391-1396.

Shiu, S.Y., Li, L., Xu, J.N., Pang, C.S., Wong, J.T.& Pang, S.F. (1999) Melatonin-induced inhibition of proliferation and G1/S cell cycle transition delay of human choriocarcinoma JAr cells: possible involvement of MT2 (MEL1B) receptor. *J Pineal Res* 27(3): 183-192.

Siu, S.W., Lau, K.W., Tam, P.C.& Shiu, S.Y. (2002) Melatonin and prostate cancer cell proliferation: interplay with castration, epidermal growth factor, and androgen sensitivity. *Prostate* 52(2): 106-122.

Sreekumar, A., Poisson, L.M., Rajendiran, T.M., Khan, A.P., Cao, Q., Yu, J., Laxman, B., Mehra, R., Lonigro, R.J., Li, Y., Nyati, M.K., Ahsan, A., Kalyana-Sundaram, S., Han, B., Cao, X., Byun, J., Omenn, G.S., Ghosh, D., Pennathur, S., Alexander, D.C., Berger, A., Shuster, J.R., Wei, J.T., Varambally, S., Beecher, C.& Chinnaiyan, A.M. (2009) Metabolomic profiles delineate potential role for sarcosine in prostate cancer progression. *Nature* 457(7231): 910-914.

Tamarkin, L., Baird, C.J.& Almeida, O.F. (1985) Melatonin: a coordinating signal for mammalian reproduction? *Science* 227(4688): 714-720.

Tan, D.X., Manchester, L.C., Reiter, R.J., Qi, W.B., Karbownik, M.& Calvo, J.R. (2000) Significance of melatonin in antioxidative defense system: reactions and products. *Biol Signals Recept* 9(3-4): 137-159.

Terraneo, L., Bianciardi, P., Caretti, A., Ronchi, R.& Samaja, M. (2010) Chronic systemic hypoxia promotes LNCaP prostate cancer growth in vivo. *Prostate* 70(11): 1243-1254.

Vaupel, P. (2004) Tumor microenvironmental physiology and its implications for radiation oncology. *Semin Radiat Oncol* 14(3): 198-206.

Wilding, G. (1995) Endocrine control of prostate cancer. *Cancer Surv* 23: 43-62.

Xi, S.C., Siu, S.W., Fong, S.W.& Shiu, S.Y. (2001) Inhibition of androgen-sensitive LNCaP prostate cancer growth in vivo by melatonin: association of antiproliferative action of the pineal hormone with mt1 receptor protein expression. *Prostate* 46(1): 52-61.

Xi, S.C., Tam, P.C., Brown, G.M., Pang, S.F.& Shiu, S.Y. (2000) Potential involvement of mt1 receptor and attenuated sex steroid-induced calcium influx in the direct anti-proliferative action of melatonin on androgen-responsive LNCaP human prostate cancer cells. *J Pineal Res* 29(3): 172-183.

Zhong, H., De Marzo, A., Laughner, E., Lim, M., Hilson, D.& Zagzag, D. (1999) Overexpression of hypoxia inducible factor 1alpha in common human cancers and their metastases. *Cancer Res* 59: 5830-5835.

Zhong, H., Semenza, G.L., Simons, J.W.& De Marzo, A.M. (2004) Up-regulation of hypoxia-inducible factor 1alpha is an early event in prostate carcinogenesis. *Cancer Detect Prev* 28(2): 88-93.

Part 2

Diagnostic Markers

6

Tumoral Markers in Prostate Cancer

Noemí Cárdenas-Rodríguez and Esaú Floriano-Sánchez
Sección de Posgrado e Investigación, Instituto Politécnico Nacional
Laboratorio de Bioquímica y Biología Molecular, Escuela Médico Militar
Laboratorio de Neuroquímica, Instituto Nacional de Pediatría
México, D.F.

1. Introduction

In Mexico, in 70% of cases, the prostate cancer (PCa) is found in advanced stage. PCa currently occupies second place in frequency of cancer in men, surpassed only by skin cancer, and is the second principal cause of death in men after of lung cancer (Hall et al., 2005).

Reactive oxygen species (ROS) such as superoxide ($O_2^{\bullet-}$) and hydrogen peroxide (H_2O_2) are found in a large number of tumors and in high levels they induce cell death, apoptosis, senescence and angiogenesis (Ushio-Fukai & Nakamura, 2008).

One of the major sources of ROS is NADPH oxidase (NOX). The NOX are a family of enzymes that are found in various tissues. The NOX receives an electron from NADPH generating $O_2^{\bullet-}$ (Bánfi et al., 2001). Xia et al, Lim et al. and Brar et al. found that some NOX isozymes increase in association with ROS-production and tumor progression in ovarian and human colon cancer and in DU-145 cells of PCa, respectively (Brar et al., 2003; Lim et al., 2005; Xia et al., 2007).

Cells have different antioxidant systems including low molecular weight antioxidant molecules and various antioxidant enzymes. Superoxide dismutase (SOD) catalyses the dismutation of $O_2^{\bullet-}$ into H_2O_2 that can be transformed into H_2O and O_2 by catalase (CAT) (Genkinger et al., 2006). Mn-SOD is the major antioxidant in the mitochondria and is essential to the vitality of mammalian cells. In many types of tumor cells has been found to contain high levels of Mn-SOD, Cu/Zn-SOD or CAT expression compared to their nonmalignant counterpart such as in human tumor cancer cells of esophageal, gastric, ovary, breast, neuroblastoma, osteosarcoma, melanoma, pleura and leukemia (Grigolo et al., 1998; Janssen et al., 2000; Starcevic et al., 2003; Qian et al., 2005, López Laur et al., 2008). However, the role of these enzymes in carcinogenesis remains unclear.

On the other hand, iNOS or NOS-2 is an inducible isoform of nitric oxide synthases (NOS). All isoforms of NOS catalyze the reaction of L-arginine, NADPH and oxygen to nitric oxide (NO•), L-citrulline and NADP. NO• is a lipophilic physiological messenger wich regulate a variety of cellular responses and may exert its cellular action by cGMP-dependent as well as by cGMP-independent pathways (Stamler, 1994). The expression of iNOS has been found to be increased in a variety of human cancers such as colon, stomach, brain and breasts cancers (Alderton et al., 2001; Church & Fulton, 2006) by multiple mechanisms that control their activity (Stamler, 1994; Friebe & Koesling, 2003).

Ciclooxygenase-1 and 2 (COX-1/2) catalyze the initial step in the formation of prostaglandins (Smith & Langenbach, 2001). Very recently their role in carcinogenesis has become more evident. They influence apoptosis, angiogenesis, and invasion, and play a key role in the production of carcinogens. Usually, a high level of COX expression is found in cancer cells (Dannenberg & Zakim, 1999). The role of COX-2 in carcinogenesis has been recently described. Multiple lines of evidence confirm that selective COX-2 inhibitors reduce prostaglandin production and the risk of colorectal, skin and other neoplasias (Sonoshita et al., 2001). COX-2 is related to the formation of carcinogens, tumor promotion and inhibition of apoptosis, angiogenesis and the metastatic process (Ebehart et al.,1994; Uefuji et al., 2000). However, the interactions and links between lipid metabolism and cancer progression remain to be elucidated.

Therefore, in the present study, we decided to evaluate and compare, for the first time, the pattern protein expression of p22 *phox* subunit of NOX, Mn-SOD, Cu/Zn-SOD, CAT, iNOS and COX-2 protein expression in patients with PCa and with BPH.

2. Patients and methods

We obtained 62 samples of prostate tissue through of various surgical procedures (transurethral resection and biopsy transrectal). Approval was obtained from the local research and ethics committee for use of tissue. Of these samples, 30 patients (48.4%) had a diagnosis of PCa, while as 32 patients (51.6%) had a diagnosis of BPH (Department of Medical Urology, Hospital Central Militar, Mexico). The sample collection was conducted from January 2006 to December 2009 and was considered inclusion, exclusion and elimination criteria.

In the PCa group the average age was of 65.3 years and the concentration of preoperative PSA was of 8.6 ng/mL. In this group, the patients were classified according to Gleason scale. The score was of 4 in 1 case (3.3%), 6 in 19 cases (63.3%), 7 in 9 cases (30%) and 8 in 1 case (3.3%). None of the patients had undergone chemotherapy or radiotherapy before surgery.

In the BPH group the average age was of 66.5 years and the concentration of preoperative PSA was of 8.7 ng/mL.

Tissues obtained (500 mg) were stored at -83°C (Revco® Legaci ULT2186 3-35 Dupont SVVA Refrigerants) until further processing.

2.1 Immunohistochemistry

For light microscopy, tissue samples of PCa and BPH were fixed by immersion in formalin (pH 7.4) and embedded in paraffin. Serial cuts of 3 mm of thickness were mounted on poli-L-lisina coated slides (Sigma, St Louis, MO). Sections were initially deparaffinized by washing in xylene and decreasing ethanol concentrations and boiled in Declere (Cell Marque, Hot Springs, AR) to unmask antigen sites. Slides were washed in phosphate buffer saline (PBS). Endogenous peroxidase activity was blocked by exposing slides to 0.6% H_2O_2 in PBS for 30 min.

After of washing in PBS, nonspecific binding was avoided by incubation with 5% blocking solution (5% normal goat serum in PBS) for 20 min. Sections were incubated overnight (16 h) with primary anti-p22 *phox* subunit NOX, anti-Mn-SOD, anti-Cu/Zn-SOD, anti-CAT, anti-iNOS and anti-COX-2 antibody (1:100 for each one). Following removal of the antibodies and repetitive rinsing with PBS, slides were incubated with a biotinylated goat anti-IgG secondary antibodies (1:500 fur each one) (Jackson ImmunoReseach, West Grove, PA). Immunocytochemical identification of positive cells was performed by the use of an avidinbiotinylated peroxidase complex (ABC-kit Vectastain, Vector Laboratories, Burlingame, CA) and diaminobenzidine (Vector Laboratories, Burlingame, CA). After of intensive washing in PBS, slides were counterstained with hematoxylin. Sections were dehydrated in graded alcohols, treated with xylene and subsequently mounted. All specimens were examined by light microscopy (Axiovert 200 M, Carl Zeiss, Germany), photographs were taken with a digital camera (Axiocam HRC, Carl Zeiss, Germany). The number of positive cells (brown) was determined with a computerized image analyzer KS-300 3.0 (Carl Zeiss, Germany). The percentage of damaged area with histopathological alterations was obtained (400x magnification). Five random fields were studied (total area 1,584,000 μ^2). The results were expressed as a percentage.

2.2 Statistics

Findings were expressed as the mean ± SD. The statistical significance of the protein expression levels of p22 *phox* subunit of NOX, Mn-SOD, Cu/Zn-SOD, CAT, iNOS and COX-2 between PCa and BPH groups glands or stroma, was determined using the software Prism version 3.32 (GraphPad Prism 4.0 Software, San Diego, CA, USA) with "student t-test". It was considered a p <0.05 as statistical difference between groups.

3. Results

The results obtained in PCa and BPH groups are summarized in Table 1. NOX, Mn-SOD, Cu/Zn-SOD and CAT protein immunohistochemistry were significantly higher (1.76, 1.7, 1.78 and 5.88 fold, respectively) in stroma and were significantly higher (3.74, 1.69, 4.76 and 1.59 fold ,respectively) in gland of patients with PCa than that in patients with BPH.

Moreover, NOX, Mn-SOD and CAT protein expressions were significantly higher in gland than in stroma, while as Cu/Zn-SOD protein expression was significantly higher in stroma than in gland in patients with BPH. NOX and Mn-SOD protein expression were significantly higher in gland than in stroma in patients with PCa.

However, iNOS and COX-2 protein expressions were significantly higher in stroma and gland of BPH (1.47 and 2.9 fold, respectively) in comparison with PCa.

Parameters	BPH (n=32) Stroma	Gland	PCa (n=30) Stroma	Gland
NOX	4.8 ± 1.9	6.7 ± 2[a]	8.45 ± 1.7[c]	25.08 ± 3.5[d,b]
Mn-SOD	11.97 ± 1.6	14.73 ± 1.4[c]	20.45 ± 2.1[c]	24.83 ± 1.7[d,b]
Cu/Zn-SOD	30.3 ± 6.6[d]	11.1 ± 1.9	54.1 ± 14.6[c]	52.8 ± 8.8[d]
CAT	9.8 ± 1.5	37.9 ± 4.5[c]	57.6 ± 15.5[c]	60.1 ± 4.5[d]
iNOS	23.3 ± 8.8[e]	24.6 ± 6.3[f]	15.9 ± 7.1	16.3 ± 4.6
COX-2	12.1 ± 1.3[g]	14.8 ± 2.1[h]	7.4 ± 0.9	5.12± 0.7

[a]P=0.0002 vs stroma BPH; [b]P<0.0001 vs stroma PCa; [c]P<0.0001 vs stroma BPH; [d]P<0.0001 vs gland BPH; [e]P=0.0072 vs stroma PCa; [f]P=0.0016 vs gland PCa; [g]P=0.0314 vs stroma PCa; [h]P=0.0072 vs gland PCa

Table 1. Mean ± SD NOX, Mn-SOD, Cu/Zn-SOD, CAT, iNOS and COX-2 protein expressions (%) in PCa and BPH group.

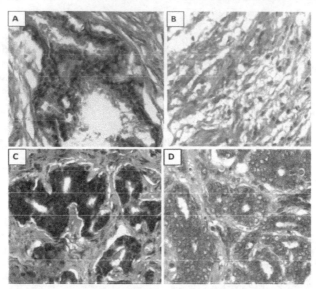

Fig. 1. Immunohistochemical determination of p22 phox subunit of NOX and Mn-SOD in BPH and PCa. (A) y (B) gland of BPH of NOX and Mn-SOD. (C) y (D) gland of PCa of NOX and Mn-SOD. In both groups was determined % area marked by field (400x) and was analized the values with significative increase in gland PCa immunoreactivity.

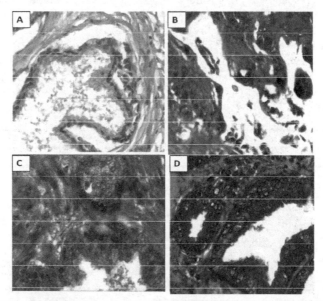

Fig. 2. Immunohistochemical determination of Cu/Zn-SOD and CAT in BPH and PCa. (A) y (B) gland of BPH of Cu/Zn-SOD and CAT. (C) y (D) gland of PCa of Cu/Zn-SOD and CAT. In both groups was determined % area marked by field (400x) and was analized the values with significative increase in gland PCa immunoreactivity.

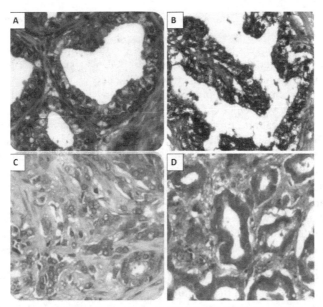

Fig. 3. Immunohistochemical determination of iNOS and COX-2 in BPH and PCa. (A) y (B) gland of BPH of iNOS and COX-2. (C) y (D) gland of PCa iNOS and COX-2. In both groups was determined % area marked by field (400x) and was analized the values with significative increase in gland PCa immunoreactivity.

4. Discussion

Recently, a new hypothesis has been proposed for prostate carcinogenesis. It suggested that exposure to environmental factors such as infectious agents and dietary carcinogens, and hormonal imbalances lead to injury of the prostate and to the development of chronic inflammation and regenerative 'risk factor' lesions, referred to as proliferative inflammatory atrophy (PIA). PCa is associated with oxidative stress, which stimulates the production of reactive oxidative species (ROS) and reactive nitrogen species. Oxidative stress derived from endogenous and exogenous sources are associated with DNA damage that occurs with aging and plays a role in carcinogenesis (Klein et al., 2006).

The results obtained, for the first time, in this study showed an increased in the expression of p22 *phox* subunit of NOX, Mn and Cu/Zn-SOD and CAT in stroma and gland of PCa.

In previous studies concluded that NOX has a role as a signaling mechanism that regulates the cell growth and apoptosis in PCa (Vignais, 2002). The exact signaling pathways of NOX are uncertain and may be tissue specific.

Angiotensin II stimulates the activity of NOX in vascular smooth muscle via protein kinase and NF-κB in the airways and in melanomas (Arnold et al., 2001). Arbiser et al. demonstrated that NOX-1-induced vascular endothelial growth factor (VEGF) and VEGF receptor expression promoting the angiogenesis and rapid expansion of the tumors (Arbiser et al., 2002). Babior BM found that the high levels of ROS are produced spontaneously in PCa and in ovarian cancer. This high production of reactive species was inhibited using an inhibitor of NOX, the diphenyl iodonium (DPI) and the inhibitor of mitochondrial electron chain, rotenone (Babior, 1999). This suggest that NOX could promote angiogenesis in the early stages of PCa.

By controlling $O_2^{\bullet-}/H_2O_2$ levels, SOD appears to be a critical enzyme in cancer progression. Bravard et al and St Clair et al suggested to the Mn-SOD as a potential tumoral suppressor that might also be involved in cellular differentiation (Zhao et al., 2001).

We suggested that any mutation or epigenetic changes in Mn-SOD gene are the cause of the high level found in the Mn-SOD expression in PCa in the mitochondria. This could have potential effects on survival and proliferation of tumor cells, a fact which has been found in other tumors with aggressive behavior and with a poor prognosis for the patient.

MnSOD polymorphisms have been investigated in several types of malignancies, such as lung, breast and skin cancer (Liu et al., 2004; Han et al., 2007; Bewick et al., 2008). There are at least two functional validated single nucleotide polymorphisms in Mn-SOD. One of these variants is a change in the amino acid codon 9 from valine (GTT) to alanine (GCT) and another is a change in the amino acid codon 16 from valine (GTT) to alanine (GCT) (Tugcu et al., 2007). These changes alter the secondary structure of the protein, affect the transport of the enzyme into mitochondria and reduce the enzymatic activity of Mn-SOD, leaving the cell vulnerable to oxidative damage.

Our results suggest that Mn-SOD probably plays an important role in resistance to treatment of various tumors or in the evolution of invasive tumors.

Brown et al demonstrated an essential role of $O_2^{\bullet-}$ in the posttranslational activation of Cu/Zn-SOD and in the ratio of active to inactive Cu/Zn-SOD, which may be relevant to various diseases, including cancer (Brown et al., 2004). Therefore, $O_2^{\bullet-}$ production by NOX could be induce protein over-expression of Cu/Zn-SOD in PCa.

CAT plays an integral role in the primary defense against oxidative stress by converting H_2O_2 into H_2O and O_2. Genetic polymorphisms of CAT can change expression levels of the protein. A $-262C \rightarrow T$ polymorphism in the promoter region of the CAT gene is associated with risk of several conditions related to oxidative stress. A transcription factor binding site search indicates that the -262 C allele is located in close proximity to several binding sites for transcription factors and could potentially influence rates of transcription. Forsberg et al. previously showed that the T allele was associated with greater CAT protein levels in some tissues than the C allele (Forsberg et al., 2001). However, different regulatory mechanism of CAT in PCa should be explained.

Our results showed different expressions in NOX, Mn-SOD, Cu/Zn-SOD and CAT in stroma and gland in PCa and BPH groups. The increase of NOX and Mn-SOD expression in gland of PCa and BPH group may have been due to excessive $O_2^{\bullet-}$ and H_2O_2 production that stimulate migration, invasion and angiogenesis of the tumor cells in response to the intracellular changes in ROS levels in this prostate component. The differences in the architecture of the prostate are most likely related to changes in the tumor invasion process

Furthermore our results suggest that exist alterations in the prooxidative-antioxidative balance in PCa, this imbalance is known to alter cellular redox processes, growth, and proliferation and cell cycles, since it is known that certain free radicals mediate the activation of cellular transduction, of transcription factors such as Fos, Jun and nuclear factor kB and an increase in mitochondrial activity in the cells. Moreover, transcription factors such as Rac1, Ref-1 and p53 regulated by ROS are involved in angiogenesis (Ushio-Fukai & Nakayama, 2008).

NO• is synthesized by three differentially gene-encoded NOS in mammals: neuronal NOS (nNOS or NOS-1), inducible NOS (iNOS or NOS-2) and endothelial NOS (eNOS or NOS-3). All three isoforms present similar structures and catalytic modes. The expression of NOS-2 is induced by inflammatory stimuli while NOS-1 and NOS-3 are more or less constitutively expressed. The active form of NOS-1 and -3 requires two NOS monomers associated with two Ca^{2+}-binding protein calmodulin and cofactors such as (6R)-5,6,7,8-tetrahydrobiopterin (BH_4), FAD, FMN and haem group and catalyze the reaction of L-arginine, NADPH and oxygen to NO•, L-citrulline and NADP (Alderton et al., 2001; Stuehr et al., 2004). NOS isoforms are differentially regulated at transcriptional, translational and post-translational levels. The intracellular localization is relevant for NOS activity. Evidence indicates that NOS are present in plasma membrane, Golgi, cytosol, nucleus and mitochondria (Oess et al., 2006; Iwakiri et al., 2006). The expression of iNOS can be transcriptionally regulated by factors such as cytokines (e.g. interferon-γ (IFN- γ), interleukin-1β (IL-1 β) and tumour necrosis factor-α (TNF-α), bacterial endotoxin (LPS) and oxidative stress (e.g. under conditions encountered during hypoxia)(Xu & Liu, 1998).

An initial study on iNOS expression in human breast cancer suggested that iNOS activity was higher in less differentiated tumours in a panel of 15 invasive breast carcinomas (Thomsen et al., 1995). Reveneau et al reported NOS activity in 27 of 40 tumours studied (Reveneau et al., 1999). Vakkala et al showed that carcinomas with both iNOS positive tumour and stromal cells had a higher apoptotic index and a higher calculated microvessel density index (Vakkala et al., 2000). Loibl et al further demonstrated that while none of the benign lesions were positive for iNOS, 67% *in situ* carcinomas and 61% invasive lesions showed iNOS tumour cell staining (Loibl et al., 2002).

In addition to breast cancer, iNOS has also been shown to be markedly expressed in approximately 60% of human adenomas and in 20-25% of colon carcinomas, while expression was either low or absent in the surrounding normal tissues (Ambs et al., 1998a). In human ovarian cancer, iNOS activity has been localized in tumour cells and not found in normal tissue (Thomsen et al., 1995). Other tumours that have demonstrated iNOS gene expression are brain, head and neck, esophagus, lung, prostate, bladder, pancreatic, and Kaposi's sarcoma (Cobbs et al., 1995; Rosbe et al., 1995; Wilson et al., 1998; Ambs et al., 1998a; Klotz et al., 1998; Hajri et al., 1998; Weninger et al., 1998; Swane et al., 1999).

In this study, we found that exist strong expression of iNOS in stroma and gland of HPB, in comparison with PCa. It Have been demonstrated that NO•- mediated up-regulation of VEGF. In the results is possible that NO• generated by iNOS in stroma may promote early new blood vessel formation by up-regulating VEGF and enhance ability of the tumour to grow and increases its invasiveness ability in gland. (Ambs et al., 1998a). Moreover, the accumulation of p53 in gland can result in down-regulation of iNOS expression by inhibition of iNOS promoter activity (Ambs et al., 1998b). On the other hand, the generation of chronic injury and irritation initiate the inflammatory response of stroma to gland (NOS-1). A subsequent respiratory burst an increase uptake of oxygen that leads to the release of reactive oxygen species (NO•, $ONOO^-$, N_2O_3, NO_2 and NO_3) from leucocytes can damage surrounding cells and drive carcinogenesis by altering targets and pathways that are crucial to normal prostate homeostasis (Coussens & Werb, 2002; Fukumura et al., 2006).

COX-1 and COX-2 regulate a key step in prostanoid (i.e., tromboxanes and prostaglandins) synthesis. Prostaglandins regulate various pathophysiological processes such as inflammatory reaction, gastrointestinal cytoprotection and ulceration (Smith & Langenbach,

2001). COX-1 is the constitutive isoform and COX-2 is the inducible isoform. COX-1 is expressed in most tissues and plays a role in the production of prostaglandins that control normal physiological processes. COX-2 is undetectable in most normal tissues (except for the central nervous system, kidneys and seminal vesicles), but is induced by various inflammatory and mitogenic stimuli (growth factors, pro-inflammatory cytokines and tumor necrosis factor) and other regulatory factors (Peppelenbosch et al., 1993; Zhang et al., 1998, Chen et al., 2001; Dempke et al., 2001). Although the mechanism of COX-2 upregulation is not fully understood, it could result from activation of Ras and mitogen-activated protein kinase (MAPK) pathway. It has been recognized that Akt/PKB activity is implicated in Ras-induced expression of COX-2. COX-2 is regulated at transcriptional and post-transcriptional levels by proinflamatory agents. These pathways lead to the activation of regulatory factors that eventually bind the promoter region of the COX-2 gene. (Sheng et al., 1998, 2000).

In this study, we found that exist strong expression of COX-2 in stroma and gland of HPB, in comparison with PCa. There are conflicting data regarding whether COX-2 is increased in the epithelial , gland or the stromal component of tumors (Horsman et al., 2010). Liu et al were the first to describe tumorigenesis induced by COX-2 over-expression. In their study, the murine COX-2 gene was inserted downstream of a murine mammary tumor virus promoter. As a consequence, hyperplasia and carcinoma of the mammary gland were observed and associated with strong COX-2 expression in mammary gland epithelial cells with increase prostaglandin E2 levels. (Liu et al., 2001). The role of COX-2 in tumor promotion is more strongly supported by previous studies in colorectal tumor models describen by Oshima et al (Oshima et al., 1996). These findings have been confirmed analyzing many tumors including pancreas, skin, gastric, bladder, lung, head, and neck cancers, suggesting that COX-2, but not COX-1, may play a pivotal role in tumor formation and growth (Thun et al., 2002). COX-2-derived prostaglandins contribute to tumor growth by inducing angiogenesis that sustain tumor cell viability and growth. COX-2 is expressed within human tumor neovasculature as well as in neoplastic cells present in human colon, breast, prostate and lung cancer biopsy tissue. (Kerbel & Folkman, 2002). The proangiogenic effects of COX-2 are mediated primarily by three products of arachidonic metabolism: Tromboxane A2, Prostaglandins I2 and E2 and selective inhibition of COX-2 activity has been shown to suppress angiogenesis *in vitro* and *in vivo* (Tsujii et al., 1998; Masferrer et al., 2000; Uefuji et al., 2000). We suggested that COX-2 overexpression in stroma inhibit apoptosis and promote angiogenesis in prostate gland.

Our results suggest that iNOS and COX-2 play a key role in tumorigenesis and indicate that iNOS and COX-2-selective inhibitors could be a novel class of therapeutic agents for PCa.

5. Conclusions

We suggested that the $O_2^{\bullet-}/H_2O_2$ balance regulated by the over-expression of NOX, Cu/Zn-SOD, Mn-SOD and CAT is actively involved in tumor environment, cell proliferation, differentiation, tumor progression and angiogenesis of PCa. On the other hand, iNOS and COX-2 may promote blood vessel formation in gland from its over-expression in stroma by multiple mechanisms that involve reactive oxygen species, transcription factors, cytokines, growth factors and tumor necrosis factor.

Moreover, we suggested that the NOX, Cu/Zn-SOD, Mn-SOD, CAT, iNOS and/or COX-2 in combination with PSA, could be a molecular markers or prognostic indicators for the early diagnosis and post-treatment monitoring of PCa.

6. Future research

Our research group is determining the gene expression and activity of nitric oxide synthases isoforms (eNOS, nNOS and iNOS), Mn-SOD, Cu/Zn-SOD, Glutathione peroxidase, Glutathione reductase, Glutathione-S-transferase, Catalase and Ciclooxygenase-2 to integrate the effect of the regulation of the antioxidant system in the development of prostate cancer and recently in breast cancer.

Actually, we begin a new line of research where we studied the gene expression and polymorphisms of some components of the cytochrome P450 system as well as its association with the risk of developing prostate cancer and breast cancer. We found a protein over-expression of CYP2W1, 4F11 and 8A1, orphans cytochromes, in prostate cancer. We hope to find a molecular marker or prognostic indicator for prostate cancer and breast cancer.

7. References

[1] Alderton, W.K.; Cooper, C.E. & Knowles, R.G. (2001). Nitric oxide synthases: structure, function and inhibition. *Journal of Biochremistry*, Vol. 357, No. 3, (August 2001), pp. 593-615, ISSN 0021-924X

[2] Ambs, S.; Merriam, W.G.; Bennett, W.P.; Felley-Bosco, E.; Ogunfusika, M.O.; Oser, S.M.; Klein, S.; Shields, P.G.; Billiar, T.R. & Harris, C.C. (1998a) Frequent nitric oxide synthase-2 expression in human colon adenomas: implication for tumor angiogenesis and colon cancer progression. *Cancer Research*, Vol. 58, No. 2, (January 1998), pp. 334-341, ISSN 1538-7445

[3] Ambs, S.; Ogunfusika, M.O.; Merriam, W.G.; Bennett, W.P.; Billiar, T.R. & Harris, C.C. (1998b). Up-regulation of inducible nitric oxide synthase expression in cancer-prone p53 knockout mice. *Proceedings of the National Academy of Sciences U S A*, Vol. 95, No. 15, (July 1998), pp. 8823-8828, ISSN 0027-8424

[4] Arbiser, J.L.; Petros, J; Klafter, R.; Govindajaran, B.; McLaughlin, E.R.; Brown, L.F.; Cohen, C.; Moses, M.; Kilroy, S.; Arnold, R.S. & Lambeth. J.D. (2002). Reactive oxygen generated by Nox1 triggers the angiogenic switch. *Proceedings of the National Academy of Sciences U S A*, Vol. 99, No 2, (January 2002), pp. 715-720, ISSN 0027-8424

[5] Arnold, R.S.; Shi, J.; Murad, E.; Whalen, A.M.; Sun, C.Q.; Polavarapu, R.; Parthasarathy, S.; Petros, .JA. & Lambeth, J.D. (2001). Hydrogen peroxide mediates the cell growth and transformation caused by the mitogenic oxidase Nox1. *Proceedings of the National Academy of Sciences U S A*, Vol. 98, No 10, (May 2001), pp. 5550-5555, ISSN 0027-8424

[6] Babior, B.M. (1999). NADPH oxidase: an update. *Blood*, Vol. 92, No. 5, (March 1999), pp. 1454-1476, ISSN 0006-4971

[7] Bánfi, B.; Molnár, G.; Maturana, A.; Steger, K.; Hegedûs, B.; Demaurex, N. & Krause, K.H. (2001). A Ca^{2+}-activated NADPH oxidase in testis, spleen, and lymph nodes. The *Journal of Biological Chemistry*, Vol. 276, No. 40, (October 2001), pp. 37594-37601, ISSN 0021-9258

[8] Bewick, M.A.; Conlon, M.S. & Lafrenie, R.M. (2008). Polymorphisms in manganese superoxide dismutase, myeloperoxidase and glutathione-S-transferase and survival

after treatment for metastatic breast cancer. *Breast Cancer Research and Treatment*, Vol. 111, No. 1, (September 2008), pp. 93-101, ISSN 0167-6806

[9] Brar, S.S.; Corbin, Z.; Kennedy, T.P.; Hemendinger, R.; Thornton, L.; Bommarius, B.; Arnold, R.S.; Whorton, A.R.; Sturrock, A.B.; Huecksteadt, T.P.; Quinn, M.T.; Krenitsky, K.; Ardie, K.G.; Lambeth, J.D. & Hoidal, J.R. (2003). NOX5 NAD(P)H oxidase regulates growth and apoptosis in DU 145 prostate cancer cells. *American Journal of Physiology.Cell Physiology*, Vol. 285, No. 2, (August 2003), pp. C353-C369, ISSN 0363-6143

[10] Brown, N.M.; Torres, A.S.; Doan Pe, & O`Halloran, T.V. (2004). Oxygen and the copper chaperone CCS regulate posttranslational activation of Cu, Zn superoxide dismutase. *Proceedings of the National Academy of Sciences U S A*, Vol. 101, No. 15, (April 2004), pp. 5518–5523, ISSN 0027-8424

[11] Chen, C.C.; Sun, Y.T.; Chen, J.J. & Chang, Y.J. (2001). Tumor necrosis factor-induced cyclooxygenase-2 expression via sequential activation of ceramide-dependent mitogenactivated protein kinases, and I_B kinase 1/2 in human alveolar epithelial cells. *Molecular Pharmacology* Vol. 59, No. 3, (March 2001), pp. 493–500, ISSN 0026-895X

[12] Church, J.E. & Fulton, D. (2006). Differences in eNOS activity because of subcellular localization are dictated by phosphorylation state rather than the local calcium environment. *The Journal of Biological Chemistry*, Vol. 281, No. 3, (October 2005), pp. 1477-1488, ISSN 0021-9258

[13] Cobbs, C.S.; Brenman, J.E.; Aldape, K.D.; Bredt, D.S. & Israel, MA. (1995). Expression of nitric oxide synthase in human central nervous system tumors. *Cancer Research*, Vol. 55, No. 4, (February 1995), pp. 727-730, ISSN 1538-7445

[14] Coussens, L.M. & Werb, Z. (2002). Inflammation and cancer. *Nature*, Vol. 420, No. 6917, (December 2002), pp. 860-867, ISSN 0028-0836

[15] Dannenberg, A.J. & Zakim, D. (1999). Chemoprevention of colorectal cancer through inhibition of cyclooxygenase-2. *Seminars in Oncology*, Vol. 26, No. 5, (October 1999), pp. 499–504, ISSN 0093-7754

[16] Dempke, W.; Rie, C.; Grothey, A. & Schmoll, H.J. (2001). Cyclooxygenase-2: a novel target for cancer chemotherapy? *The Journal of Cancer Research of Clinical On*cology, Vol. 127, No. 7, (July 2001), pp. 411–417, ISSN 0171-5216

[17] Eberhart, C.E.; Coffey, R.J.; Radhika, A.; Giardiello, F.M.; Ferrenbach, S. & DuBois, R.N. (1994) Up-regulation of cyclooxygenase 2 gene expression in human colorectal adenomas and adenocarcinomas. *Gastroenterology*, Vol. 107, No. 4, (October 1994), pp. 1183–1188, ISSN 0016-5085

[18] Forsberg, L.; Lyrenas, L.; de Faire, U. & Morgenstern, R. (2001). A common functional C-T substitution polymorphism in the promoter region of the human catalase gene influences transcription factor binding, reporter gene transcription and is correlated to blood catalase levels. *Free Radical Biology & Medicine*, Vol. 30, No. 5, (March 2001), pp. 500 –505, ISSN 0891-5849

[19] Friebe, A. & Koesling, D. (2003). Regulation of nitric oxide-sensitive guanylyl cyclase. *Circulation Research*, Vol. 93, No. 2, (July 2003), pp. 96-105, ISSN 00097330

[20] Fukumura, D.; Kashiwagi, S. & Jain, R.K. (2006). The role of nitric oxide in tumour progression. *Nature Reviews Cancer*, Vol. 6, No. 7, (July, 2006), pp. 521-534, ISSN 1474-175X

[21] Genkinger, J.M.; Platz, E.A.; Hoffman, S.C.; Strickland, P.; Huang, H.Y.; Comstock, G.W. & Helzlsouer, K.J. (2006). C47T polymorphism in manganese superoxide dismutase (MnSOD) antioxidant intake and survival. *Mechanisms of Ageing and Development*, Vol. 127, No. 4, (April 2006), pp. 371-377, ISSN 0047-6374

[22] Grigolo, B.; Lisignoli, G.; Toneguzzi, S.; Mazzetti, I. & Facchini, A. (1998). Copper/zinc superoxide dismutase expression by different human osteosarcoma cell lines. *Anticancer Research*, Vol. 18, No. 2A, (March-April 2008), pp. 1175-1180, ISSN 0250-7005

[23] Hajri, A.; Metzger, E.; Vallat, F.; Coffy, S.; Flatter, E.; Evrard, S.; Marescaux, J. & Aprahamian, M. (1998). Role of nitric oxide in pancreatic tumour growth: in vivo and in vitro studies. *British Journal of Cancer*, Vol. 78, No. 7, (October 1998), pp. 841-849, ISSN 0007-0920.

[24] Hall, S.E.; Holman, C.D.; Wisniewsk, Z.S. & Semmens, J. (2004).Prostate cancer: socio-economic, geographical and private-health insurance effects on care and survival *British Journal of Urology*, Vol.95, No. 1, (January 2005), pp. 51-58, ISSN 0007-1331

[25] Han, J.; Colditz, G.A. & Hunter, D.J. (2007). Manganese superoxide dismutase polymorphism and risk of skin cancer (United States). *Cancer Causes Control*, Vol. 18, No. 1, (February 2007), pp. 79-89, ISSN 0957-5243

[26] Horsman, M.R.; Bohn, A.B. & Busk, M. (2010). Vascular targeting therapy: potential benefit depends on tumor and host related effects. *Experimental Oncology*, Vol. 32, No. 3, (September 2010), pp. 143-148, ISSN 1812-9269

[27] Iwakiri, Y.; Satoh, A.; Chatterjee, S.; Toomre, D.K.; Chalouni, C.M.; Fulton, D.; Groszmann, R.J.; Shah, V.H. & Sessa, W.C. (2006). Nitric oxide synthase generates nitric oxide locally to regulate compartmentalized protein S-nitrosylation and protein trafficking. *Proceedings of the National Academy of Sciences U S A*, Vol. 103, No. 52, (December 2006), pp. 19777-19782, ISSN 0027-8424

[28] Janssen, A.M.; Bosman, C.B.; van Duijn, W.; Oostendorp-van de Ruit, M.M.; Kubben, F.J.; Griffioen, G.; Lamers, C.B.; van Krieken, J.H.; van de Velde, C.J. & Verspaget, H.W. (2000). Superoxide dismutases in gastric and esophageal cancer and the prognostic impact in gastric cancer. *Clinical Cancer Research*, Vol. 6, No. 8, (August 2000), pp. 3183-3192, ISSN 1078-0432

[29] Kerbel, R. & Folkman, J. (2002). Clinical translation of angiogenesis inhibitors. *Nature Reviews Cancer*, Vol. 2, No. 10, (October 2002), pp. 727–739, ISSN 1474-175X

[30] Klein, E.A.; Casey, G. & Silverman, R. (2006). Genetic susceptibility and oxidative tress in prostate cancer: integrated model with implications for prevention. *Urology*, Vol. 68, No 6, (December 2006), .pp. 1145–1151, ISSN 0090-4295

[31] Klotz, T.; Bloch, W.; Volberg, C.; Engelmann, U. & Addicks, K. (1998). Selective expression of inducible nitric oxide synthase in human prostate carcinoma. *Cancer*, Vol. 82, No. 10, (May 1998), pp. 1897-903, ISSN 1097-0142

[32] Lim, S.D.; Sun, C.; Lambeth, J.D.; Marshall, F.; Amin, M.; Chung, L.; Petros, J.A. & Arnold, R.S. (2005) Increased Nox1 and hydrogen peroxide in prostate cancer. *Prostate*, Vol. 62, No. 2, (February 2005), pp. 200–207, ISSN 0270-4137

[33] Liu, C.H.; Chang, S.H.; Narko, K.; Trifan, O.C.; Wu, M.T.; Smith, E.; Haudenschild, C.; Lane, T.F. & Hla, T. (2001). Over-expression of cyclooxygenase-2 is sufficient to induce tumorigenesis in transgenic mice. The *Journal of Biological Chemistry*, Vol. 276, No. 1, (January 2001), pp. 18563–18569, ISSN 0021-9258

[34] Liu, G.; Zhou, W.; Park, S.; Wang, L.I.; Miller, D.P.; Wain, J.C.; Lynch, T.J.; Su, L. & Christiani, D.C. (2004). The SOD2 Val/Val genotype enhances the risk of non small cell lung carcinoma by p53 and XRCC1 polymorphisms. *Cancer*, Vol. 101, No. 12, (December 2004), pp. 2802-2808, ISSN 0008-543X

[35] Loibl, S.; von Minckwitz, G.; Weber, S.; Sinn, H.P.; Schini-Kerth, V.B; Lobysheva, I.; Nepveu, F.; Wolf, G.; Strebhardt, K. & Kaufmann, M. (2002). Expression of endothelial and inducible nitric oxide synthase in benign and malignant lesions of the breast and measurement of nitric oxide using electron paramagnetic resonance spectroscopy. *Cancer*, Vol. 95, No. 6, (September 2002), pp. 1191-1198, ISSN 1097-0142

[36] López Laur, J.D.; Abud, M.; López Fontana, C.; Silva, J.; Cisella, Y.; Pérez Elizalde, R. & Ortiz, A. (2008). Antioxidant power and cellular damage in prostate cancer. *Archivos Españoles de Urología*, Vol. 61, No. 5, (June 2008), pp. 563-569, ISSN 0004-0614

[37] Masferrer, J.L.; Leahy, K.M.; Koki, A.T.; Zweifel, B.S.; Settle, S.L.; Woerner, B.M.; Edwards, D.A.; Flickinger, A.G.; Moore, R.J. & Seibert, K. (2000). Antiangiogenic and antitumor activities of cyclooxygenase-2 inhibitors. *Cancer Research*, Vol. 60, No. 5, (March 2000), pp. 1306–1311, ISSN 1538-7445

[38] Oess, S.; Icking, A.; Fulton, D.; Govers, R. & Müller-Esterl, W. (2006). Subcellular targeting and trafficking of nitric oxide synthases. *Journal of Biochremistry*, Vol. 396, No. 3, (June 2006) pp. 401-409, ISSN 0021-924X

[39] Oshima, M.; Dinchuk , J.E.; Kargman, S.L.; Oshima, H.; Hancock, B.; Kwong, E.; Trzaskos, J.M.; Evans, J.F. & Taketo, M.M. (1996). Suppression of intestinal polyposis in *Apc*-knockout mice by inhibition of cyclooxygenase-2 (COX-2). *Cell*, Vol. 87, No. 5, (November 1996), pp. 803–809, ISSN 0092-8674

[40] Peppelenbosch, M.P.; Tertoolen, L.G.; Hage, W.J. & de Laat, S.W. (1993). Epidermal growth factor-induced actin remodeling is regulated by 5-lipoxygenase and cyclooxygenase products. *Cell*, Vol. 74, No. 3, (August, 1993), pp. 565–575, ISSN 0092-8674

[41] Qian, Y.; Zheng, Y.; Abraham, L.; Ramos, K.S. & Tiffany-Castiglioni, E. (2005). Differential profiles of copper-induced ROS generation in human neuroblastoma and astrocytoma cells. *Brain Research. Molecular Brain Research*, Vol. 134, No 2, (April 2005), pp. 323-332, ISSN 0169-328X

[42] Reveneau, S.; Arnould, L.; Jolimoy, G.; Hilpert, S.; Lejeune, P.; Saint-Giorgio, V.; Belichard, C. & Jeannin, J.F. (1999). Nitric oxide synthase in human breast cancer is associated with tumor grade, proliferation rate, and expression of progesterone receptors. Laboratory Investigation, Vol. 79, No. 10, (October 1999), pp. 1215-25, ISSN 0023-6837

[43] Rosbe, K.W.; Prazma, J.; Petrusz, P.; Mims, W.; Ball, S.S. & Weissler, M.C. (1995). Immunohistochemical characterization of nitric oxide synthase activity in squamous cell carcinoma of the head and neck. *Otolaryngology: Head and Neck Surgery*, Vol.113, No. 5, (November 1995), pp. 541-549, ISSN 01945998

[44] Sheng, H.; Shao, J. & Dubois, R.N. (2001). K-Ras-mediated increase in cyclooxygenase 2 mRNA stability involves activation of the protein kinase B. *Cancer Research*, Vol. 61, No. 6, (March 2001), pp. 2670–2675, ISSN 1538-7445

[45] Sheng, H.; Shao, J.; Dixon, D.A.; Williams, C.S.; Prescott, S.M.; DuBois, R.N. & Beauchamp, R.D. (2000). Transforming growth factor-1 enhances Ha-ras-induced expression of cyclooxygenase-2 in intestinal epithelial cells via stabilization of

mRNA. The *Journal of Biological Chemistry*, Vol. 275, No. 9, (March 2000), pp. 6628–6635, ISSN 0021-9258

[46] Smith, W.L. & Langenbach, R. (2001). Why there are two cyclooxygenase isozymes. *The Journal of Clinical Investigation*, Vol. 107, No. 12, (June 2001), pp. 1491-1495, ISSN 0021-9738

[47] Sonoshita, M.; Takaku, K.; Sasaki, N.; Sugimoto, Y.; Ushikubi, F.; Narumiya, S. & Oshima, M. (2001). Acceleration of intestinal polyposis through prostaglandin receptor EP2 in Apc-knockout mice. *Nature Medicine*, Vol. 7, No. 9, (September 2001), pp. 1048–1051, ISSN 1078-8956

[48] Stamler, J.S. (1994). Redox signaling: nitrosylation and related target interactions of nitric oxide. *Cell*, Vol. 78, No. 3, (September 1994), pp. 931-936, ISSN 0092-8674

[49] Starcevic, S.L.; Diotte, N.M.; Zukowski, K.L.; Cameron, M.J. & Novak, R.F. (2003). Oxidative DNA damage and repair in a cell lineage model of human proliferative breast disease (PBD). *Toxicological Sciences (U.S.)*, Vol. 75, No.1, (September 2003), pp. 74-81, ISSN 1096-6080

[50] Stuehr, D.J.; Santolini, J.; Wang, Z.Q.; Wei, C.C. & Adak, S. (2004). Update on mechanism and catalytic regulation in the NO synthases. *The Journal of Biological Chemistry*, Vol. 279, No. 35, (May 2004), pp. 27257-27562, ISSN 0021-9258

[51] Swana, H.S.; Smith, S.D.; Perrotta, P.L.; Saito, N.; Wheeler, M.A. & Weiss, R.M. (1999). Inducible nitric oxide synthase with transitional cell carcinoma of the bladder. *Journal of Urology*, Vol. 161, No. 2, (February 1999), pp. 630-634, ISSN 0022-5347

[52] Thomsen, L.L.; Miles, D.W.; Happerfield, L.; Bobrow, L.G.; Knowles, R.G. & Moncada, S. (1995). Nitric oxide synthase activity in human breast cancer. *British Journal of Cancer*, Vol. 72, No. 1, (July 1995), pp. 41-44, ISSN 0007-0920

[53] Thun, M.J.; Henley, S.J. & Patrono, C. (2002). Nonsteroidal anti-inflammatory drugs as anticancer agents: mechanistic, pharmacologic, and clinical issues," *Journal of the National Cancer Institute*, Vol. 94, No. 4, (February 2002), pp. 252-266, ISSN 0027-8874

[54] Tsujii, M.; Kawano, S.; Tsuji, S.; Sawaoka, H; Hori, M. & DuBois, R.N. (1998). Cyclooxygenase regulates angiogenesis induced by colon cancer cells. *Cell*, Vol. 93, No. 5, (May 1998), pp. 705–716, ISSN 0092-8674

[55] Uefuji, K.; Ichikura, T. & Mochizuki, H. (2000). Cyclooxygenase-2 expression is related to prostaglandin biosynthesis and angiogenesis in human gastric cancer. *Clinical Cancer Research*, Vol. 6, No. 1, (January 2000), pp. 135–138, ISSN 1557-3265

[56] Tugcu, V.; Ozbek, E.; Aras, B.; Arisan, S.; Caskurlu, T. & Tasci, A.I. (2007). Manganese superoxide dismutase (Mn-SOD) gene polymorphisms in urolithiasis. *Urological Research*, Vol. 35, No 5, (October 2007), pp. 219-224, ISSN 0300-5623

[57] Uefuji, K.; Ichikura, T. & Mochizuki, H. Cyclooxygenase-2 expression is related to prostaglandin biosynthesis and angiogenesis in human gastric cancer. *Clinical Cancer Research*, Vol. 6, No. 1, (January 2000), pp. 135–138, ISSN 1557-3265

[58] Ushio-Fukai, M. & Nakamura, Y. (2008). Reactive oxygen species and angiogenesis: NADPH oxidase as target for cancer therapy. *Cancer Letters*, Vol. 266, No. 1, (July 2008), pp. 37-52, ISSN 0304-3835

[59] Vakkala, M.; Kahlos, K.; Lakari, E.; Paakko, P.; Kinnula, V. & Soini, Y. (2000). Inducible nitric oxide synthase expression, apoptosis, and angiogenesis in in situ and invasive breast carcinomas. *Clinical Cancer Research*, Vol. 6, No. 6, (June 2000), pp. 2408-2416, ISSN 1557-3265

[60] Vignais, P.V. (2002). The superoxide-generating NADPH oxidase: structural aspects and activation mechanism. *Cell and Molecular Life Sciences*, Vol. 59, No. 9, (September 2002), pp. 1428–1459, ISSN 1420-682X

[61] Weninger, W.; Rendl, M.; Pammer, J.; Mildner, M.; Tschugguel, W.; Schneeberger, C.; Stürzl, M. & Tschachler, E. (1998). Nitric oxide synthases in Kaposi sarcoma are expressed predominantly by vessels and tissue macrophages. *Laboratory Investigation*, Vol. 78, No. 8, (August 1998), pp. 949-955, ISSN 0023-6837

[62] Wilson, K.T.; Fu, S.; Ramanujam, K.S. & Meltzer, S.J. (1998). Increased expression of inducible nitric oxide synthase and cyclooxygenase-2 in Barrett s esophagus and associated adenocarcinomas. *Cancer Research*, Vol. 58, No. 14, (July 1998), pp.:2929-2934, ISSN 1538-7445

[63] Xia, C.; Meng, Q.; Liu, L.Z.; Rojanasakul, Y.; Wang, X.R. & Jiang, B.H. (2007). Reactive oxygen species regulate angiogenesis and tumor growth through vascular endothelial growth factor. *Cancer Research*, Vol. 67, No. 22, (November 2007), pp. 10823-10830, ISSN 0008-5472

[64] Xu, W. & Liu, L. (1998). Nitric Oxide: from a mysterious labile factor to the molecule of the Nobel Prize. Recent progress in nitric oxide research. *Cell Research*, Vol. 8, No. 4, (December 1998), pp. 251-258, ISSN 1001-0602

[65] Zhang, F.; Subbaramaiah, K.; Altorki, N. & Dannenberg, A.J. (1998). Dihydroxy bile acids activate the transcription of cyclooxygenase-2. The *Journal of Biological Chemistry*, Vol. 273, No. 4, (January 1998), pp. 2424-2428, ISSN 0021-9258

[66] Zhao, Y.; Kiningham, K.K.; Lin, S.M. & St Clair, D.K. (2001). Overexpression of MnSOD protects murine fibrosarcoma cells (FSa-II) from apoptosis and promotes a differentiation program upon treatment with 5-azacytidine: involvement of MAPK and NFkappaB pathways. *Antioxidants & Redox Signaling*, Vol. 3, No. 3, (June 2001), pp. 375–386, ISSN 1523-0864

7

Cancer Detection from Transrectal Ultrasound Guided Biopsy in a Single Center

Selvalingam S., Leong A.C., Natarajan C., Yunus R.[1] and Sundram M.
Department of Urology, General Hospital Kuala Lumpur
[1]Department of Pathology, General Hospital Kuala Lumpur
Malaysia

1. Introduction

Transrectal ultrasound-guided biopsy of the prostate is the mainstay in the diagnosis of prostate cancer. Cancer detection rates varies from centre to centre and is dependent on various factors including technique, number of cores, prostate volume, PSA levels and digital rectal examination findings.

There are also differences in various ethnic groups with regards to prostate cancer incidence especially in the west where African Americans have a higher incidence. In Malaysia there are three major ethnic groups; Malays (65%), Chinese(25%) and Indians (8%). There is no evidence as yet to show any differences in prostate cancer detection among the three ethnic groups

The Malaysian National Cancer Registry published in 2006[1], ranks prostate cancer as the 4th most common cancer in Malaysian men after large bowel, lung and nasopharyngeal cancer. It constitutes 7.3% of all cancers in men. The overall prostate cancer incidence per 100 000 population (CR) was 7.3 and Age Standardised Incidence (ASR) was 12. By ethnicity Malays had the lowest ASR , 7.7 followed by Indians, 14.8 and Chinese 15.8. In fact Prostate Cancer is the fifth most common cancer among Malay men, fourth among Chinese and the second most common cancer among the Malaysian Indians. Overall , the Age Specific Incidence per 100 000 population increased from 9.7 among men in their 50s to 60.4 in men in their 60s

In an observation by Lim et al[1] from the Malaysian Clinical Research Center, Malaysian Indians have a higher incidence compared to Indians from Chennai, Malaysian Malays have a lower incidence compared to Singapore Malays and Malaysian Chinese have the highest incidence compared to Chinese in other Asian countries. These findings will need to be verified by further research.

It is also postulated that Asians prostate are generally smaller than western counterparts but volume for volume Asians have a higher PSA and part of the reason may be due to higher level of inflammation in Asian prostates.

2. Aims and objectives

The primary objective of this study is to look at a single centre's cancer detection rate and to determine the various factors that may influence cancer detection namely age, PSA levels, number of cores and prostate volume. The study also aims to determine if cancer detection is higher in Chinese and Indian patients compared to Malay patients as reflected by the national Age Standardised Incidence in the three ethnic groups.

2.1 The secondary objectives include

To determine the detection of prostate inflammation and PIN and its correlation with age, PSA levels , prostate volume and ethnic group within this small cohort of patients.

To evaluate if prostates with malignancy have a strong association with inflammation and PIN.

To determine if malignancy in older patients is more aggressive as reflected by a higher Gleason sum and higher PSA.

3. Materials and methods

671 patients who underwent TRUS biopsies of the prostate from January 2009 to August 2010 were analyzed and the various parameters associated with each biopsy documented. These included patient demographics such as age, race, PSA and previous biopsy history. Prostate parameters included size, digital rectal examinations findings and number of cores taken. The histological parameters looked at were Gleason primary and secondary scores and total percentage of tumour.

Transrectal Ultrasound Guided biopsies were performed by various operators ranging from urological trainees to consultants. There was variablility in the number of cores taken where a few operators were following the Vienna nomogram and others were doing a standard 12 core biopsy. Patients who had more than 12 cores were either having a repeat biopsy or had additional targeted biopsies based on ultrasound findings. 95.8% of patients evaluated were undergoing their first biopsy. Prostate volume was assessed transrectally using the BK Hawk Ultrasound. Prostate volume was available for analysis only from January 2010 onwards.

Statistical analysis was with SPSS version 18, Chi square test was used for categorical data and independent t test used to compare means.

4. Results

Between January 2009 to August 2010, a total of 671 TRUS biopsy results were analysed. The mean age of patients presenting for TRUS biopsy at our centre was 68.38 +/- 7years. Overall median PSA was 9 +/- 132.9 ng/mL .The ethnic distribution of patients included 48.1% Malays, 36.7% Chinese, 13.1% Indians and 1.6% of other ethnic origin. Compared to the national demographics there were less Malays and more Chinese and Indians in this cohort of patients. 50.5% of our patients presented with a prostate specific antigen (PSA) level of between 4 to 10ng/mL and 24.7% presented with levels higher than 20 ng/mL.

The majority of patients had a reasonably high prostate volume; 41.6% had a volume of more than 50g while only 17.5% had a prostate volume less than 30g. Overall Malay and Indian patients presented with larger prostates. 90% of Malay and Indian patients presented with prostate volume of more than 30g compared to 66.7% of Chinese patients.

There is an increasing trend of prostate volume and PSA level with age. None of the patients less than 50 years old had a prostate volume of more than 50g, while 48% of patients older than 70 years old had volume more than 50g. (Table 1)

Population age group

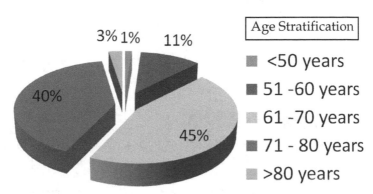

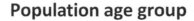

Fig. 1. Stratification of age groups among patients who were biopsied.

Prostate volume (g)	Age stratification (% Patients)			
	<50	50-60	61-70	71-80
<20	0%	17.6 %	4.2 %	2.3 %
20-29	0%	23.5%	8.5%	15.9 %
30-39	100%	5.9%	21.1%	18.2%
40-49	0%	23.5%	25.4 %	15.9%
>50	0%	29.4%	40.8%	47.7%

Table 1. Increasing Prostate Volume seen with Increasing Age

The median PSA of patients younger than 50 years old was 6.8 +/- 4.7 ng/mL , patients 51 to 60 years, 7.96 +/- 177 ng/mL, patients 61 to 70 years , 7.89 +/- 124 ng/mL, patients 71 to 80 years old, 11.0 +/- 127 ng/mL and patients older than 80 years, 26.5 +/- 163ng/mL. (Figure 2) With regards to race, the Malay patients had a median PSA 10 +/- 138.4ng/mL , Chinese patients median PSA 8.55 +/- 113.8 ng/mL and Indians had the lowest median PSA 7.6 +/- 167 ng/mL.

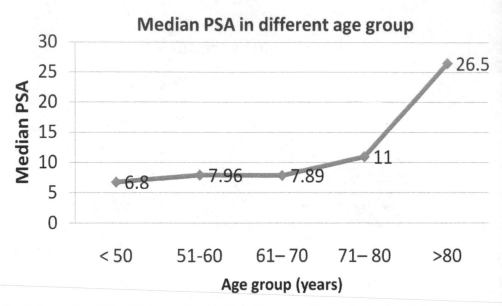

Fig. 2. Increasing PSA with increasing Median Age among the patients biopsied

In a separate cross sectional study done among Malaysian community in 2005[2], as part of a prostate awareness campaign, the mean PSA of men in their 50s was 1.4 +/- 6.3 ng/mL , men in their 60s, 2.3 +/- 3.8 ng/mLand above 70, 4.3 +/- 11 ng/mL. In the similar study Malays had a mean PSA 2.3 +/- 8.3 ng/mL, Chinese 1.8 +/- 3 ng/mL and Indians 1.3 +/- 1.9 ng/mL.

This ethnic variation in PSA in Malaysia is contrary to a separate study by Chia et al [3] from Singapore who did not find any PSA variation between the three ethnic groups, however in that study 92.8% of participants were Chinese.

From the 671 biopsies analysed, 29.1% had 6 to 10 cores taken, 46.8% had 12 cores, and 24.1% had more than 12 cores. The TRUS biopsy cancer detection rate at our center was 25.6% and it was almost similar in all the major ethnic groups (Malay-24%, Chinese- 26.2%, Indian 24.4%)(p> 0.05). Prostate inflammation was identified in 16.8% of our patients, while PIN was seen in 9%. Prostate inflammation was fairly similar in the Malay and Chinese population (Malay-17.4%, Chinese-17.8%) but the Indian population had a lower inflammation rate of 12.8%.

Of the patients who had malignancy, 34.2% had 6 to 10 cores taken, 46.2% had 12 cores and 19.6% had more than 12 cores taken. When compared with patients who were diagnosed with benign disease, the distribution of cores taken was similar;26.5% with 6 to 10 cores taken, 51.6% with 12 cores and 21.9% with more than 12 cores.

Cancer detection was 0 % in patients < 50 years, 17.6% in those 51 to 60 years old, 20.2% in patients 61 to 70 years old, 32.4% for those 71 to 80 years old and 50% for patients older than 80 years. There was no PIN seen in patients < 50 years old, 4.1% in patients 51 to 60 years old, 11.1 % for those 61 to 70 years old, and 8.3% above the age of 70 years. Prostate inflammation was seen in all age groups ranging from 11% to 19% and lowest (8.3%) in patients older than 80 years (Figure 3)

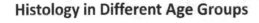

Histology in Different Age Groups

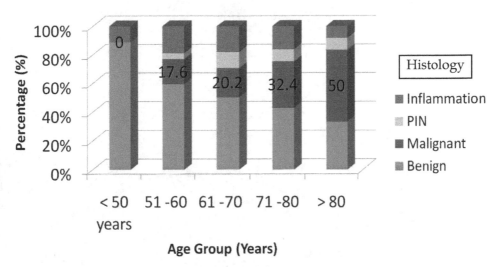

Fig. 3. Variability of biopsy histology based on age stratification. Increasing detection of malignancy with increasing age.

With regards to PSA at presentation, malignancy was detected in 15.3% of patients with PSA 0 to 10ng/ml, 16.2% with PSA 11 to 20ng/ml, 39% with PSA 21 to 50ng/ml and 77.9% with PSA >50ng/ml. Inflammation was seen in 13.8% of patients with PSA 0 to 10ng/ml, 27% with PSA 11 to 20ng/ml,24.7% with PSA 21 to 50ng/ml and 6.5% with PSA more than 50ng/ml. PIN was seen in 11% of patients with PSA 0 to 10ng/ml, 12.6% with PSA 11 to 20ng/ml, 3.9% with PSA 21 to 50ng/ml and 0% with PSA more than 50ng/ml (Figure 4)

As expected, patients diagnosed with malignancy had a higher median PSA of 26.6 +/- 230ng/ml as compared with benign disease (7.3 +/- 82ng/mL,) inflammation (11.7 +/- 23.7ng/mL) and PIN (8.2 +/- 7.1ng/mL). In our study, the PSA level did not show any correlation with prostate volume.

The higher the prostate volume, the lower the cancer detection. 60% of prostates weighing less than 20g were found to be malignant, 35.3% malignant for volume 20 to 29g, 24% for volume 30 to 39g, 21.4% for volume 40 to 49g and 14.5% for volume more than 50g. PIN was generally not seen in prostates less than 40g. Inflammation however, was seen in 14 to 17% of cases regardless of the prostate volume.

Of the 25.6% of patients with malignancy, 28% of them had a Gleason sum of 6, 24.8% with Gleason 7, 22.4% with Gleason 8, 24.2% with Gleason 9 and 0.6% with Gleason 10. Gleason sum 7 was seen in 30.8%, 19.3% and 28.6% of patients in their 6th, 7th and 8th decade of life respectively. Gleason sum 8 and above was seen in 60.6%, 43.9% and 43.1% of patients in their 6th,7th and 8th decade of life respectively. Patients above 80 years presented with significantly higher grade disease. 83.3% had gleason sum 8 and above.

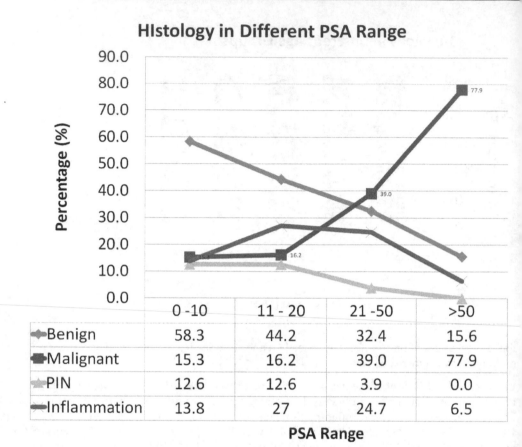

PSA Range	0 -10	11 - 20	21 -50	>50
Benign	58.3	44.2	32.4	15.6
Malignant	15.3	16.2	39.0	77.9
PIN	12.6	12.6	3.9	0.0
Inflammation	13.8	27	24.7	6.5

Fig. 4. Line graph shows the probability of detecting various histological diagnosis based on range of PSA at presentation, it acts as a useful guide for the clinician who is doing the biopsy.

5. Conclusion

Cancer detection rate in our center was 25.6% and it appears to be the same among the 3 major ethnic groups. It was noticed that Malay patients presented with a higher median PSA and this is not explained by a large prostate volume as the Indian patients had similarly large prostates but presented with a lower PSA level. Prostate inflammation among Malay patients was similar with that of the Chinese patients. Therefore, it is possible that there may be other factors that could be contributing to the higher PSA among Malays . It was also interesting to note that despite presenting with a higher PSA level, Malay patients had similar cancer detection rate as the other two ethnic groups.

There appears to be variation in PSA among the various ethnic groups , however this is an area that will require further research as there may be other confounding factors that would contribute to the differences seen.

The distribution of the number of cores taken was similar between patients diagnosed with malignancy and benign disease. 65.8% patients diagnosed with malignancy had 12 or more biopsies taken compared to 73.5% in patients diagnosed with benign disease. (p>0.05) Therefore in this analysis, the number of cores taken did not influence cancer detection rates.

Wether the operator performing the biopsy is an independent factor predicting cancer detection rate was not studied in this analysis. Nathan et al [4]suggested significant differences in operators performing transrectal biopsy in the detection of prostate cancer.

It is evident that cancer detection was much better in the smaller prostates, especially when the volume was less than 20g. The diagnosis of malignancy decreases with increasing prostate volume. This is supported by many other studies including a study by Remzi et al [5] suggesting a repeat biopsy in prostates with total volume more than 20 mls with a negative first biopsy.This is probably due to easier detection in a smaller volume prostate undergoing biopsy. Reitbergen et al [6] found that most important factor responsible for the failure of diagnosis of prostate cancer at the primary screening was prostate volume. Another hypothesis is the higher probability of a smaller prostate with elevated PSA harbouring cancer as compared to a larger sized prostate gland. However, although Chinese patients generally presented with smaller prostates, their cancer detection rate was no higher than the other ethnic groups. It is also interesting to note that PIN was only identified in prostates more than 40g. Inflammation was observed at equal rates in small and large prostates (14 to 17%).

As expected, the cancer detection rate increased with increasing PSA ranging from 15.3% detection for PSA 0 to 10ng/ml to 77.9% for PSA more than 50ng/ml. There was a significant rise in cancer detection with a PSA > 20ng/mL. Prostate inflammation detection was 14%-27% among patients with PSA< 50ng/mL but was significantly less (6.5%) in patients with PSA more than 50ng/ml. This finding does not suggest any correlation between prostate inflammation and malignancy in this cohort of patients . Terekawa et al [7] found an inverse relationship between histologic inflammation and prostate cancer in men with PSA 10-50 ng/mL undergoing prostate biopsy.

Detection of PIN was significantly higher in patients with PSA 0 to 20ng/ml compared to higher PSA levels. Within this range of PSA , 12% of biopsies had PIN . The incidence of isolated PIN in prostate biopsies varies in the literature. In urological practice, incidence varies between 4.4-25% [8]

Cancer detection increased with increasing age averaging 30 to 50% in patients above 70 years old. Patients below 50 years who were biopsied did not have cancer and none had PIN, however 11.1% had prostate inflammation and the rest had benign disease. The lowest incidence of prostate inflammation was seen in patients older than 80 years. These patients also had the highest cancer detection rate.

This study also showed the expected trend of a rising prostate volume with increasing age. From the age of 50 years onwards, there was a 10g increase in prostate volume in every decade and this trend stabilises after the 8th decade of life. Median PSA also notably increased with age. Men older than 80 years old had the highest median PSA, 26.5 ng/mL and when diagnosed with malignancy had a significantly higher grade cancer.

From this preliminary study it appears that there could be some differences in the presentation of prostate disease and PSA distribution in Asian patients as compared to their western counterpart. The patients in this cohort were detected with malignancy at a higher PSA compared to their western counterparts. Further research would be required to explore these differences and to further study the PSA variation between the various ethnic groups.

6. Acknowledgement

Dr Teo Swi Han, Dr Nurul Hayati bt Abu Hassan and Dr Khalid bin Othman for their effort in tracing all the patient records.

Keywords: TRUS, Prostate Cancer, Inflammation

7. References

[1] Lim TC, Norraha AR, 2006, *Natioanal Cancer Registry*
[2] Sothilingam S et al 2010 , *Prostate Cancer Screening, Malaysian Perspective*, Urologic Oncology- Seminars and Original Investigations; 28 670-72
[3] Chia et al , 2007, *PSA levels among Chinese, Malays and Indians in Singapore from a community based study.* Asian Pac J Cancer Prev Jul-Sept; 8(3): 375-8
[4] Nathan et al , 2009, *Operator is an Independent Predictor of Detecting Prostate Cancer at Transrectal Ultrasound Guided Prostate Biopsy.*, J Urol: 182, 2659-2663.
[5] Remzi et al, 2003, *Can Total and Transition Zone Volume of Prostate determine whether to perform a repeat biopsy*, Urology; 61(1): 161-6
[6] Reietbergen et al , 1998 , *Repeat screening for prostate cancer after 1 year followup in 984 biopsied men*: Clinical and pathological factors in detecting cancer., J Urol: 160-2121-5.
[7] Terekawa et al , 2008, *Inverse Association between Histologic Inflammation in Needle Biopsy specimens and Prostate Cancer in men with serum PSA 10-50 ng/mL,* , Urology: 1194-1197.
[8] Jonian et al , 2005,*Prostatic Intraepithelial Neoplasia (PIN): Importance and Clinical Management .* European Urology 48 , 379-385.

8

Elderly and Early Prostate Cancer

K. Stamatiou

Urology department Tzaneion General Hospital of Pireas
Greece

1. Introduction

Prostate cancer (PC) is the second most frequent malignant disease and the second-leading cause of cancer deaths among men in the United States [1]. Both evidence and epidemiologic studies have shown that PC is rare in men younger than 50 years of age, but thereafter the risk of incident prostate cancer increases significantly with increasing age [2]. After the introduction and widespread use of the prostate-specific antigen (PSA) blood test, PC incidence has increased and it is expected that this disease is likely to become a more prominent and pressing problem in many countries as the percentage of elderly men increases [3]. Actually declines in mortality at younger ages, medical advances, and better health care have resulted in longer life expectancy in both the developing and the developed world the last three decades. Statistics compiled by the United Nations showed that in 1999, 10% of the world population was 60 years and older [4]. By 2050, this percentage will rise to 22%. In Hong Kong, where the proportion of elderly is even higher, it is estimated to rise to 40%. Regarding male gender, the population over 65 years is expected to increase 4-fold worldwide by 2050 [5]. Achievements of the 20th century have changed the world's demographic proportions without altering the epidemiology of PC. Indeed, PC still remains a disease of elderly men and thus, increased PC incidence could be partly attributed to the steadily growing ageing population [6].

While the majority of elderly PC patients in the past were diagnosed with local advanced or metastatic disease, a rising number of elderly men are now diagnosed with early stage PC. It is not known whether and if this is due to the effective utilization of health care resources or to the widespread use of PSA testing worldwide. Several studies however showed that after the introduction of PSA, additionally to the increase in the PC detection rate, an eventual shift towards earlier pathological stage was occurred also [3]. The increased life expectancy enjoyed by the world population also means that the life span beyond age 60 is much longer than demographers have previously envisaged. Currently, a large proportion of the population remains active beyond the age of 70 and lives beyond the age of 80. Since many of them are healthy, the number of elderly men who will be diagnosed with PC and may require treatment will further increase in the coming years [7].

The aim of present study is to discuss the issue of screening for PC in elderly individuals as well as to review the current data on the treatment of early stage PC in elder males. A secondary aim is to examine whether or not advanced age impacts on PC risk. The impact of life expectancy on the choice of treatment in both patients and health care providers has been investigated also.

2. Methods

We identified studies published from 1990 onwards by searching the MEDLINE database of the National Library of Medicine. Initial search terms were localized prostate cancer, early stage prostate cancer, combined with elderly patients, life expectancy, palliative, curative, quality of life, watchful waiting, radical prostatectomy, brachytherapy and external beam radiotherapy. References in the selected publications were checked for relevant publications not included in the Medline/Pubmed search.

3. Results

3.1 How ageing can increase the risk of prostate cancer?

A definitive cause of PC has not been identified and the specific mechanisms that lead to the development of the disease are still unknown. Although several risk factors have been proposed, the only risk factors that can be considered established are age, race and family history. Evidence suggests that an association between the above risk factors through a common pathogenic mechanism exists. On one hand, development and function of the prostate gland is endocrine controlled and androgen/estrogen synergism is necessary for the integrity of the normal human prostate. On the other hand androgen action is critical to the development, progression and cure of PC. Under those circumstances, it could be expected that ageing facilitate PC development through androgenic action. In fact, androgens undergo a significant age-dependent alteration: with ageing the production of testosterone by the testes is decreasing leading thus in a significant reduction of the endogenous testosterone levels. DHT activity decreases in the epithelium while in the stroma it remains constant over the whole age range. The age-dependent decrease of the DHT accumulation in epithelium and the concomitant increase of the estrogen accumulation in stroma lead to a tremendous increase of the estrogen/androgen ratio in the human prostate. Although, the specific pathway remains partially investigated, it is widely accepted that these alterations promote the initiation of benign prostatic hypertrophy, the most common disease of the ageing prostate. Similarly to benign prostatic hypertrophy, PC incidence increases with age: it seldom develops before the age of 40 and is chiefly a disease found in men over the age 65 years. Epidemiological evidence from autopsy studies show that while a very high proportion of elderly men has histological evidence of the disease, a much smaller proportion actually develop clinically apparent PC however, most of the impalpable cancers likely to progress and become clinically significant (advanced Gleason score, greater volume) are found in older individuals ([8]). However, age-related increase in the prevalence of prostate cancer found in autopsy is not similar worldwide. Variations in the reported incidence of PC between different racial groups suggest that some populations are either more susceptible to PC-promoting events or are exposed to different promoting agents ([9]). Take the above in consideration it could be speculated that ageing may promote clonal transformation events of pathogenetic importance for the initiation of PC. These clonal transformation events may be boosted by genetic predisposing factors. Although the exact pathways remain unknown, evidence suggests that they involving the androgen receptor (AR). The AR is a structurally conserved member of the nuclear receptor superfamily and signalling via the AR is critical for carcinogenesis and progression of the disease. The AR´s amino-terminal domain is required for transcriptional activation and contains a region of polyglutamine encoded by CAG trinucleotide repeats. As androgen influences prostate cancer growth, expansion of CAG repeats in the AR affect the risk of developing prostate cancer in a race and age depending matter [10].

Age-dependent clonal transformation events that affect the risk of developing prostate cancer may also occur to the Insulin-like Growth Factor-II (IGF-II) gene. The IGF-II gene is an auto- paracrine growth stimulator that is an important positive modulator of cancer development. IGF-II losses of imprinting, as well as increased IGF-II expression resulting from age-dependent changes in DNA methylation, have been recently associated with increased risk for PC development [11].

3.2 The issue of screening for prostate cancer in elderly individuals

A major consideration for cancer screening is to weigh up the possibility someone will have needless treatment against saving lives. PC can develop into a fatal, painful disease, but it can also develop so slowly that it will never cause problems during the man's lifetime. Actually, although none of the existing screening tools can accurately distinguish between lethal and indolent PC, the use of PSA has been shown to increase the PC detection rate with a shift to detection at earlier and therefore curable stages [12]. This fact generated also concerns about over-diagnosis and over-treating and arguments both for and against the efficacy of screening. Under the light of this evidence it became clear why the issues of over-diagnosis and over-treating are of outmost importance when deciding to screen elderly individuals [13].

Data from US Cancer of the Prostate Strategic Urological Research Endeavor shows that most of the patients diagnosed with prostate cancer the last two decades in the US had low or intermediate disease at diagnosis [14]. Moreover, between 20 and 30% of PCs found in radical prostatectomy specimens of men with PSA-detected disease are non palpable, potentially indolent cancers (Gleason <6, tumor volume <0,5cm3) [15,16]. Since doubling time of high and intermediate differentiated prostatic carcinomas reaches 7 and 5 years respectively, a small tumor (<0,5cm3) poses little threat for the life of older individuals (from the perspective that needs enough time to became life threatening). In confirmation to the above, Albertsen and colleagues demonstrated that men with prostate biopsy specimens showing Gleason score 2 to 4 disease faced a minimal risk of death from prostate cancer within 15 years from diagnosis [17]. Given that life expectancy of American males at the age of 65 is 16 years [18] and the mean time to cancer-specific death of apparently clinically localized prostate cancer is 17 years [19], it became obvious why PC screening and treatment of PSA detected PCs in elderly patients is a controversial issue. Most doctors however argue against PSA testing for men who are in their 70s or older, because even if prostate cancer were detected, most men would be dead of something else before the cancer progressed [20]. This is true only in part. As previously mentioned, today a large proportion of the population lives beyond age 70 and many are healthy. These men have several reasons –the belief in the benefit of early diagnosis, the need to have trust, and a desire for reliable screening resembling women- to undergo testing for prostate cancer. Yet, patient's anxiety increase the likelihood of getting the screening test, by acting powerfully on the screening decisions of physicians, whose clinical judgment would otherwise make them least, inclined to order the test [21].

At the moment, PC screening is being performed unofficially in elderly patients visiting outpatient departments of general hospitals and consulting rooms. The exact magnitude of this opportunistic screening is not known however it is believed that reaches high numbers worldwide. Hoffman and associates and Walter and colleagues found a 56% and 50% PSA screening rate in their cohort of elderly men in 2003 and 2010, respectively [22,23]. Bowen and co-workers found that PC screening rates among men at the age of 80 and older are even higher than that of men in the age range of 50 to 64 years (64% versus 56%)[24]. Similarly, in a study by D'Ambrosio and colleagues, the highest yearly exposure to PSA screening and the highest frequency of repeat testing were observed in the age range of 70 to the 79 years [25]. In contrast, Zeliadt and associates demonstrated that PSA testing among men older than 75 years has declined slightly following the recommendations by the US Preventive Services Task Force in 2008 and is still continuing to decline (15). Aus and colleagues found that restrictions in the use of PSA test in individuals over 75 years resulted in PC incidence falls after peaking at the age of 75 [26]. Interestingly, evidence suggests that PSA testing may be useful in diagnosis of aggressive early PC in a subset of elderly patients. A current study by Brassell and colleagues showed that as men age, parameters consistent with more aggressive disease become more prevalent [27] a fact that was confirmed by the findings of an autopsy study demonstrating that a proportion of elderly men with histologically apparent disease may develop lethal PC (21). Therefore it is not surprising that older individuals with clinically apparent PC usually die from PC. These data may have implications for future screening and treatment recommendations. Currently, age plays an important role in both screening decision and treatment choice and thus elderly patients are less likely to undergo PSA test and receive local therapy.

Data from US Cancer of the Prostate Strategic Urological Research Endeavor shows a significant reduction of risk of death from metastatic prostate cancer and a decrease in prostate carcinoma-specific mortality the last two decades in the US (14). As yet it is not possible to say what proportion of the fall in mortality is the result of improvements in treatment, changes in cancer registration coding, the attribution of death to PC, and the effects of PSA testing. Accumulative evidence however suggests that early screening of PC in asymptomatic men reduce their risk of death from metastatic disease. Interestingly, the recently published results of the European Randomised Study for Screening of Prostate Cancer (ERSPC) reported a relative PC mortality reduction of at least 20% by PSA-based population screening [28] while Goel and Kopec reported an even higher reduction of risk of death from metastatic PC among men who were not screened regularly as part of a screening program [29].

Given that PSA screening mainly diagnoses early PC, it may be justifiable for otherwise healthy elderly men to undergo PSA test. This is of outmost importance since older patients are more likely to have high-risk prostate cancer at diagnosis and lower overall survival. In fact, under-use of potentially curative local therapy among older men with high-risk disease may explain, at least in part, the observed differences in cancer-specific survival across age strata.[30]. Taking in consideration these findings along with observations of Brassell and co-workers (27) it became obvious that evidence supports making decisions regarding screening on the basis of disease risk and life expectancy rather than chronologic age.

Currently, no standard recommendation for PC screening exists. Recently, the American Urological Association recommends PC screening to men aged 40 years or older. In contrast, screening is presently discouraged by the EC Advisory Committee on Cancer Prevention for its negative effects are evident and its benefits still uncertain [31]. According to the U.S. Preventive Services Task Force, evidence is insufficient to recommend in favour of, or against routine PC screening (23). The abovementioned professional organizations and health agencies as well as most of medical experts agree that it is important that the benefits and risks of diagnostic procedures and treatment be taken into account when considering whether to undertake PC screening. On the other hand, treatment recommendations are now recognizing that older men with PC should be managed according to their individual health status, which is mainly driven by the severity of associated comorbid conditions, and not according to chronological age. According to the International Society of Geriatric Oncology Prostate Cancer Task Force, it is possible, based on a rapid and simple evaluation, to classify patients into four different groups: 1) "Healthy" patients (controlled comorbidity, fully independent in daily living activities, and no malnutrition) should receive the same treatment as younger patients; 2) "Vulnerable" patients (reversible impairment) should receive standard treatment after medical intervention; 3) "Frail" patients (irreversible impairment) should receive adapted treatment; 4) Patients who are "too sick" with "terminal illness" should receive only symptomatic palliative treatment.(30) The same rapid and simple evaluation may help physicians who perform PSA screening to decide who to screen.

3.3 Treatment options and treatment decision making

The main treatment options include radical prostatectomy (RP), radiotherapy (external beam radiotherapy and brachytherapy), watchful waiting (WW) and androgen deprivation therapy (ADT). Other include, cryotherapy (freezing the prostate), high-intensity focused ultrasound (HIFU), radiofrequency interstitial tumour ablation (RITA) and non-hormonal therapy (cytotoxic agents). Radical prostatectomy, brachytherapy and external beam radiotherapy are considered curative, while watchful waiting and hormone-therapy palliative. All treatments have risks of complications, although frequency and severity may vary. The primary goal of treatment is to target the men most likely to need intervention in order to prevent prostate cancer death and disability while minimizing intervention-related complications. However, whereas the standard oncologic evaluation works reasonably well in most other populations, in elderly PC patients, tends to overestimate possible harms associated with radical treatment and underestimate patients ability to withstand treatments side effects. In accordance to the above, various studies have demonstrated that potentially curative therapy (radical prostatectomy or radiotherapy) is applied less often in older PC patients (32,33,34,35,36). Traditionally, PC is considering a slow progressive disease that needs enough time to become life threatening for an elder individual and this possibly explains the above observation. However, a multivariate analysis of the SEER database revealed significantly decreased odds of receiving cancer directed surgery in the elderly patient with lung, liver, breast, pancreas, esophageal, gastric cancers, sarcoma and rectal cancer while other studies have demonstrated under use of cancer directed radiation and chemotherapy (37,38,39). These findings are posing justifiable concern about under-treatment of the elderly cancer patient and raise the provocative question if this is due to judicious, evidence based selection or discrimination based only on age (40). The reasons for the observed under use of cancer directed treatment in the elderly remain elusive. However, discrimination -if present- reflects the stereotypes that older people are physically frail, unfit for curative treatment, indisposed to accept treatment related complications, impatient and uninterested in prolonging survival. With regard to PC treatment decision making, increasing age is definitely a risk factor for receiving inadequate treatment (41). Harlan et al demonstrated that advantaged age is- still- considering as important as PSA, clinical stage and Gleason score while other demonstrated that age is the predominant factor influencing treatment decision making: Alibhai and colleagues generated an age-stratified random sample of 347 men from a cohort of patients with newly diagnosed prostate carcinoma in the Ontario Cancer Registry. Patients who were younger than 60 years were more likely to receive radical prostatectomy than radiation therapy or no therapy. Men between 60 and 69 years of age were more likely to receive radiation therapy than radical prostatectomy. Men between 70 and 79 years were most likely to receive no therapy, and nearly all men over 80 years received no therapy [42]. Basically, although age plays a key role in treatment decision making, age itself is not predictive of outcome in an elderly cancer patient. In contrast, treatment outcome is strictly associated with clinical parameters such as the tumor stage, tumor grade or Gleason score and PSA level and therefore, treatment selection should be balanced between clinical stage and remaining life expectancy. It should be noticed however that the 10-year rule currently used to estimate life expectancy in elderly PC patients has demonstrated limited predictive validity and its use in clinical decision-making doesn't decrease the likelihood of receiving inappropriate treatment in elderly individuals [31].

Regarding localized PC, available treatment options include established therapies such as WW, RP, brachytherapy and external beam radiotherapy and non established therapies such as minimal invasive techniques and early hormone-therapy [43]. RP is considering the gold standard for the treatment of localized PC and in fact it is the most common treatment with approximately 60,000 operations performed annually in the US [44]. However, only a small number of elderly patients with early stage PC are treated with RP [45]. The reason why advanced age is an unfavorable predictor of the probability of surgical treatment is not known [46]. Actually, the fact that elderly individuals have lower life expectancy as well as the belief that elderly patients with localized disease are considering more prone to die with PC than of it, partly explain why PR is the less popular treatment of early PC in elderly patients. Moreover, elderly patients are often being considering fragile enough to receive surgical treatment. Whether and if age increase surgical risk is a controversial issue and for this reason several investigators claim that it is co-morbidity that actually increases the surgical risk and not ageing itself [47]. Although, co-morbid illness has demonstrated increasing importance as a prognostic factor, its role is poorly defined. It is generally accepted that co-morbidity limits the generalization of results to older and sicker patients however; the widespread integration of co-morbidity into clinical practice has yet to be realized.

Reported differences in PC specific survival across age strata may be associated with under use of potentially curative local therapy among older men. In fact, PC mortality increases with ageing, peaks at the age of 70-75 and no significant decrease occurs thereafter (table 1). According to the SEER database, younger men (under age 65) with localized prostate cancer had 25-year prostate cancer mortality rates of approximately 19% for Gleason 6 disease, 37% for Gleason 7 disease, and 50% for Gleason 8-10 disease [48]. Given that the survival advantage of surgery is most pronounced in men with higher stage disease, it became obvious that elderly PC patients with aggressive disease and life expectancy >10 years are likely to die from progressive prostate cancer [49]. Worth mentioning, Bechis et al. studied men in the Cancer of the Prostate Strategic Urologic Research Endeavor (CaPSURE) database with complete risk, treatment, and follow-up information. They found that older patients are more likely to have high-risk prostate cancer at diagnosis and less likely to receive local therapy [30]. In confirmation to the above, Dahm et al.showed that risk of death from PC for elderly PC patients treated with PR is significantly lower when compared with

AGE	DEATHS	% RATE
15-19	0	0
20-24	1	0,0
25-29	2	0,0
30-34	1	0,0
35-39	4	0,0
40-44	20	0,1
45-49	71	0,3
50-54	233	0,9
55-59	722	2,8
60-64	1738	6,9
65-69	3123	12,5
70-74	4636	18,5
75-79	5337	21,4
80-84	4536	18,2
> 85	4625	18,1

Table 1. Age and PC specific mortality (US Public service 1989).

that of elderly PC patients treated with watchful waiting ([50]). Results from other studies showed that surgical therapy can achieve excellent oncologic results in selected elderly patients but they didn't found significant differences in overall survival ([51],[52]). According to the results of the Scandinavian Prostate Cancer Group (SPCG) study, radical prostatectomy is associated with less deaths from prostate cancer (10 vs.15%), less deaths from any other cause (24 vs 30%) and less metastases (14 vs. 23%) in a median follow-up of 8.2 years. However, benefit in cancer specific survival is limited to patients younger than 65 years.

On the other hand there are several facts supporting WW (deferring intervention until the advent of symptoms) as an ideal treatment of early PC in elderly patients: Epidemiological evidence from autopsy studies show that while a very high proportion of elderly men has histological evidence of the disease, a much smaller proportion actually develop clinically apparent PC ([53]). Several authors demonstrated that elderly patients with localized PC have a favorable outlook following WW ([54],[55]) and other showed that WW results in similar overall survival when compared with RP ([56]). In a pooled analysis of 828 case records from six nonrandomized studies, of men treated conservatively for clinically localized prostate cancer, Chodak et al, found an impressive 87% five years disease-specific survival rate ([57]), however other found that disease specific survival is better in patients who had undergone surgery and some authors argue that WW simply postpone the final treatment ([58],[59],[60],[61]).

Notably, there are no randomized clinical trials comparing surgery with radiation therapy in elderly PC patients, however an observational study, by Albertsen and colleagues showed that surgery is superior to radiation in localized prostate cancer in terms of prolonging overall and disease-specific survival ([62]).

The truth is that the preferred management of clinically localized prostate cancer is not known, due in large part to the paucity of randomized controlled trials comparing the effectiveness and harms across primary treatment options. It seems that age itself is the main determinant of treatment selection: according to the Swedish Cancer Register in men with localized tumors expectant treatment was much more commonly used in those aged > or =75 years than in those aged <75 years ([63]). It is also clear that WW is an adequate approach for the treatment of early stage PC in patients suffering of live threatening diseases, unfit for radical treatment, however, it remains unclear whether and if treatment can be delayed until absolutely necessary with no detriment to curability in otherwise healthy elderly PC patients. Interestingly, Wong et al found no survival advantage associated with expectant treatment for localized PC in elderly men aged 65 to 80 years [64]. Certainly observational data cannot completely adjust for potential selection bias and confounding, however these results clearly shows that specific factors other than tumor stage may contribute to WW failure. Given that PC exhibits a wide range of biologic behaviour, it could be assumed that disease specific survival outcomes in patients with localised PC following WW are associated with Gleason score or baseline PSA level: In the study of Johansson, only the 6% of patients with well differentiated PC, died of PC while mortality rates for intermediate and poorly differentiated cancers were 17% and 56% respectively (54). Soloway and associates reported an 85% treatment-free rate at 5 years on a small cohort of patients diagnosed with 'low-risk' prostate cancer managed by WW [65]. Sandblom et al found also a great influence on survival and suggest the grade of malignancy to be taken into account when deciding on therapy (55).

The major risk of watchful waiting is that without treatment, prostate cancer can grow and spread outside the prostate capsule. In fact, even small, slow-growing tumors may become rapidly growing tumors and sometimes prostate cancer that appears to be small and slow growing may be larger and more aggressive than originally thought. Identification of patients who have a low probability of disease progression could be based on strict clinical and pathologic criteria such as Gleason score of 6 or less, a PSA level of 10 ng/ml or less, and stage T1c–T2a disease [66]. Again, although patients with these characteristics have a much more favourable natural history and progression rate than those who have a higher Gleason grade or PSA level, in a substantial proportion of men tumours will still progress to advanced, incurable prostate cancer and death [67].

These data suggest that it is of outmost importance to distinguish between patients who are at higher risk and need active therapy and patients who are at low risk for disease progression and support making decisions regarding treatment on the basis of disease risk and life expectancy rather than on chronologic age [68,69].

It therefore became clear that a comprehensive health status assessment is the key in distinguishing between frail and healthy elderly patients and in developing appropriate management approaches for these individuals. The geriatric assessment differs from a standard medical evaluation as it focuses on elderly individuals with complex problems and emphasizes functional status, co-morbidity and quality of life. Most importantly, comprehensive geriatric assessment frequently takes advantage of an interdisciplinary team of providers (urologists, radiation oncologists, medical oncologists and geriatricians).

Recently, the SIOG has developed a proposal of recommendations in this setting based on a systematic bibliographical search focused on screening, diagnostic procedures and treatment options for localised, locally advanced and metastatic prostate cancer in senior adults. Specific aspects of the geriatric approach were emphasised, including evaluation of health status (nutritional, cognitive, thymic, physical and psycho-social) and screening for vulnerability and frailty [70]. According to the above elderly PC patients are classified in 4 groups. In Group 1 (no abnormality), patients are 'fit' and should receive the same treatment as younger patients; patients in Group 2 (one impairment in IADL or one uncontrolled comorbidity or at risk of malnutrition) are 'vulnerable' and should receive standard treatment after medical intervention; patients in Group 3 (one impairment in ADL or more than one uncontrolled comorbidity or severe malnutrition) are 'frail' and should receive adapted treatment; patients in Group 4 (dependent) should receive only symptomatic palliative treatment (32).

4. Conclusions

Actually, health status is more reliable prognostic factor for survival and treatment related outcomes in oncology than patient age and with this modern approach should be adapted in order to screening senior adults. Age, PSA level, histological grade, and comorbidities should be carefully balanced before making a treatment decision, in elderly men suffering from prostate cancer. Elderly men with limited life expectancy due to other significant life-limiting medical conditions, such as chronic obstructive pulmonary disease and advanced coronary artery disease, are less likely to benefit from aggressive treatment and are candidate for a palliative approach Therefore, it is reasonable to withhold early detection through PSA screening in these patients thus avoiding the associated risks and impact on quality of life. In selected cases of healthy elderly patients and long life expectancy, PSA screening and curative treatment of undifferentiated prostate cancers could be considered as a rational choice.

5. References

[1] Jemal A, Thomas A, Murray T, Thun M. Cancer statistics, 2002. CA Cancer J Clin 2002;52:23-47.

[2] Levy I. Prostate cancer: the epidemiology perspective. Can J Oncol 1994;4 Suppl 1:4-7.

[3] United Nations Economic and Social Council.Concise report on world population (2000). Report of the Secretary-General to the 33rd session of the Commission on Population and Development, 27-31 March 2000 available at:
    http://www.un.org/documents/ecosoc/cn9/2000/ecn92000-3.pdf.

[4] Siegel R, Ward E, et al. Cancer statistics, 2007. CA Cancer J Clin 2007;57:43-66.

[5] Jemal, A; Cheung FM. Ageing population and gender issues. In: Yeung YM, ed. New challenges for development and modernization: Hong Kong and the Asia-Pacific region in the new millennium. Hong Kong: Chinese University Press; 2002:207-23.

[6] Crawford, ED. Epidemiology of prostate cancer. Urology 2003;62(6):3–12.

[7] AIRTUM Working Group. Italian cancer figures, Report 2010: Cancer prevalence in Italy. Patients living with cancer, long-term survivors and cured patients. Epidemiol Prev. 2010;34 (5-6 Suppl 2):1-188.

[8] Schutze U. Latent prostatic carcinoma -an autopsy study of men over 50 years of age. Zentralbl Allg Pathol. 1984;129(4):357-64.

[9] Breslow N, Chan CW, Dhom G, Drur-y RA, Franks LM, Gellei B et al. Latent carcinoma of prostate in seven areas. Int J Cancer 1977;20:680–688.

[10] Hardy DO, Scher HI, Bogenreider T, Sabbatini P, Zhang ZF, Nanus DM, Catterall JF. Androgen receptor CAG repeat lengths in prostate cancer: correlation with age of onset. J Clin Endocrinol Metab. 1996;81:4400-4405

[11] Fu VX, Dobosy JR, Desotelle JA, Almassi N, Ewald JA, Srinivasan R, Berres M, Svaren J, Weindruch R, Jarrard DF.Aging and cancer-related loss of insulin-like growth factor 2 imprinting in the mouse and human prostate. Cancer Res. 2008;68(16):6797-802.

[12] Smith DS, Catalona WJ, Herschman JD. Longitudinal screening for prostate cancer with prostate-specific antigen. JAMA. 1996;276:1309-1315.

[13] Woolf HS. Screening for prostate cancer with prostate- specific antigen: an examination of evidence. N Engl J Med 1995;333:1401-5.

[14] Cooperberg, MR; Lubeck, DP; Mehta, SS; Carroll, PR. Time trends in clinical risk stratification for prostate cancer: implications for outcomes (data from CaPSURE). J Urol. 2003;170(6 Pt 2):S21-S25.

[15] Epstein JI, Walsh PC, Carmichael M, Brendler CB. Pathologic and clinical findings to predict tumor extent of nonpalpable (stage T1c) prostate cancer. JAMA. 1994;271:368-374.

[16] Johansson, JE. Expectant management of early stage prostatic cancer: Swedish experience. J Urol. 1994;152:1753-1756.

[17] Albertsen PC, Hanley JA, Gleason DF, Barry MJ. Competing risk analysis of men aged 55 to 74 years at diagnosis managed conservatively for clinically localized prostate cancer. JAMA. 1998;280:975-980.

[18] Minino A, Smith BL. Deaths: preliminary data for 2000. Natl Vital Stat Rep. 2001;49:1-40 No author listed. US Public service, National Statistics Division. "Prostate cancer" National Statistics. Washton D.C.1983.

[19] Horan AH, McGehee M. Mean time to cancer-specific death of apparently clinically localized prostate cancer: policy implications for threshold ages in prostate-specific antigen screening and ablative therapy. BJU Int. 2000;85:1063-1066

[20] Scales C, Curtis L, Norris R, Schulman K, Albala D, Moul J. Prostate specific antigen testing in men older than 75 years in the United States. J Urol 2006;176(2):511-4.

[21] Haggerty J, Tudiver F, Brown JB, Herbert C, Ciampi A, Guibert R. Patients' anxiety and expectations. How they influence family physicians' decisions to order cancer screening tests. Can Fam Physician. 2005;51(12):1659.

[22] Hoffman RM, Barry MJ, Stanford JL, Hamilton AS, Hunt WC, Collins MM. Health outcomes in older men with localized prostate cancer: results from the Prostate Cancer Outcomes Study. Am J Med. 2006;119(5):418-25.

[23] Walter LC, Bertenthal D, Lindquist K, Konety BR. PSA screening among elderly men with limited life expectancies. Nat Clin Pract Urol. 2007;4(10):532-3.

[24] Bowen DJ, Hannon PA, Harris JR, Martin DP. Prostate cancer screening and informed decision-making: provider and patient perspectives. Prostate Cancer Prostatic Dis. 2011[Epub ahead of print].

[25] D'Ambrosio GG, Campo S, Cancian M, Pecchioli S, Mazzaglia G. Opportunistic prostate-specific antigen screening in Italy: 6 years of monitoring from the Italian general practice database. Eur J Cancer Prev. 2010;19:413-6.

[26] Aus G, Robinson D, Rosell J, Sandblom G, Varenhorst E, for the South-East Region Prostate Cancer Group. Survival in prostate carcinoma–outcome from a prospective, population-based cohort of 8887 men with up to 15 years of follow-up:

results from three counties in the population-based National Prostate Cancer Registry of Sweden. Cancer. 2005;103:943–951.

[27] Brassell SA, Rice KR, Parker PM, et al. Prostate cancer in men 70 years old or older, indolent or aggressive: clinicopathological analysis and outcomes. J Urol. 2011;185:132-7.

[28] Schröder FH, Hugosson J, Roobol MJ, Tammela TL, Ciatto S, Nelen V, Kwiatkowski M, Lujan M, Lilja H, Zappa M, Denis LJ, Recker F, Berenguer A, Määttänen L, Bangma CH, Aus G, Villers A, Rebillard X, van der Kwast T, Blijenberg BG, Moss SM, de Koning HJ, Auvinen A; ERSPC Investigators. Screening and prostate-cancer mortality in a randomized European study. N Engl J Med. 2009;360(13):1320-8

[29] Kopec JA, Goel V, Bunting PS, Neuman J, Sayre EC, Warde P, Levers P, Fleshner N. Screening with prostate specific antigen and metastatic prostate cancer risk: a population based case-control study. J Urol. 2005;174(2):495-9

[30] Bechis SK, Carroll PR, Cooperberg MR. Impact of age at diagnosis on prostate cancer treatment and survival. J Clin Oncol. 2011;29:235-41.

[31] Advisory Committee on Cancer Prevention. Position paper. Recommendations on cancer screening in European Union. Eur J Cancer 2000;36:1473–8

[32] Bennett CL, Greenfield S, Aronow H, Ganz P, Vogelzang NJ, Elashoff RM. Patterns of care related to age of men with prostate cancer. Cancer 1991;67(10):2633-41.

[33] Harlan LC, Potosky A, Gilliland FD, Hoffman R, Albertsen PC, Hamilton AS, Eley JW, Stanford JL, Stephenson RA. Factors associated with initial therapy for clinically localized prostate cancer: prostate cancer outcomes study. J Natl Cancer Inst. 2001;93(24):1864-71.

[34] Samet, J; Hunt, WC; Key, C, et al. Choice of cancer therapy varies with age of patient. JAMA 1986;255:3385–3390.

[35] Lu-Yao, GL; McLerran, D; Wasson, J; Wennberg, JE. An assessment of radical prostatectomy. Time trends, geographic variation, and outcomes. The Prostate Patient Outcomes Research Team. JAMA. 1993;269:2633–2636.

[36] Sverson, RK; Montie, JE; Porter, AT; Demers, RY. Recent trends in incidence and treatment of prostate cancer among elderly men. J Natl Cancer Inst. 1995;87:532–534.

[37] Schrag D, Cramer LD, Bach PB, Begg CB. Age and adjuvant chemotherapy use after surgery for stage III colon cancer. J Natl Cancer Inst 2001;93:850 –7.

[38] Mahoney T, Kuo YH, Topilow A, Davis JM. Stage III colon cancers: why adjuvant therapy is not offered to elderly patients. Arch Surg 2000;135:182-5.

[39] O'Connell JB, Maggard MA, Ko CY. Cancer-directed surgery for localized disease: decreased utilization in the elderly. Ann Surg Oncol 2004;962–969.

[40] Fuchshuber P. Age and Cancer Surgery: Judicious Selection or Discrimination? Ann Surg Oncol. 2004;11(11):951–952

[41] Krahn, MD; Bremner, KE; Asaria, J, et al. The ten-year rule revisited: accuracy of clinicians' estimates of life expectancy in patients with localized prostate cancer. Urology. 2002;60:258–263.

[42] Alibhai, SMH; Krahn, MD; Cohen, MM, et al. Is there age bias in the treatment of localized prostate carcinoma? Cancer. 2004;100:72–81.

[43] Anandadas CN, Clarke NW, Davidson SE, O'Reilly PH, Logue JP, Gilmore L, Swindell R, Brough RJ, Wemyss-Holden GD, Lau MW, Javle PM, Ramani VA, Wylie JP, Collins GN, Brown S, Cowan RA; North West Uro-oncology Group. Early prostate cancer--which treatment do men prefer and why? BJU Int. 2011 Jun;107(11):1762-8. doi: 10.1111/j.1464-410X.2010.09833.x. Epub 2010 Nov 17

[44] Healthcare Cost and Utilization Project (U.S.). United States Agency for Healthcare Research and Quality. http://www.ahrq.gov/data/hcup/hcupnet.htm. Accessed December 2006.)

[45] Schwartz KL, Alibhai SM, Tomlinson G, Naglie G, Krahn MD. Continued undertreatment of older men with localized prostate cancer. Urology. 2003 Nov;62(5):860-5.

[46] Carter HB, Epstein JI, Partin AW. Influence of age and prostate-specific antigen on the chance of curable prostate cancer among men with non palpable disease. Urology. 1999;53(1):126-30.

[47] Roberts CB, Albertsen PC, Shao YH, Moore DF, Mehta AR, Stein MN, Lu-Yao GL. Patterns and correlates of prostate cancer treatment in older men. Am J Med. 2011 Mar;124(3):235-43

[48] Wong YN, Wan F, Mitra N, et al. Treatment of localized prostate cancer: a survival analysis using SEER-Medicare data. Program and abstracts of the American Urological Association 2006 Annual Meeting; May 20-25, 2006; Atlanta, Georgia. Abstract 658.

[49] Inman BA, Slezak JM, Kwon ED, et al. 25-year outcomes of radical prostatectomy for the treatment of all stages of non-metastatic prostate cancer. Program and abstracts of the American Urological Association 2006 Annual Meeting; May 20-25, 2006; Atlanta, Georgia. Abstract 646.

[50] Dahm P, Silverstein AD, Weizer AZ, Crisci A, Vieweg J, Paulson DF. When to diagnose and how to treat prostate cancer in the "not too fit" elderly. Crit Rev Oncol Hematol. 2003;48(2):123-31

[51] Wilt TJ, Brawer MK, Barry MJ, Jones KM, Kwon Y, Gingrich JR, Aronson WJ, Nsouli I, Iyer P, Cartagena R, Snider G, Roehrborn C, Fox S. The Prostate cancer Intervention Versus Observation Trial:VA/NCI/AHRQ Cooperative Studies Program #407 (PIVOT): design and baseline results of a randomized controlled trial comparing radical prostatectomy to watchful waiting for men with clinically localized prostate cancer. Contemp Clin Trials. 2009;30(1):81-7.

[52] Thompson RH, Slezak JM, Webster WS, Lieber MM. Radical prostatectomy for octogenarians: how old is too old? Urology. 2006 Nov;68(5):1042-5. Epub 2006 Nov 7.

[53] Pienta K, Esper PS, Risk Factors for Prostate Cancer Ann Int Med 1993; 118(10):793-803

[54] Johansson JE, Holmberg L, Johansson S, Bergström R, Adami HO. Fifteen-year survival in prostate cancer. A prospective, population-based study in Sweden. JAMA. 1997;277(6):467-71.

[55] Sandblom G, Dufmats M, Varenhorst E. Long-term survival in a Swedish population-based cohort of men with prostate cancer. Urology 2000;56(3):442-7

[56] Iversen P, Madsen PO, Corle DK. Radical prostatectomy versus expectant treatment for early carcinoma of the prostate. Twenty-three year follow-up of a prospective randomized study. Scan J Urol Nephrol Suppl 1995;172:65-72.

[57] Chodak GW, Thisted RA, Gerber GS, Johansson JE, Adolfsson J, Jones GW, Chisholm GD, Moskovitz B, Livne PM, Warner J. Results of conservative management of clinically localized prostate cancer. N Engl J Med. 1994;330(4):242-8

[58] Bill-Axelson A, Holmberg L, Filen F, et al. Radical prostatectomy versus watchful waiting in localized prostate cancer: The Scandinavian Prostate Cancer Group-4 randomized trial. J Natl Cancer Inst 2008;100:1144-54.

[59] McLaren DB, Watchful waiting or watchful progression? Prostate specific antigen doubling times and clinical behavior in patients with early untreated prostate carcinoma. Cancer. 1998;82:342-348

[60] Stattin P, Holmberg E, Bratt O, Adolfsson J, Johansson JE, Hugosson J; National Prostate Cancer Register. Surveillance and deferred treatment for localized prostate cancer. Population based study in the National Prostate Cancer Register of Sweden. J Urol. 2008;180(6):2423-9

[61] Makarov MV, Partin AW. Conflicting insights into the role of watchful waiting in the management of adenocarcinoma of the prostate Rev Urol. 2006;8(4):232-234

[62] Albertsen PC, Hanley JA, Penson DF, Fine J. Ten year outcomes following treatment for clinically localized prostate cancer: a population based study. Program and abstracts of the American Urological Association 2006 Annual Meeting; May 20 25, 2006; Atlanta, Georgia. Abstract 652.

[63] Adolfsson J, Garmo H, Varenhorst E, Ahlgren G, Ahlstrand C, Andrén O, Bill-Axelson A, Bratt O, Damber JE, Hellström K, Hellström M, Holmberg E, Holmberg L, Hugosson J, Johansson JE, Petterson B, Törnblom M, Widmark A, Stattin P. Clinical characteristics and primary treatment of prostate cancer in Sweden between 1996 and 2005. Scand J Urol Nephrol. 2007;41(6):456-77.

[64] Wong YN, Mitra N, Hudes G, Localio R, Schwartz JS, Wan F, Montagnet C, Armstrong K. Survival associated with treatment vs observation of localized prostate cancer in elderly men. JAMA. 2006; 296(22):2683-93.

[65] Soloway MS, Soloway CT, Williams S, Ayyathurai R, Kava B, Manoharan M. Active surveillance; a reasonable management alternative for patients with prostate cancer: the Miami experience. BJU Int. 2008;101(2):165-9.

[66] Epstein JI, Chan DW, Sokoll LJ, Walsh PC, Cox JL, Rittenhouse H, Wolfert R, Carter HB. Nonpalpable stage T1c prostate cancer: prediction of insignificant disease using free/ total prostate specific antigen levels and needle biopsy findings. J Urol 1998;160: 2407-2411

[67] Thaxton CS, Loeb S, Roehl KA, Kan D, Catalona WJ. Treatment Outcomes of Radical Prostatectomy in Potential Candidates for 3 Published Active Surveillance Protocols. Urology. 2010;75(2):414-8.

[68] Klotz L. Active surveillance with selective delayed intervention: using natural history
     to guide treatment in good risk prostate cancer. J Urol. 2004 Nov;172(5 Pt 2):S48-
     50.
[69] Berglund A, Garmo H, Tishelman C, Holmberg L, Stattin P, Lambe M. Comorbidity,
     treatment and mortality: a population based cohort study of prostate cancer in
     PCBaSe Sweden. Urol. 2011;185(3):833-9
[70] Droz JP, Balducci L, Bolla M, Emberton M, Fitzpatrick JM, Joniau S, Kattan MW,
     Monfardini S, Moul JW, Naeim A, van Poppel H, Saad F, Sternberg CN.
     Background for the proposal of SIOG guidelines for the management of prostate
     cancer in senior adults. Crit Rev Oncol Hematol. 2010 Jan;73(1):68-91.

9

Improving Prostate Cancer Classification: A Round Robin Forward Sequential Selection Approach

Sabrina Bouatmane[1], Ahmed Bouridane[2,3],
Mohamed Ali Roula[4] and Somaya Al-Maadeed[5]

[1]Département d'Electronique, Faculté des Sciences de l'Ingénieur, Université de Jijel, Jijel
[2]Departemt of Computer Science, King Saud University, Riyadh
[3]School of Computing, Engineering and Information Sciences
Northumbria University at Newcastle, Pandon Building
[4]Faculty of Advanced Technology, University of Glamorgan, Pontypridd
[5]Department of Computer Science & Engineering Qatar University, Doha
[1]Algérie
[2]Saudi Arabia
[3,4]UK
[5]Qatar

1. Introduction

Over the last decade prostate cancer has become one of the most common cancer in male population with an estimated 1.37 million people diagnosed and 200,000 annual death rate worldwide (Stewart & Kleihues, 2003). Biopsies are often advised after a Prostate Specific Antigen (PSA) test reveals high levels of PSA in the blood which usually indicate high risks of Prostatic Carcinoma (PCa). The biopsy is needed because high PSA levels can also be caused by other benign conditions like Benign Prostatic Hyperplasia (BPH) (Kronz, Westra & Epstein, 1999)

Biopsy of the prostate, usually stained by Hematoxylin and Eosin (H&E) technique, is the key step for confirming the diagnosis of malignancy and grading treatment. By viewing the microscopic images of biopsy specimens, pathologists can determine the histological grades. In December 1999, a study of more than 6,000 patients by Johns Hopkins researchers found that up to two out of every 100 people who come to larger medical centers for treatment, following a biopsy, are given a diagnosis that is "totally wrong". The results suggested that second opinion pathology examinations not only prevent errors, but also save lives and money. Human assessment is time consuming and very subjective due to inter- and intra-observer variations. At present, most diagnosis of cancer is still done by visual examination of radiological images, microscopy of biopsy specimens, direct observation and so on. These views are typically interpreted in a qualitative manner by clinicians trained to classify abnormal features such as structural irregularities. A more quantitative and reproducible approach for analyzing images is highly desired. Therefore, how to develop a more objective computer-aided technique to automatically and correctly classify prostatic carcinoma is the goal of this research study. The aim here is to use automatic classifiers as a diagnosis aid along with human expertise by applying image processing and computer vision techniques to perform quantitative measurements of relevant features that can discriminate between different types of tissues that occur in biopsies. In the case of the prostate gland, four major classes of tissues have to be recognized and labeled by the pathologist (Figure 1 shows some samples of each class):

1. *stroma*: STR (normal muscular tissue);
2. *benign prostatic hyperplasia*: BPH (a benign condition);
3. *prostatic intraepithelial neoplasia*: PIN (a precursor state for cancer);
4. *prostatic carcinoma*: PCa (abnormal tissue development corresponding to cancer).

Numerous investigations have been carried out using different approaches such as morphology, texture analysis, and others for the classification of prostatic samples (Bartels et al., 1998; Clark et al., 1987). The Gleason grading system (Gleason & Tannenbaum, 1977) is a well known method. In this grading system, the prostate cancer can be classified into five tumor grades represented by a number ranging from 1 to 5 with five being the worst grade possible (O'Dowd et al., 2001). Tabech et al. proposed (Tabesh et al., 2005) an automatic two-stage system for prostate cancer diagnosis with the Gleason grading. The color, morphometric and texture features are extracted from prostate tissue images in their system. Then, linear and quadratic Gaussian classifiers were used to classify images into tumor/non tumor classes and further categorized into low/high grades for cancer images. Huang et al. proposed (Huang & Lee, 2009) two feature methods based on fractal dimension to analyze the variations of intensity and texture complexity in the regions of interest. Each image can be classified into an appropriate grade by using Bayesian, KNN, and support vector machine (SVM) classifiers, respectively. Leave on out and k fold cross-validation procedures were used to estimate the correct classification rates.

However, all these studies have been performed using a color space that is limited either to gray-level images, or to the standard RGB channels. In both cases, the color sampling process results in a loss of a considerable amount of spectral information, which may be extremely valuable in the classification process. High throughput liquid crystal tunable filters (LCTF) have recently been used in pathology, enabling a complete high resolution optical spectrum to be generated at every pixel of a microscope image. Studies suggest that multispectral images can capture relevant data not present in conventional RGB images. In (Liu et al., 2002) the authors used a large set of multispectral texture features for the detection of cervical cancer. In (Barshack et al., 1999), spectral morphometric characteristics were used on specimen of breast carcinoma cells stained with haematoxylin and eosin (H&E). Their analysis showed a correlation between specific patterns of spectra and different groups of breast carcinoma cells. Larsh et al. (Larsh et al., 2002) suggested that multispectral imaging can improve the analysis of pathological scenes by capturing patterns that are transparent both to the human eye and the standard RGB imaging.

In (Boucheron et al., 2007) Boucheron et al a comparison is performed between multispectral and RGB data for nuclei classification of breast tissue. Using SVM classifiers, the authors have concluded that multispectral bands do not contain much more discriminatory spectral information than the RGB bands for nuclei classification. However, the research was concerned with the classification of single pixels and it was limited to the classification of nuclei of histological breast images. Masood & Rajpoot (Masood & Rajpoot, 2008) present a study based on the comparison of two approaches: 3D spectral/spatial analysis and 2D spatial analysis. They have compared the results using a textural analysis on single hyperspectral band against 3D spectral spatial analysis of histological colon images. However, the classification features were not extracted from multispectral data but rather from segmented 2D images obtained from multispectral data. Roula et al have described a novel approach, in which additional spectral data is used for the classification of prostate needle biopsies (Roula, 2002, 2003) which reduced overall error rate from 11.6% to 5.1%.

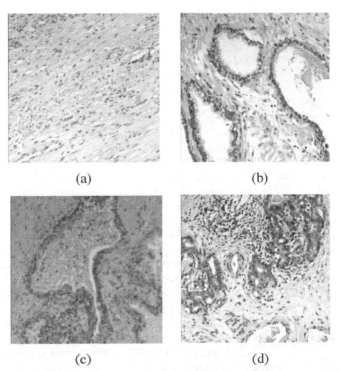

(a)   (b)

(c)   (d)

Fig. 1. Images showing representative samples of the four classes. (a) Stroma. (b) BPH. (c) PIN. (d) PCa.

The major problem arising in using multispectral data is high-dimensional feature vector size (> 100). The number of training samples used to design the classifier is small relative to the number of features. For such a high dimensionality problem, pattern recognition techniques suffer from the well-known curse-of-dimensionality (Jain et al., 2000): keeping the number of training samples limited and increasing the number of features will eventually result in badly performing classifiers. One way to overcome this problem is to reduce the dimensionality of the feature space. While a precise relationship between the number of training samples and the number of features is hard to establish, a combination of theoretical and empirical studies has suggested the following rule of thumb regarding the ratio of the sample size to dimensionality: the number of training samples per class should be greater than or equal to five times the features used (Dash & Liu, 1997). For example, if we have a feature vector of dimension 20, then we need at least 100 training samples per class to design a satisfactory classifier.

Another way to reduce the dimensionality of the feature space is by using feature selection methods. The term feature selection refers to the selection of the best subset of the input feature set. These methods used in the design of pattern classifiers have three goals: (1) to reduce the cost of extracting the features, (2) to improve the classification accuracy, and (3) to improve the reliability of the estimation of the performance, since a reduced feature set requires less training samples in the training procedure of a pattern classifier (Jain et al., 2000). Feature selection produces savings in the measuring features (since some of the features are discarded) and the selected features retain their original physical interpretation.

In previous papers (Bouatmane et al., 2007), we addressed the high input dimensionality problem by selecting the best-subset of sequential forward selection SFS followed by a classification using a nearest neighbour classifier (1NN) technique. Although, this approach produced results superior to previously reported methods (Roula, 2002,2003) , the classification accuracy can be further improved by decomposing this multiclass problem into a number of simpler two-class problems. In this case, each subproblem can be regarded separately and solved using a suitable binary classifier. The outputs of this collection of classifiers can then be combined to produce the overall result for the original multiclass problem. In this paper, we propose a Round-Robin (RR) classification algorithm using a sequential forward selection/nearest neighbor (SFS/1NN) classifier to improve the classification accuracy. Round Robin classification is a technique which is suitable for use in multiclass problems. The technique consists of dividing the multiclass problem into an appropriate number of simpler binary classification problems (Furnkranz, 2002). Each binary classifier is implemented as an SFS/1NN classifier, and the final outcome is computed using majority voting technique. A key characteristic of this approach is that, in a binary class, the classifier attempts to find the features that only distinguish that particular class. Thus, different features are selected for each binary classifier, resulting in an overall increase in the classification accuracy. In contrast, in a multiclass problem, the classifier tries to find those features that distinguish all classes at once.

The remainder of this chapter is organized as follows: Sect. 2 gives a description of the dataset used including texture and structural features. Section 3 is concerned with feature selection problem and describes the RR approach followed by the probability estimate for the classifier outputs and error estimation. Sect. 4 describes the image acquisition and dataset. Sect. 5 gives the results obtained and their analysis and discussion including a performance comparative study. Sect. 6 analyses the features selected and sect. 7 gives ROC curves and finally sect. 8 gives a summary of the chapter.

2. Images features

Over the last years, the most prolific and promising works in the area of cancer classification have been in the area of texture analysis of the nucleus (Tabesh et al., 2005; Liu et al., 20). This is not surprising since pre-cancerous abnormalities are manifested in visual and subvisual changes in cell characteristics. In fact, it is generally believed that the initial signs of cell neoplasia appear in the nucleus. Because nuclear chromatin and its spatial arrangement can be viewed as a type of texture and whether tissue samples are examined at low, medium or high magnification, texture is a key element in the differentiation between normal and malignant tissue patterns.

However, texture features are not sufficient to classify all the groups. The complex structures present in BPH, PIN and also PCa need a higher level description. Thus, structural features, based on segmentation, have been computed for different spectral bands and consolidated in a large feature vector. The features used are described in the following subsections.

2.1 Texture feature

To identify prostatic patterns, texture features are needed as a discriminative measurement for the samples. Haralick (Haralick, 1979) assumed that texture information is sufficiently identified by a matrix indexed by grey levels and where the elements represent the frequency of having two defined grey levels separated by a defined distance in a defined direction. This matrix is called grey level co-occurrence matrix (GLCM):

$$co(i, j, d, \theta) = \alpha \tag{1}$$

The above equation means that there are α pairs of pixels having i and j respectively, as grey levels and separated by the cylindrical co-ordinate $[d, \theta]$. The values of d, for which the GLCM is computed, depend on the nature of the texture. Small d values are suitable for fine textures, whereas larger distances are needed to measure coarse textures.

For an image of 256 grey levels (Ng=256), there would be 65536 feature elements to use as a measure for the texture. Therefore, the direct use of the co-occurrence matrix is computationally intensive and as such is not practical. Instead, the texture features are represented by deriving some more meaningful measurements. A set of features was proposed by Haralick to characterise the homogeneity, the coarseness, the periodicity and the linearity of textures. These features are defined as follows:

Angular Second Moment

$$ASM = \sum_{i=1}^{N_g} \sum_{j=1}^{N_g} P(i, j)^2 \tag{2}$$

Contrast or difference moment

$$CON = \sum_{i=1}^{N_g} \sum_{j=1}^{N_g} (i - j)^2 P(i, j) \tag{3}$$

Dissimilarity

$$DIS = \sum_{i=1}^{N_g} \sum_{j=1}^{N_g} |i - j| P(i, j) \tag{4}$$

Correlation

$$COR = \sum_{i=1}^{N_g} \sum_{j=1}^{N_g} \left[(i - \mu_x)(j - \mu_y) P(i, j)^2 \right] / (\sigma_x \sigma_y) \tag{5}$$

Where $\mu_x, \mu_y, \sigma_x, \sigma_y$ are the means and the variances of the row sums and column sums of the co-occurrence matrix respectively.

Entropy or randomness

$$ENT = -\sum_{i=1}^{N_g} \sum_{j=1}^{N_g} P(i, j) \log P(i, j) \tag{6}$$

Inverse difference Moment:

$$IDM = -\sum_{i=1}^{N_g} \sum_{j=1}^{N_g} \frac{P(i, j)}{(1 + (i - j)^2)} \tag{7}$$

2.2 Structural features

The use of texture features alone is not sufficient to capture the complexity of the patterns in prostatic neoplasia. Although, the classification of stroma is relatively simple because of its homogenous nature at low resolution, BPH and PCa present more complex structures, as both can contain glandular areas and nuclei clusters as well. The glandular areas are smaller in regions exhibiting PCa while the nuclear clusters are much larger. The PIN pattern is an intermediate state between the BPH and PCa. It appears that accurate classification requires the quantification of these differences. Segmenting the glandular and the nuclear areas can achieve this quantification, as the glandular areas are lighter compared to the surrounding tissue, while the nuclear clusters are darker (Larsh et al., 2002; Roula et al., 2002).

Figure 2 summarises the segmentation scheme. From the segmented images 1 and 2, two features, f1 and f2 can be computed

$$f_1 = N/_{W^2} \tag{8}$$

$$f_2 = G/_{W^2} \tag{9}$$

Where G and N are the number of pixels segmented as glandular area and classified as nuclear area, respectively. W is the size of the analysis window. These two features allow the quantification of how much nuclear clusters and glandular areas are present in the samples.

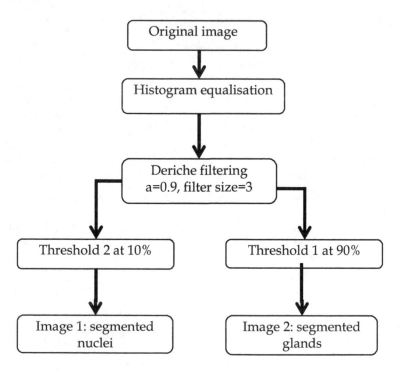

Fig. 2. Segmentation of nuclei and glandular areas

3. Classification of prostate cancer using round robin approach

3.1 Feature selection problem

As discussed in Section 1, the major problem arising from multispectral data is related to the feature vector size. Typically, with 16 bands and 8 features in each band, the feature vector size is 128. For such a high dimensionality problem, pattern recognition techniques suffer from the well-known curse-of-dimensionality problem: keeping the number of training samples limited and increasing the number of features will eventually result in badly performing classifiers (Jain et al., 2000; Jimenez, & Landgrebe, 1998).

PCA (a well-known unsupervised feature extraction method) has been used by Roula et al. on the large resulting feature vectors to reduce its dimensionality to a manageable size. In their work, Roula et al. used PCA and a linear discrimination function on significant PCA components for the classification.

Another technique to reduce the dimensionality of the feature space is by using feature selection methods. The term feature selection refers to the selection of the best subset of the input feature set. This results in a feature selection producing a smaller set of features (since some of the features are discarded) with the selected features retaining their original physical interpretation. This feature selection problem can be viewed as a multiobjective optimization problem since it involves minimizing the feature subset while maximizing classification accuracy.

Mathematically, the feature selection problem can be formulated as follows: Suppose Y is an original feature vector with cardinality n, $X \subseteq Y$, $J(X)$ is the selection criterion function for the new feature vector X. The goal is to optimize $J(X)$. The choice of an algorithm for selecting the features from an initial set depends on n. The feature selection problem is said to be of small scale, medium scale, or large scale accordingly as n belongs to the intervals [0,19], [20,49], or [50,+∞], respectively (Duda et al., 2001; Kudo & Sklansky, 2000).

Generally, feature selection algorithms have two components: a selection algorithm that generates proposed subsets of features and attempts to find an optimal subset; and an evaluation algorithm which determines how 'good' a proposed feature subset is, by returning some measure of goodness to the selection algorithm. However, without a suitable stopping criterion the feature selection process may run exhaustively or forever through the space of subsets. Stopping criteria can be: (i) whether addition (or deletion) of any feature does not produce a better subset; and (ii) whether an optimal subset according to some evaluation function is obtained. Ideally, a feature selection method searchs through the subsets of features, and tries to find the best one among all the competing candidate subsets according to some evaluation function. However, this procedure is exhaustive as it tries to find only the best one. It may be too costly and practically prohibitive, even for a medium-sized feature set size. Other methods based on heuristic or random search methods; attempt to reduce computational complexity by compromising performance (Davies & Russell, 1994).

In (Dash & Liu, 1997) different feature selection methods are categorized into two broad groups (i.e., filter and wrapper) depending on the type of classification algorithm used for the selection of the subset. For example, the filter methods do not require a feedback from the classifier and estimate the classification performance by some indirect assessments, such as distance measures which reflect how well the classes separate from each other. On the other hand, the wrapper methods are classifier-dependent. Based on the classification accuracy, the methods evaluate the "goodness" of the selected feature subset directly, which should intuitively lead to a better performance. Currently, many experimental results reported so far use the wrapper methods.

In this work, an SFS algorithm, which is simple and empirically successful, is proposed for feature selection. It starts with an empty subset of features and performs a hill-climbing deterministic search. At each iteration, a feature not yet selected is individually incorporated in the subset to calculate a criterion. Then the feature which yields the best criterion value is included in the new subset. This iteration will not be stopped until no improvement of the criterion value is achieved. SFS is used as a wrapper approach, therefore the criterion employed to carry out the search is based on error estimation by the selected features using 1NN classifier. In addition, we propose another scheme in which the multiclass problem is addressed using Round Robin (RR) classification approach where the classification problem is decomposed into a number of binary classes. The key point is that it is then possible to design simpler and more efficient binary classifiers as will be demonstrated in the next Section.

3.2 Round robin method

The RR or pairwise class binarization transforms a c-class problem into $c(c - 1)/2$ two-class problems i, j with one for each set of classes i, j ($i = 1, \ldots, c - 1, j = i + 1, \ldots, c$). A binary classifier for problem i, j is trained with examples of classes i and j, whereas examples of classes $k \neq i, j$ are ignored for this problem (Furnkranz, 2002). Figure 3 illustrates a multiclass (four-class) learning problem where one classifier (SFS/1NN classifier in this study) separates all classes. Figure 4 shows Round Robin learning with $c(c - 1)/2$ classifiers. For a four-class problem, the Round Robin trains six classifiers, one for each pair of classes. Each class is trained using a feature selection algorithm based on the SFS/1NN classifier.

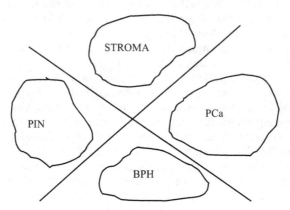

Fig. 3. Multiclass learning

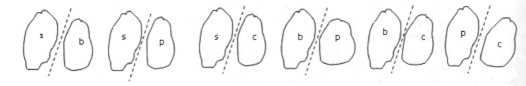

Fig. 4. Round Robin learning. p: PIN. c: PCa. b: BPH. s: STR.

The objects are then classified by applying a combination rule on the set of decisions. One strategy is to use voting where the object is labeled to the class with the highest number of votes. When classifying an unknown new sample, each classifier (1NN in this case) determines to which of its two classes the sample is more likely to belong. In this case, we are faced with the possibility of ties. To avoid these ties, a probability estimate value for each classification has to be used.

In pattern recognition, 1NN is one of the simplest and most widely used algorithms. Given a query sample x, a 1NN algorithm determines the closest neighbor of x in the training nodes using some distance metric (e.g. Euclidean distance in our study) and predicts the class label of the nearest node. In contrast to other statistical classifiers, 1NN needs no model to fit. This property simplifies the structure of the training process by avoiding model training, thus training with a 1NN classifier only requires selecting the appropriate features.

For the sake of probability estimates, probabilistic outputs of the classifier were required rather than label prediction. For 1NN, objects are assigned to the class of the nearest object in the training set. Posterior probabilities are estimated by comparing the nearest neighbor distances for all classes (Duin & Tax, 1998). A RR ensemble converts a c-class problem into a series of two-class problems by creating one classifier for each pair of classes. New items are classified by submitting them to the $c(c-1)/2$ binary predictors. The final prediction is achieved by a majority voting. The probability of a query q belonging to a class c can be calculated as follows (Grimaldi et al., 2003) (equation 10):

$$p(c|q) = \frac{\sum_{m \in M} P_m(c|q) \cdot 1_{(m_c = c)}}{\sum_{m \in M} P_m(c|q)} \tag{10}$$

where M is the set of ensemble members, mc is the class predicted by m and $P_m(c|q)$ is the posterior probability given by ensemble predictor m (the binary classifiers). If m does not involve class c, then $P_m(c|q) = 0$. The probability estimates of the binary classifiers will be combined using the maximum rule; therefore the instances are assigned to the class with the maximum output given by equation (10). Clearly, RR is a problem decomposition technique. However, there are some aggregation benefits as each class is focused on by c-1 classifiers.

3.3 Error estimation

Given a small set of samples, appropriate strategies for learning and testing become very critical to avoid over-fitting. Leave-one-out (LOO) and k-fold cross-validation are two popular error estimation procedures to reduce bias in machine learning and testing problems especially with small sample size (sss) (Jain et al., 2000). The procedure of LOO method is to take one out of n observations and use the remaining n-1 observations as the training set for deriving the parameters of the classifier. The classifier is then used to classify the removed observation. This process is repeated for all n observations in order to obtain the estimation of the classification accuracy. In the case of k-fold cross-validation method, the entire sample set is randomly partitioned into k disjoint subsets of equal size, where n is the total number of samples in the entire set. Then, k -1 subsets are used to train the classifier and the remaining subset is used to test for accuracy estimation. This process is repeated for all distinct choices of k subsets and the average of correct classification rates is calculated. Notice that k -fold cross-validation is reduced to LOO if k=n.

When referring to the performance of a classification model, we are interested in the model's ability to correctly predict or separate the classes. When looking at the errors made by a classification model, the confusion matrix used in this paper gives the full picture. The confusion matrix shows how accurate the predictions are made by the model. The rows correspond to the known class of the data, i.e. the labels in the data while the columns correspond to the predictions made by the model. The value of each of element in the matrix is the number of predictions made with the class corresponding to the column, for example, with the correct value as represented by the row. Thus, the diagonal elements show the number of correct classifications made for each class, and the off-diagonal elements show the errors made.

Accuracy is the overall correctness of the model and is calculated as the sum of the correct classifications divided by the total number of classifications. Precision is a measure of the accuracy provided that a specific class has been predicted. It is defined by:

$$Precision = \frac{tp}{tp + fp} \tag{11}$$

where tp and fp are the numbers of true positive and false positive predictions for the considered class. Recall is a measure of the ability of a prediction model to select instances of a certain class from a data set. It is also commonly called sensitivity, and corresponds to the true positive rate and can be written as:

$$Recall = Sensitivity = \frac{tp}{tp + fn} \tag{12}$$

where tp and fn are the numbers of true positive and false negative predictions for the considered class. tp+ fn is the total number of test examples of the considered class.

4. Sample preparation, image acquisition and datasets description

Entire tissue samples were taken from prostate glands. Sections 5-µm thick were extracted and stained using the widely used H&E stains. These samples were routinely assessed by two experienced pathologists and graded histologically as showing STR, BPH, PIN, and PCa. From these samples, whole subimage sections were captured using a classical microscope and CCD camera. An LCTF (VARISPECTM) was inserted in the optical path between the light source and a CCD camera. The LCTF has a bandwidth accuracy of 5 nm. The wavelength is controllable through the visible spectrum (from 400 to 720 nm). This allowed for the capture of multispectral images of the tissue samples by using different spectral frequencies. Figure 5 shows a prostatic tissue sample viewed at different magnification.

In order to offset any bias due to the different range of values for the original features, the input feature values are normalized over the range [1,11] using equation (13) (Raymer et al., 2000). Normalizing the data is important to ensure that the distance measure allocates equal weight to each variable. Without normalization, the variable with the largest scale will dominate the measure:

$$x'_{i,j} = \left(\frac{x_{i,j} - \min_{k=1...n} x(k,j)}{\max_{k=1...n} x(k,j) - \min_{k=1...n} x(k,j)} \times 10 \right) + 1 \tag{13}$$

where x^i_j is the jth feature of the ith pattern, $x^t_{i,j}$ is the corresponding normalized feature and n is the total number of patterns.

The data were taken from a total of 10 different patients with typically 3-6 biopsies per patient (from different areas in the prostate) and 8-12 images were taken from each samples (from different areas in the image). The dataset consists of textured multispectral images taken at 16 spectral channels (from 500 to 650 nm) (Roula et al., 2002). Five hundred and ninety-two different samples (multispectral images) of size 128 × 128 have been used to carry out the analysis. The samples are examined at low power (40 x objective magnifications) by the two highly experienced independent pathologists and labelled into four classes: 165 cases of Stroma, 106 cases of BPH, 144 cases of PIN, and 177 cases of PCa.

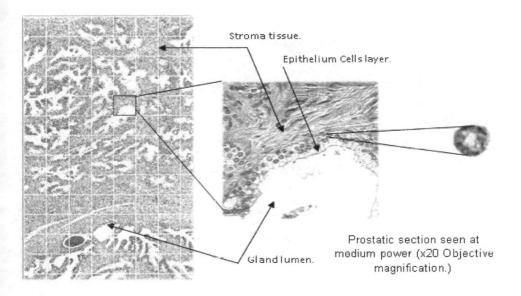

Stroma tissue.

Epithelium Cells layer.

Prostatic section seen at medium power (x20 Objective magnification.)

Gland lumen.

Fig. 5. Prostatic tissue sample viewed at low and medium magnifications

5. Experiments and discussion

The assessment of the classification performance has been made using three procedures: 4-fold cross-validation, 10 cross-validation and leave-one-out (LOO) which was applied patient-wise. To obtain a k-fold cross-validation estimate of the classification performance, the dataset was randomly split into k sets of a roughly equal size. Splitting was carried out such that the proportion of samples per class was roughly equal across the sets. Each run of the k-fold cross-validation algorithm consisted of a classifier design on k-1 dataset subsets (training) while testing was performed on the remaining subset. The optimal feature subset for each cross-validation run was determined as the subset with the highest LOO accuracy estimate on the corresponding training set.

The first aim was to determine the optimum number of features to obtain the best achievable classification performance. Therefore, the feature selection algorithm SFS described in section 3 with a 1NN classifier was used. Figure 6 shows the results obtained using LOO error estimation. The curve representing the results from the feature selection shows a strong increase in performance for small subsets followed by slight increase up to medium sized subsets. Large subsets cause a drop in the recognition rate.

For k-fold cross-validation the results show that using SFS with different training sets does not yield identical feature subsets. This is illustrated by the diagram in Figure 7 which shows the fraction of how often a feature was selected divided by the total number of simulations using 4 cross-validation method. One can see that the selected features originate from different spectral bands.

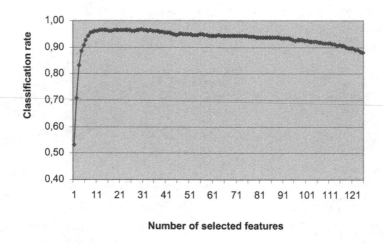

Number of selected features

Fig. 6. Recognition rate of SFS algorithm

The accuracies of the selected features subsets are given in Table 1. The combination of the binary classifiers' results generated by proposed Round Robin algorithm is performed using two methods: the voting rule using the resulted classes (Tahir & Bouridane, 2006) and the maximum probability obtained using equation (10). For all the cross validation estimations, the RR SFS/1NN with the maximum probability gives the best classification accuracy. As shown in Table 1, RRSFS algorithm using LOO error estimation achieves the lowest error rate. The overall classification error has been reduced from 3.37% to 0.17%. To gain an insight into the classification of different classes of prostate cancer, the confusion matrix of the multiclass SFS/1NN and the proposed Round Robin learning using SFS/1NN are also given. Table 2 depicts the results using the LOO error estimation where Table 3 gives the corresponding results using 4 cross-validations. Note that in all the cases, BPH and PIN classes present the highest error rate in terms of classification but the use of Round Robin algorithm reduces significantly the error rate in these classes.

Bagging is a general method of combining classifiers that can be applied to any base method. It is a relatively simple idea: n datasets are created by sampling the patterns with replacement from the original training set. Each of the n datasets has the same number of patterns as the original training set. A classifier is then trained on each dataset by combining the outputs using simple voting. Bagging has obtained impressive error reductions with decision trees such as CART (Breiman, 1996) and C4.5 (Freund & Schapire, 1996; Quinlan, 1996) on a wide range of datasets.

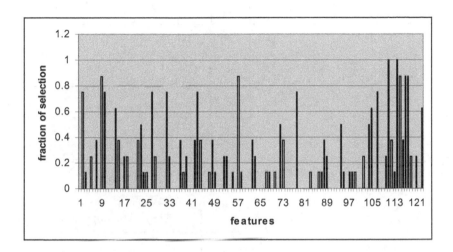

Fig. 7. Subsets yielded by application of the SFS from 4 cross-validations

	4 cross-validation error estimation %	10 cross validation error estimation %	Leave-one-out error estimation %
1NN classifier	13.34	12.18	12
SFS/1NN classifier	10.22	7.41	3.37
Round robin SFS/1NN (voting rule)	10.98	9.62	2.87
Round robin SFS/1NN (maximum probability rule)	8.91	7.26	0.17

Table 1. Comparison of error classification rate

In Boosting, the classifiers in the ensemble are trained serially, with the weights on the training instances set adaptively according to the performance of the previous classifiers. If the classifier does not directly support weighted instances, this can be simulated by sampling from the training set with a probability proportional to an instance weight. The main idea is that the classification algorithm should concentrate on the difficult instances.

SFS/1NN multiclass learning						Round Robin SFS/1NN learning				
Classified as:	BPH	PCa	PIN	Stroma	Error (%)	BPH	PCa	PIN	Stroma	Error (%)
BPH	101	0	0	5	4.71	106	0	0	0	0
PCa	1	174	2	0	1.69	0	177	0	0	0
PIN	0	2	137	5	4.86	0	0	143	1	0.69
Stroma	5	0	0	160	3.03	0	0	0	165	0
overall					3.37					0.17

Table 2. Classification Error by multiclass and round robin learning using SFS/1NN and loo error estimation

Round Robin SFS/1NN learning						SFS/1NN multiclass learning				
Classified as:	BPH	PCa	PIN	Stroma	Error (%)	BPH	PCa	PIN	Stroma	Error (%)
BPH	96	0	0	10	9.43	93	3	2	8	12.26
PCa	1	164	8	4	7.43	2	163	11	1	7.90
PIN	0	13	129	2	10.41	3	8	122	11	15.27
Stroma	8	1	5	151	8.48	5	1	3	156	5.45
overall					8.91					10.22

Table 3. Classification error by multiclass and round robin learning using SFS/1NN and 4cross-validation

C4.5			Nearest neighbor			
C4.5	Bagging	Boosting	NN	Bagging	Boosting	RR-SFS
91.6	93.2	95.4	88.0	89.2	88.1	99.83

Table 4. Classification accuracy (%) using various ensemble techniques

Table 4 shows the comparison between the RR-SFS/1NN versus Bagging and AdaBoost. Decision Tree (C4.5) (Quinlan, 1993) and NN classifiers are used as base classifiers for bagging and boosting.

Unfortunately, bagging and boosting are unable to improve the classification accuracy when an NN classifier is used as a base classifier (Yongguang et al., 2004). This fact is clearly seen from Table 6 where the classification accuracy is degraded while using AdaBoost, and only minor improvements are achieved when using bagging. However, the classification accuracy is improved by using bagging and boosting when C4.5 is used as base classifier. Furthermore, it is clear from the table that the proposed Round Robin ensemble technique using TS/1NN has outperformed both bagging and boosting ensemble-design techniques.

A key characteristic of the proposed Round Robin approach is that different features are captured and used for each binary classifier in the four-class problem, thus producing an overall increase in the classification accuracy. In contrast, in a multiclass problem, the classifier tries to find those features that distinguish all four-classes at once. Furthermore, the inherent curse-of-dimensionality problem, which arises in a multispectral data, is also resolved by the RR SFS/1NN classifiers since each classifier is trained to compute and use only those features that distinguish its own binary classes.

Table 5 shows the number of features used by the ensemble of binary classifiers. Different numbers of features have been used by the various binary classifiers producing an overall increase in the classification accuracy. Fc represents those features that are common in two or more different binary classifiers. The total number of features in the proposed Round Robin technique is comparable with the multiclass SFS/1NN with lower error rate, but the number of features used by each binary classifier is smaller than that used in other methods. Consequently, multispectral data is better utilized by using a Round Robin technique since the use of more features means more information is captured and used in the classification process. Furthermore, simple binary classes are also useful for analyzing features and are extremely helpful for pathologists in distinguishing various patterns such as BPH, PIN, STR, and PCa.

	Feature selection method		Features used
	SFS/1NN	Multi-class	13
1 2 3 4 5 6	SFS/1NN	Binary-class (stroma-Bph) Binary-class (Stroma-Pin) Binary-class (stroma-PCa) Binary-class (Bph-Pin) Binary-class (Bph-PCa) Binary-class (Pin-PCa)	4 1 4 1 1 4
	SFS/1NN	Round Robin	$\sum_{i=1}^{6} F - F_c = (15 - 3) = 12$

Table 5. Number of Features Used By Different Classifiers

Figure 8 shows the results of Recall and Precision measures for different algorithms including the results of Round Robin tabu search RR TS/1NN (Tahir & Bouridane, 2006). From the graphs presented one can observe that for both Precision and Recall, the values of RR SFS/1NN are very high for different classes of prostate cancer. In addition, one can notice from equations (11) and (12) that the values for FP and FN tend to zero when the Precision and Recall tend to 100%. Thus, the false positives and especially false negatives are almost null with our approach. This clearly demonstrates the efficiency of our proposed RR technique.

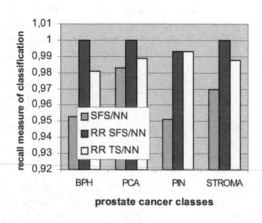

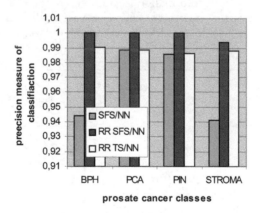

Fig. 8. Precision and recall measures of classification

6. Analysis of the selected features

Very often, it is interesting to know if the difference in the mean values for a given feature between two groups is accidental or due to an inherent difference between the groups regarding a specific feature. For example, the mean of a given image feature can be numerically different for normal and cancer prostate cells. But does this difference reflect a real physical dissimilarity between the two groups or is it due to those specific samples? And in the case where it is a real physical difference, what is the level of confidence when making such statements?

In this work, Student t-test (Montgomery, 1997) was used as a statistical test of significance for mean difference of each class pair for all the selected features. Table 6 and 7 show the selected features for SFS/1NN classifier and RR SFS/1NN method using LOO, respectively. The asterisk (*) in the table shows that this feature exhibits a significant difference in means for all group pairs of cancer (Stroma, BPH, PIN, PCa) with 95 % confidence (p-value<0.05) while (**) shows confidence in difference of means higher than 99% (p-value<0.01). For the round robin method, t-test was run only for the binary classes.

In Table 6, for 9 out of the 13 features selected, the p-value exhibits values lower than 0.05, i.e. yields confidence levels in difference between groups >95%. Three features exhibit a confidence level in the mean difference superior to 99%.

It was observed that dissimilarity, inverse difference moment, entropy and contrast are the texture features selected. They are all measures of homogeneity of grey level texture. This indicates that prostatic tissues display a clear visual difference in terms of texture. Consequently, neighboring pixels were more likely to have larger grey level differences for different grades of malignancy. Note that the features which have not asterisks exhibit significant difference in means, but not for all the pairs of classes.

Rank	Selected features	Spectral band
1	Inverse difference moment *	13
2	structural (f2) *	9
3	Structural (f1)	8
4	Dissimilarity *	3
5	Contrast	7
6	Structural (f1) **	7
7	Structural (f2)	5
8	Dissimilarity	11
9	Contrast *	4
10	Entropy **	8
11	Contrast **	6
12	Inverse difference moment	8
13	Structural (f1) *	11

Table 6. Selected features by SFS/1NN Classifier

Binary classifiers	Selected features	Spectral band
(Stroma-Bph) classifier	Structural (f2)**	11
	Dissimilarity **	15
	Dissimilarity **	13
	Angular second moment **	13
(Stroma-Pin) classifier	Contrast **	15
(Stroma-PCa) classifier	Structural (f2) **	9
	Structural (f1)**	3
	Inverse difference moment **	5
	Dissimilarity **	4
(Bph-Pin) classifier	Structural (f1)**	14
(Bph-PCa) classifier	Structural (f1)**	14
(Pin-PCa) classifier	Inverse difference moment **	10
	Contrast **	2
	Dissimilarity **	4
	Structural (f2)**	9

Table 7. Selected features By RR-SFS/1NN Classifier

For the RR SFS/1NN method, all the features presented in Table 7 exhibit a confidence level in mean difference superior to 99% for all the binary classes. This can be explained by the fact that the RRSFS/1NN method selects the features that distinguish only that class. In contrast, in multiclass SFS/1NN, the classifier tries to find those features that distinguish all classes at once.

The presence of structural features can be observed, especially to discriminate BPH and PCa from the other classes. This is because BPH is first characterised by a conspicuous glandular presence. For the PCa, this is due to the predominance of nuclei clusters and the total absence of glands, which makes it easy to detect using the structural features. We note also that the texture features selected are all measures of homogeneity. Contrast is selected alone by Stroma-Pin classifier without the structural features since the glands are totally absent from Stroma. PIN, which is an intermediate state between PCa and BPH may or may not contain lumen glands. Correlation is totally absent from the two tables thus indicating that correlation is a poor discriminant feature. It can be concluded that the joint use of texture and structural features is an efficient method to classify all groups together.

Finally, it is important to see the impact of the multispectral dimension on the classification; the features selected in both methods are from different bands. This shows that the satisfactory results obtained previously are not only due to the adequate choice of features but to the contribution of the multispectral information which characterizes the different classes.

7. ROC curve

ROC curve (receiving operating characteristic) analysis has been widely used as a method for medical decisions making. It is a plot of false positive rate (X-axis) versus true positive rate (Y-axis) of a binary classifier. ROC is commonly used for visualizing and selecting classifiers based on their performance. The true positive rate (TPR) is defined as the ratio of the number of correctly classified positive cases to the total number of positive cases. The false positive rate (FPR) is defined as the ratio of incorrectly classified negative cases to the total number of negative cases (Fawcett, 2003).

ROC curves help researchers focus on classification rules with low false positive rates, which are most important for early detection of cancer.

The diagonal line y = x corresponds to a classifier which predicts a class membership by randomly guessing it. Hence, all useful classifiers must have ROC curves above this line.

We assume that one of the classes is the class of interest and the objects labeled in this class will be called 'positive'. This achieved by considering the BPH as the negative diagnosis while Pca and PIN form the positive diagnosis outcome.

The classifier gives a continuous valued output given by equation (10) which is cut at a certain threshold. All objects for which the classifier output exceeds the threshold are labeled as positive while the remaining results are labeled as negative. By varying the threshold value from the minimum to the maximum value of the classifier output, one can construct a ROC curve. Figure 9 illustrates the ROC curves obtained with the two methods RRSFS/1NN and SFS/1NN using 4 cross-validation and an independent test set. The test set is obtained by splitting the dataset onto two equal sets, training set and test set. For cross-validation, given the test sets generated from 4 cross-validation, we can simply merge the instances together by their assigned scores into one large test set and we then plot the result.

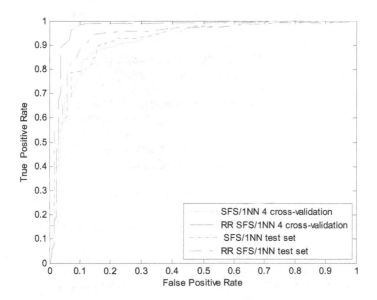

Fig. 9. ROC curves for SFS/1NN and RR-SFS/1NN classifier

The results are comparable or better than those obtained in other recent studies (Taher & Bouridane, 2006); this further demonstrates that our new proposed Round Robin technique results in an improved ability to distinguish cancer prostate tissues from healthy ones. It is clear from the figure that RRSFS/1NN algorithm performs better than simple SFS/1NN with high TPR rate.

8. Conclusion

In this chapter, a Round Robin SFS/1NN algorithm is proposed for the classification of prostate needle biopsies using multispectral imagery. To achieve this, a set of features was computed over a wide range of visible wavelength and the results have indicated a significant increase in the classification accuracy with Round Robin technique with high TPR. A key characteristic of the proposed Round Robin approach is that different features are used for each binary classifier from multispectral images, thus producing an overall increase in the classification accuracy. In contrast, in a multiclass problem, the classifier tries to find only those features that distinguish all classes at once. RR SFS/1NN has also demonstrated the effectiveness of some texture and structural features to make difference between different classes which can be helpful for the pathologist. Finally, the algorithm is generic and can be used for different datasets from other pattern recognition areas.

9. References

Barshack, I.; Kopolovic, J.; Malik, Z. & Rothmann, C. (1999)Spectral morphometric characterization of breast carcinoma cells. *Brit. J. Cancer*, vol. 79, no. 9–10, pp. 1613–1619.

Bartels, P. H et al. (1998). Nuclear chromatin texture in prostatic lesions: IPIN and adenocarcinoma. *Anal. Quant. Cytol. Histol.*, vol. 20, no. 15,pp. 389–396.

Bouatmane, S.; Nekhoul, B.; Bouridane, A. & Tanougast C. (2007). Classification of Prostatic Tissues using Feature Selection Methods. *IFMBE Proceedings*, vol 16, pp 843-846.

Boucheron, L. ;Bi Z.; Harvey, N.; Manjunath, B. & Rimm, D. (2007). Utility of multispectral imaging for nuclear classification of routine clinical histopathology imagery. *BMC Cell Biology*, 8(Suppl. 1):S8.

Breiman, L. (1996). Bagging predictors. *Machine Learning*, vol. 24 , 123-140.

Clark T. D.; Askin, F. B. & Bagnell, C. R (1987). Nuclear roundness factor: A quantitative approach to grading in prostate carcinoma, reliability of needle biopsy tissue, and the effect of tumor stage on usefulness. *Prostate*. vol. 10, no. 3, pp. 199-206.

Dash, M. Liu, H. (1997). Feature Selection for Classification. *Intelligent Data Analysis*, vol. 1, no. 3, pp. 131- 156.

Davies, S. & Russell, S. (1994). NP-completeness of searches for smallest possible feature sets. *Proc. AAAI Fall Symp Relevance*, pp.37–39.

Duda, R. O. Hart, P. E. & Stork, D.G. (2001). *Pattern Classification*. Hoboken, NJ: Wiley-Interscience.

Duin, R.P.W. & Tax, D.M.J. (1998). Classifier conditional posterior probabilities. *Lecture Notes in Computer Science*, vol. 1451, Springer, Berlin, 611-619.

Fawcett, T. (2003). ROC graphs: Notes and practical considerations for researchers. *Tech Report HPL-2003-4, HP Laboratories*.

Freund, Y. & Schapire, R. E. (1996). Experiments with a new boosting algorithm. Machine Learning, Proceedings *of the Thirteenth International Conference*, pp. 325-332.

Furnkranz, J. (2002). Round robin classification. *J. Mach. Learn. Res.*, vol. 2,pp. 721-747.

Gleason, D. F. & Tannenbaum, M. (1977). The veteran's administration cooperative urologic research group: Histologic grading and clinical staging of prostatic carcinoma, in *Urologic Pathology: The Prostate*. Philadephia, PA: Lea Febiger, , pp. 171-198.

Grimaldi, M.; Cunningham, P. & Kokaram, A. (2003). An evaluation of alternative feature selection strategies and ensemble techniques of classifying music. *Workshop in Multimedia Discovery and Mining* at ECML/PKDD.

Haralick, R. M. (1979). Statistical and structural approaches to texture. *Proc. Of the IEEE*, vol. 67, pp.786-804.

Huang, P.W. & Lee, C.H. (2009) automatic classification for pathological prostate images based on fractal analysis, *IEEE transactions on medical imaging*, VOL. 28, NO. 7, pp.1037-1050.

Jain, A. K.; Duin, R. P. W. & Mao, J. *(2000). Statistical pattern recognition: A review. IEEE Trans. Pattern Anal. Mach. Intell.*, vol. 22, no. 1, pp. 4-37.

Jimenez, L. O. & Landgrebe, D. A. (1998). Supervised classification in high dimensional space: Geometrical, statistical, and asymptotical properties of multivariate data. *IEEE Trans. Syst., Man, Cybern. C, Appl. Rev.*, vol. 28, no. 1, pp. 39-54.

Kronz, J. D; Westra, W. H & Epstein, J. I. (1999). Mandatory second opinion Surgical Pathology at a Large Referral Hospital, Cancer, vol. 86, no. 11, pp. 2426-2435.

Kudo, M. & Sklansky, J. (2000). Comparison of algorithms that select features for pattern classifiers. *Pattern Recognit.*, vol. 33, pp. 25-41.

Larsh, P.; Cheriboga, L. Yee, H. & Diem, M. (2002). Infrared spectroscopy of humans cells and tissue: Detection of disease. *Technol. Cancer Res. Treat.*, vol. 1, no. 1, pp. 1-7.

Liu, Y.; Zahoa, T. & Zhang, J. (2002) Learning multispectral texture features for cervical cancer detection. *Proc IEEE Int Symp. Biomed. Imaging*, Washington, DC, pp. 169-172.

Masood, K.& Rajpoot N. (2008). Colon biopsy classification Annals of the BMVA Vol. 2008, No. 4, pp 1-16.

Montgomery, D. (1997). *Design and analysis of experiments*. John Wiley & Son, 4th Ed.

O'Dowd, G. J.; Veltri, R. W.; Miller, M. C. & Strum, S. B.(2001). The Gleason score: A significant biologic manifestation of prostate cancer aggressiveness on biopsy, *Prostate Cancer Res. Inst.: PCR Insights*, vol. 4, no. 1, pp. 1-5.

Quinlan, J. R. (1996). Bagging, Boosting, and C4.5. *Proceedings of the Thirteenth National Conference on Arti_cial Intelligence*, 725-730.

Quinlan, R. (1993). *C4.5: Programs for Machine Learning*. San Mateo, CA: Morgan Kaufmann,.

Raymer, M. L. et al. (2000)Dimensionality reduction using genetic algorithms. IEEE Trans. Evol. Comput., vol. 4, no. 2, pp. 164-171.

Roula, M. A.; Diamond, J.; Bouridane, A.; Miller, P. & Amira, A. (2002). A multispectral computer vision system for automatic grading of prostatic neoplasia. *Proc. IEEE Int. Symp. Biomed. Imaging* , pp. 193-196.

Roula, M.; A. Bouridane, A. & Miller, P. (2003) A quadratic classifier based on multispectral texture features for prostate cancer diagnosis. *Proc. 7th Int. Symp. Signal Process. Appl.*, Paris, France, pp. 37-40.

Stewart, B. W. & Kleihues, P. (2003). World Cancer Report World Health Organization, *International Agency for Research on Cancer*.

Tabesh, A.; Kumar, V.; Pang, H.; Verbel, D. Kotsianti, A.; Teverovskiy M. & Saidi, O. (2005). Automated prostate cancer diagnosis and Gleason grading of tissue microarrays, *Proc. SPIE Med. Imag.*, vol. 5747, pp.58–70.

Tahir, M.A. & Bouridane, A. (2006). Novel Round-Robin Tabu Search Algorithm for Prostate Cancer Classification and Diagnosis Using Multispectral Imagery. *IEEE transactions on information technology in biomedicine*, Vol. 10, No. 4.

Yongguang, B. Ishii, N. & Du, X. (2004). Combining multiple k-nearest neighbour classifiers using different distance functions. *Lectures Notes in Computer Science (LNCS 3177), 5th Int. Conf. Intell. Data Eng. Autom. Learn.*, U.K.

Part 3

Therapeutic Novelties

10

New Selenoderivatives as Antitumoral Agents

Carmen Sanmartín, Juan Antonio Palop,
Beatriz Romano and Daniel Plano
Department of Organic and Pharmaceutical Chemistry, University of Navarra
Spain

1. Introduction

Prostate cancer (PC) is the most common male malignancy in Western countries and the second most common urological malignancy (Knudsen & Vasioukhin, 2010). In 2008 the estimated new cases for PC in the European Union were 382.000 (Ferlay et al. 2010). The possibility of early detection is attractive to clinicians and potential patients in spite of the fact that until recently concrete evidence that screening would influence PC mortality was lacking (Schröder, 2010). There are many risk factors for PC occurrence. The family history, genetic and environmental factors and their interaction can contribute to develop PC (Colloca & Venturino, 2011). Other risk factors are age, ethnic-racial-geographic factors, named constitutional factors, though it is not possible to know what percentage of these neoplasms are a result of these risk factors (Ferris-i-Tortajada et al. 2011). The polymorphisms in genes associated with PC probably represent the most part of familial PC burden. The recent advances in genomic research have made it possible to identify several new genomic based biomarkers for PC. These markers are easy to measure and stable over time but only one biomarker, prostate specific antigen (PSA), is used in the clinical today (Aly et al. 2011). The PSA screening allows to detect PC years before the emergence of clinically evident disease, which usually represents locally advanced or metastatic cancer (Gjertson & Albertsen, 2011). Treatment options for advanced PC – including hormone ablation therapy, radiation and surgery – do not offer cure but delay the inevitable recurrence of the lethal hormone-refractory disease. Chemotherapy using available anticancer drugs, with the exception of the taxane drug docetaxel, for late stage PC does not offer any survival benefit. All of these treatments are costly and have significant side effects including impotence and incontinence, which negatively affect the quality of life of the patients. Prevention is an important strategy for limiting PC morbidity and mortality. Pharmacological and dietary interventions have potentials functions in reduction of incident cases and in inhibition of disease progression and recurrence (Silberstein & Parsons, 2010). 5-alpha reductase inhibitors remain the predominant therapy to reduce the future risk of a PC diagnosis. Dutasteride and finasteride are currently the only proven agents for PC risk reduction (Strope & Andriole, 2010). Among the potential dietary intervention efforts to use of the micro-nutrient selenium (Se) in PC clinical trials is emerging as an important highlight and the outcomes indicate that Se is a promising treatment. Furthermore, Se inhibits PC through multiple mechanisms, and it is beneficial in controlling the development of this disease (Abdulah et al. 2011). Se is an essential trace element for humans, animals and some bacteria and it is important for many cellular processes, cardiovascular disease, central nervous system pathologies and may prevent cancer (Dennert et al. 2011). The evidence that Se is a cancer preventive agent includes that from geographic, animal, prospective and intervention studies (Tabassum et al. 2010, Schmid et al. 2011).

Furthermore, literature reports have consistently shown that the different effects of different chemical forms and dose of Se (Algotar et al. 2011) on signaling and expression of transcripts in PC cells might have important implications in the outcome of ongoing PC prevention clinical trials. These include the forms of Se present in the diet and in the body, their functions and mechanisms of action, and methods employed in assessing an individual's Se nutritional status – both in general and in epidemiological studies into the risk of cancer in relation to diet, as well as in connection with long-term trials for investigating the disease-preventive potential of selenium supplementation. Several mechanisms have been suggested to mediate the anticancer effects of Se. The major ones are reduction of DNA damage; oxidative stress; inflammation; induction of phase II conjugating enzymes that detoxify carcinogens; enhancement of immune response; incorporation into selenoproteins; alteration in DNA methylation status of tumor suppressor genes; inhibition of cell cycle and angiogenesis and induction of apoptosis. The specific mechanisms for PC are the inhibition of androgen receptor (AR) signaling, reduction in the mRNA, and protein levels of the AR, recruitment of corepressors to the AR elements in the promoters of androgen responsive genes, inhibition of signaling pathways like NF-κB, IL-6, Stat3, and induction of apoptosis (Nadiminty & Gao, 2008) (Figure 1).

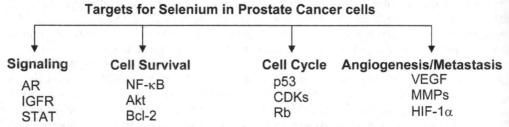

Targets for Selenium in Prostate Cancer cells

Signaling	Cell Survival	Cell Cycle	Angiogenesis/Metastasis
AR	NF-κB	p53	VEGF
IGFR	Akt	CDKs	MMPs
STAT	Bcl-2	Rb	HIF-1α

Fig. 1. Schematic representation of cellular processes targeted by Se and some specific molecular targets in each pathway. Figure from Nadiminty & Gao, 2008 with permission from John Wiley and Sons.

The rapid advance in the knowledge of different selenoproteins and their biological functions has opened up new possibilities to increase our understanding of the biological effects of Se supplementation (Rebsch et al. 2006). Selenoprotein deficiency leads to the accelerated development of lesions associated with PC progression, implicating selenoproteins in cancer risk and development and raising the possibility that Se prevents cancer by modulating the levels of these selenoproteins. Recently, it has been reported that the new discovered selenoprotein, SEP15, which is highly expressed in the prostate, may play a role either independently or by modifying the effects of Se in PC survival (Penney et al. 2010). Moreover, further research and additional trials of this type are needed to define the benefits and risks of different types and doses of Se supplements that in the future may be implemented for public health reasons. Another necessary focus for future research is a better understanding of the mechanisms by which Se interferes with the carcinogenic processes. The direction of future studies lies in clarifying the effects of these products and exploring the biological mechanisms responsible for the prevention of prostate cancer (Fairweather-Tait et al. 2011). This chapter includes information on twenty eight general chemical structures containing Se that have shown either anticancer, chemopreventive or apoptotic activities. Thus, Se derivatives emerge as promising downstream candidates for cancer therapy.

2. Selenoderivatives against prostate cancer

2.1 Methylseleninic acid, sodium selenite and sodium selenate

Some studies have shown that the selenium-based compound methylseleninic acid (MSeA, Figure 2) can disrupt AR signaling in PC cells by reaction with reduced glutathione within the PC cell (Husbeck et al., 2006). On the other hand, it was observed that a combination of MSeA with bicalutamide produced a robust downregulation of PSA through the identification of hTERT/telomerase as an important AR target. Telomerase activation has been reported in >90% of prostate cancer samples, but not in normal or benign prostatic hyperplasia tissues. Telomerase activation play an essential role in cell survival and oncogenesis, and inhibition of telomerase has been shown to suppress growth and tumorigenic potential of PC (S.A. Liu et al., 2010). Other mechanisms have demonstrated that the growth inhibitory effect could be attributed to cell cycle modulation and apoptosis induction provoked by MSeA by activation the forkhead box O1 (FOXO1) (H.T. Zhang et al., 2010). This compound has shown efficacy in transgenic adenocarcinoma of mouse prostate model (Wang et al., 2009). Too, it has been investigated in mice model treated with this Se form and were observed changes in its proteome (Zhang et al., 2011). In addition, MSeA exerted a dose-dependent inhibition of DU145 xenograft growth without genotoxic properties (Li et al., 2008). Moreover, in advanced and hormone refractory prostate cancer the efficacy of MSeA is based on down regulating hypoxia inducible factor 1α (HIF-1α) accompanied of a reduction of vascular endothelial growth factor (VEGF) and glucose transporter 1 (GLUT1) (I. Sinha et al., 2011). On the other hand, MSeA inactivated protein kinase C (PKC), particularly the promitogenic and prosurvival epsilon isoenzyme, acting through a redox modification of vicinal cysteine sulfhydryls in the catalytic domain of PKC (Gundimeda et al., 2008). Some metabolites of MSeA such as methylselenol may contribute to their anticancer activities. For example, an upregulation of cyclin dependent kinase inhibitor (CDKI) proteins p21Cip 1 and/or p27Kip 1 was observed in DU145 prostate cancer cells (Wang et al., 2010). Too, a novel mechanism of Se action has been proposed for methylselenol due to its ability to inhibit histone deacetylase (HDAC) (Kassam et al., 2011). Recently, speciation analysis showed that MSeA was completely transformed during the incubations while metabolic conversion of the other Se compounds was limited (Lunoe et al., 2011).

Sodium selenite (Figure 2) is another compound that has been studied in relation to PC and it may modulate the androgen receptor through the repression of interleukin-6 (IL-6) (Gazi et al., 2007). Too, it was observed that selenite decreased HDAC activity and increased levels of acetylated lysine 9 on histone H3, but decreased levels of methylated H3-Lys 9 (Xiang et al., 2008). Other mechanisms of action have been postulated such as an increase of the activity of the tumor suppressor protein (PTEN) and of the thioredoxin reductase (TR) (Berggren et al., 2009). Too, selenite is able to induce cell death and apoptosis by production of superoxide in mitochondria in LNCaP cells (Xiang et al., 2009). In 2010 was reported that sodium selenite inhibited the lipopolysaccharide (LPS)-induced TLR4-NF-kB signaling in PC-3 (Pei et al., 2010). Sodium selenite can act alone or in combination with other treatments for PC. So, this compound significantly enhances the effect of radiation on well established hormone-independent prostate tumors and does not sensitize the intestinal epithelial cells to radiation. These results suggest that may increase the therapeutic index of radiation therapy (Tian et al., 2010). In addition, the effectiveness on PC treatment of the association between sodium selenite and docetaxel has resulted as a new strategy in PC therapeutic approach (Freitas et al., 2011). Too, combination of genistein and selenite has shown synergistic effects on apoptosis, cell cycle arrest associated signaling pathways in p53 expression (Zhao et al., 2009). Actually, other inorganic forms of Se as sodium selenate (Figure 2), where Se is in oxidation state + 6, are in Phase I studies and have shown antiangiogenic properties (Corcoran et al., 2010).

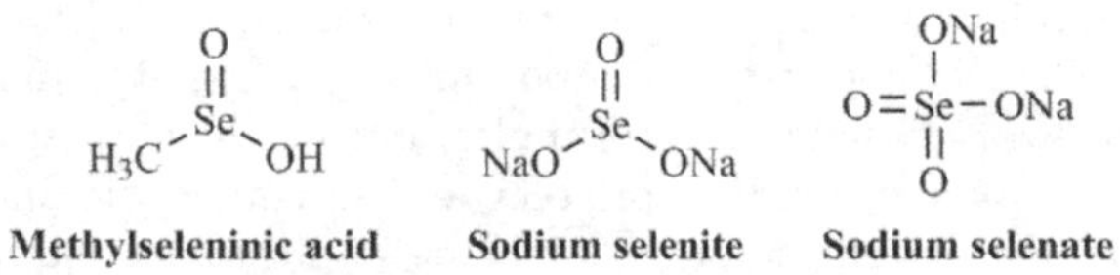

$$\underset{\textbf{Methylseleninic acid}}{H_3C \overset{\overset{\textstyle O}{\|}}{\underset{\textstyle }{\diagdown}} \overset{Se}{} \diagup OH} \qquad \underset{\textbf{Sodium selenite}}{NaO \overset{\overset{\textstyle O}{\|}}{\diagdown} \overset{Se}{} \diagup ONa} \qquad \underset{\textbf{Sodium selenate}}{O = \overset{\overset{\textstyle ONa}{|}}{\underset{\underset{\textstyle O}{\|}}{Se}} - ONa}$$

Fig. 2. Methylseleninic acid, sodium selenite and sodium selenate structures.

2.2 Methylselenocysteine and selenomethionine

Se may exert its beneficial effects through incorporation into selenoproteins including, glutathione peroxidases, selenoprotein P, iodothyronine deiodinases and thioredoxin reductases. There are more than 30 selenoproteins that have been identified in humans and they are involved in a range of cellular functions including immune function and protection against lipid and DNA damage. The cancer preventive mechanisms of action of methylselenocysteine (MeSeCys) (Figure 3) in human prostate cells are variable. A mechanism of action proposed for MeSeCys is that can alter the expression of several types of collagen gene and protein expression and thus may impact on the extracellular matrix and alter prostate cell progression and invasion (Hurst et al., 2008). Other authors affirm that the effect is due to methylselenol, a metabolite active in a study carried out in the transgenic adenocarcinoma mouse prostate model by oral administration of MeSeCys (J. Zhang et al., 2010). This hypothesis has been reinforced and completed in 2011 with the inclusion of new metabolites, the α-keto acids analogues of MeSeCys (Pinto et al., 2011). Related to selenomethionine (SeMet) (Figure 3) one of the mechanism that is gaining interest is the HDAC inhibition by metabolites of SeMet accompanied of redox signaling proteins modulation (J.I. Lee et al., 2009). Too, in combination with genistein induced growth arrest with modulation of expression of matrix metalloproteinase-2 (MMP-2) (Kumi-Diaka et al., 2010). On the other hand, this compound has been employed in order to reduce the toxic effects of di(2-ethylhexyl)phthalate (DEHP), an abundant plasticizer environmental contaminant that causes alterations in endocrine and spermatogenic functions mediated by induction of reactive oxygen species (ROS) and activation of nuclear p53 and p21 proteins in LNCaP cells. The SeMet supplementation reduced ROS production with modulation of intracellular redox status that is related to response against testicular toxicity (Erkekoglu et al., 2011). If we consider the possibility of combination between SeMet and other compound for modulating PC development the results are drug dependent. So, SeMet and alpha-tocopherol do not inhibit prostate carcinogenesis in the testosterone plus estradiol treated NBL rat model (Ozten et al., 2010). However, the selected combination of silymarin and SeMet significantly reduced two markers of lipid metabolism known associated with PC progression (Vidlar et al., 2010). In order to improve the activity and safety inorganic and organic hybrid nanoparticles are potentially useful in biomedicine, mainly for tumor treatments (Choi et al., 2010). Se nanoparticles are safer compared with SeMet isolated and was observed an inhibition of the growth of prostate LNCaP cancer cells partially through caspases mediated apoptosis, Akt kinase modulation and by disrupting AR (Kong et al., 2011).

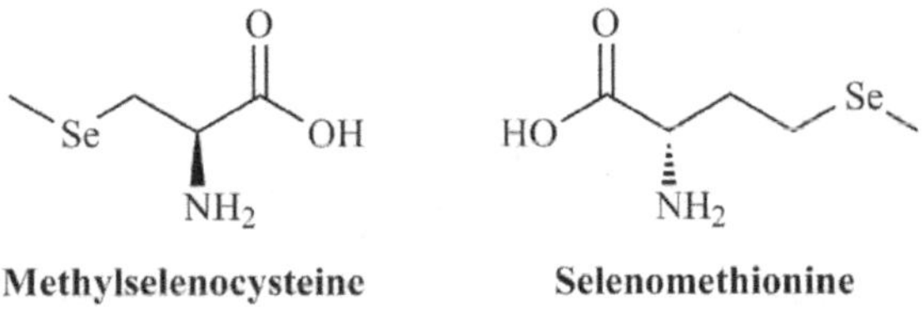

Methylselenocysteine   **Selenomethionine**

Fig. 3. Methylselenocysteine and selenomethionine structures.

2.3 Selenocyanate derivatives

The first selenocyanate described was 1,4-phenylenebis(methylene)selenocyanate (p-XSC) (Figure 4). The most recent studies postulate that this compound is capable of altering cofilin-2, single-stranded mitochondrial DNA binding protein, chaperonin 10, nucleoside diphosphate kinase 6 and chain A Horf 6 human peroxidase enzyme in LNCaP cells and in its androgen independent clone (AI) (R. Sinha et al., 2008). Too, this compound can induce apoptosis, inhibits AR expression and decreases Akt phosphorylation (Facompre et al., 2010). Other organic selenocyanates have emerged during the last years. So phenylalkyl isoselenocyanates (Figure 4), isosteric selenium analogues of naturally occurring phenylalkyl isothiocyanates, have shown a reduction in tumor size associated to apoptosis. The structure activity relationship studies concluded that an increase in the alkyl chain length is critical for the activity being n = 4, named ISC-4, the optimal (Sharma et al., 2008). In 2011, these same authors have reported that ISC-4 activates prostate apoptosis response protein 4 (Par-4) (Sharma et al., 2011). As a continuation of the synthesis of novel alkyl selenocyanates in 2010 was described the synthesis of substituted naphthalimide based organoselenocyanates (Figure 4) with the alkyl chain length n = 5 and investigated their systematic toxicity profile in mice by consideration changes in body weight, hepatotoxicity and nephrotoxicity resulting less toxic than other selenium forms but retaining the efficacy (Roy et al., 2010). Numerous studies have been conducted to elucidate the mechanism underlying the antitumor effects associated with cyclooxygenase 2 (COX-2) inhibitors. However, this mechanism has not yet been clearly defined. Nonsteroidal anti-inflammatory drugs (NSAIDs) have been shown to retard the progression of PC in men and NSAIDs have been used in clinical trials for prostate cancer. Celecoxib (Celebrex), a specific COX-2 inhibitor, reduces prostate tumors in experimental models mainly through cell cycle regulation and angiogenesis. However, the growth inhibitory properties of Celecoxib may be COX-2 independent. Considering this possible effect a novel strategy has been proposed based on to combine selenium and COX-2 inhibitor. Considering that sulfonamide moiety and pyrazole ring are important for the proapoptotic activity of Celecoxib against PC, the Selenocoxib-1 (Figure 4) was synthesized. The structural modifications introduced were the replacement of the trifluoromethyl group by methyleneselenocyanate fragment and the elimination of the methyl group. The study carried out against PAIII cells derived from a metastatic prostate tumor that arose spontaneously in a Lobund-Wistar (LW) rat. In addition, human metastatic prostate cancer cells, PC-3M, were tested for antitumor effect of Selenocoxib-1 *in vitro*. Selenocoxib-1 induced apoptosis in a dose-dependent manner in the PAIII cells and resulted more effective against PC than Celecoxib (Desai et al., 2010a). Other modulations have been introduced maintaining the methyl group in order to obtain Selenocoxib-2 (Figure 4) but it has not been studied as antitumoral yet (Desai et al., 2010b).

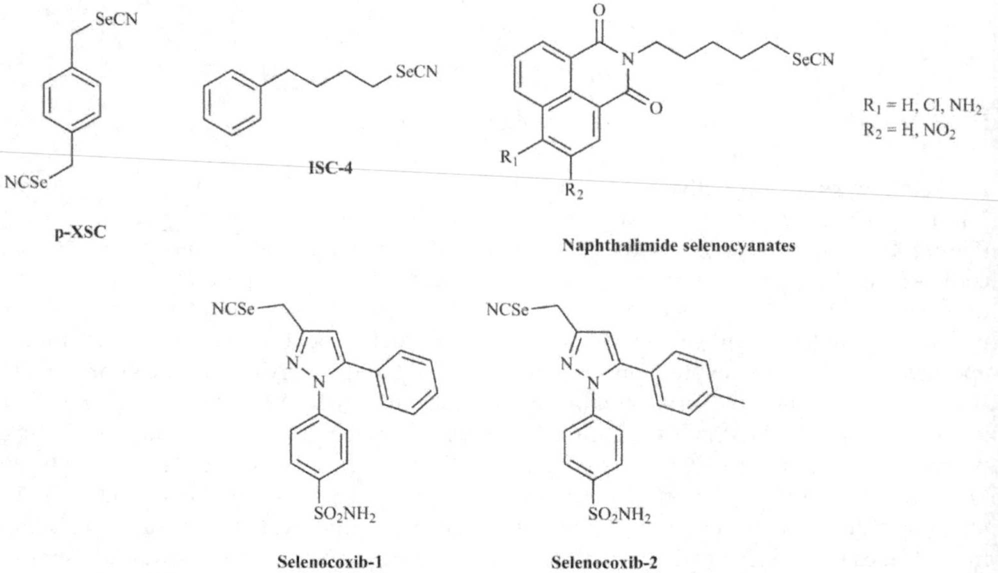

Fig. 4. Chemical structures for selenocyanate derivatives.

2.4 Heterocycles containing selenium

Ebselen (Figure 5) is one of the most relevant heterocyclic compounds derived from selenium. Ebselen is a glutathione peroxidase mimetic seleno-organic compound that attenuates the H_2O_2 level. In this process a hydroxylamine spin trap reacts with oxygen-centered radicals, including superoxide. It was seen that this compound blocked the expression of the disintegrin and metalloprotease ADAM9 in LNCaP or C4-2 PC cells through inhibition of ROS production (Sung et al., 2006). In other studies Ebselen was used as an external agent for reverting biochemical processes such as glycolysis. For example, ABC transporters like P-glycoprotein (P-gp/ABCB1), that are membrane proteins responsible for the transport of toxic compounds out of non-malignant cells and tumor tissue can be modified in their expression by coincubation with ebselen (Wartenberg et al., 2010). Too, it has been used for protecting PC-3 cells against apoptosis induction provoked by curcumin, a potent anticancer agent (Hilchie et al., 2010). On the other hand, ebselen has been reported as a covalent inactivator of α-methylacyl coenzyme A racemase (AMACR), a metabolic enzyme whose overexpression has been shown to be a diagnostic indicator of prostatic adenocarcinoma and other solid tumors and has been employed as reference drug for screening of approximately 5000 unique compounds as AMACR inhibitors (Wilson et al., 2011). In structural relation with ebselen is the organoselenium compound 1,2-bis-[1,2-benzisoselenazolone-3(2H)-ketone]ethane (BBSKE) (Figure 5), which has shown an inhibitory effect on the growth of a variety of human cancer cells, provokes S phase arrest accompanied by increases in the protein levels of cyclin A, E and p21 and decreases in levels of cyclin B1, D1 and Cdk4 (Shi et al., 2003a, 2003b). A recent study carried out in rats affirms that the metabolites of BBSKE can act as antitumoral agents (Zhou et al., 2010). Too, in association with cisplatin increases the sensitivity of the colon cancer cell line LoVo towards cisplatin via regulation of G_1 phase and reversal of G_2/M phase arrest (Fu et al., 2011). The formulation as copolymer micelles allows the accumulation into tumor efficiently due to an increase in water solubility (M. Liu et al., 2010).

D-501036, 2,5-bis(5-hydroxymethyl-2-selenienyl)-3-hydroxymethyl-N-methylpyrrole (Figure 5), has been identified as a novel antineoplastic agent with a broad spectrum of antitumoural activity against several human cancer cells and has an IC_{50} value in the nanomolar range. This compound induces cell death associated with the DNA damage-mediated induction of ataxia telangiectasia-mutated activation without interfering with topoisomerase-I and topoisomerase-II function (Juang et al., 2007). Another mechanism that has been proposed for the activity of D-501036 is angiogenesis inhibition. Although anti-angiogenesis strategies have generated a great deal of enthusiasm for therapeutic applications, it is still unknown whether these systems would be feasible for prevention. The possibility of interfering very early in tumour progression by modulating the cancer angiogenic switch is appealing, though there is increasing evidence for close correlation between inflammation, the micro-environment and tumour-associated neo-angiogenesis causing the adverse outcomes of prostate cancer (Araldi et al., 2008).

In 2010, a new series of heterocyclic organoselenium compounds were synthesized and evaluated as possible chemopreventive agents in human prostate cancer LNCaP cells. Two of this 3-selena-1-dethiacephem derivatives (Figure 5) strongly activated nuclear factor E2-related factor 2 (Nrf2)/ antioxidant response element (ARE) signaling that regulate expression of phase II antioxidant and detoxifying enzymes such as glutathione peroxidase (GPX), γ-glutamylcysteine synthetase (γ-GCS), heme oxygenase-1 (HO-1), NADPH quinone oxidoreductase (NQO-1), and glutathione S-transferase (GST) expression. These two compounds also possessed a potent antioxidant activity. Furthermore, both compounds were capable of inhibiting cell growth via cell cycle arrest. Related to structure activity relationship the presence of the exo-olefin (carbon–carbon double bond) as well as the aliphatic substitution at the imine part is critical for these compounds to activate Nrf2/ARE signaling (Terazawa et al., 2010). Other interesting derivatives are 2-substituted selenazolidine-4(R)-carboxylic acids (Figure 5). There are numerous studies that concern the induction of a protective hepatic enzyme related to gluthathione-S-tranferase and gluthathione peroxidase and it seemed of interest to evaluate these compounds in PC cells (El-Sayed et al., 2007, Poerschke & Moos 2011).

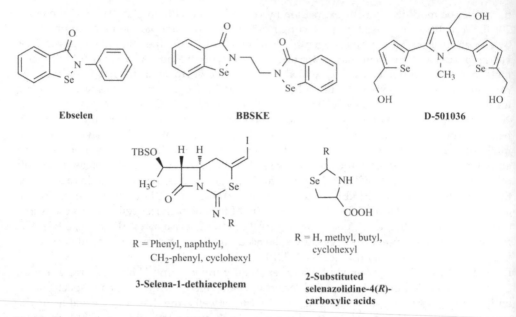

Fig. 5. Chemical structures for heterocycles containing selenium.

2.5 Selenide and diselenide derivatives

The selenide function is present in a lot of organoselenium compounds. Many of the above described derivatives possess this type of bond (i.e. MeSeCys, SeMet,). One compound does not described in the above sections is *p*-xylylbis(methylselenide) (*p*-XMS) (Figure 6), a organoselenium compound that modifies the growth, secretion of PSA and the intracellular redox status and genomic profiles (Pinto et al., 2007). Too, the selenide function is present linked to nucleosides. The natural nucleosides may be used as Se-carriers. The synthesis and antitumor activity of novel nucleosides derivatized from uridine and thymidine (Figure 6), with a selenomethyl group at various positions has been described. In general, the activity against PC cells is position-dependent. Compounds with the selenomethyl group in position 5′ are more active than the corresponding in 2′ or 3′. The probable explanation is that it is easier to metabolize the Se-nucleoside containing the primary selenomethyl than the secondary selenomethyl, thereby generating more methylselenol (Lin et al., 2009). The natural products continue to be a rich source of new promising substances for cancer therapy. Sesquiterpene lactones (SQLs) are a class of naturally occurring plant terpenoids of Asteraceae family, known for their various biological activities such as cytotoxicity against different tumor cell lines. Many authors have linked this activity mainly to the α-methylene-γ-lactone functionality, which is prone to react with suitable nucleophiles, e.g., sulfhydryl groups of cysteine, in a Michael addition mechanism. These reactions are nonspecific, leading to the inhibition of a large number of enzymes or factors involved in key biological in spite of it is well known, however, that the α-methylene-γ-lactone moiety is not an absolute requirement for cytotoxicity. In this context emerge other interesting compounds such as the alpha-santonin derivatives (Figure 6) a sesquiterpene lactone isolated from *Artemisia santonica*. The compounds with higher activity showed as common structural feature the presence of an alpha-methylidene-gamma-butyrolactone moiety in their structures (Arantes et al., 2009). This hypothesis has been corroborated in other tumoral cell lines. In addition, the bioactive α-santonin derivatives are selective against cancer cells (Arantes et al., 2010).

It is well established that various human diseases, including PC, are associated with a disturbed intracellular redox balance and oxidative stress (OS). Se based agents (Figure 6) turn the oxidizing redox environment present in certain cancer cells into a lethal cocktail of reactive species that push these cells over a critical redox threshold and ultimately kill them through apoptosis. The main advantage is that this kind of toxicity is highly selective: normal, healthy cells remain largely unaffected, since changes to their naturally low levels of oxidizing species produce little effect though the biochemical pathways triggered by these agents need to be studied in more detail such as redox modulator like cysteine-containing Bcl proteins, which control apoptosis at an early stage, certain caspases, which execute apoptotic mechanisms further downstream, are also redox sensitive (Jamier et al., 2010).

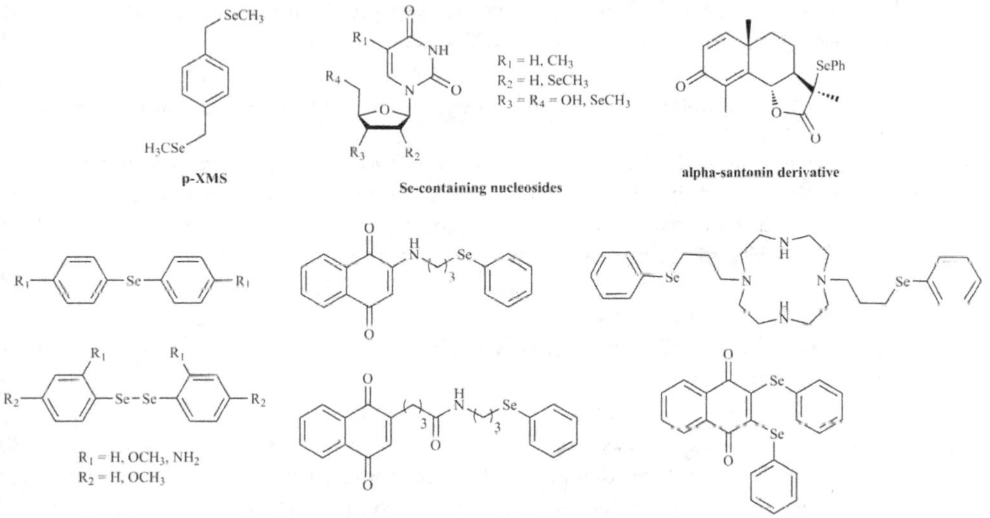

Fig. 6. Chemical structures for selenide and diselenide derivatives.

2.6 Selenium and metal complexes

Selenium- and sulfur-containing compounds have been widely studied as potential antioxidants for the prevention or reduction of oxidative DNA damage and the organoselenium compounds are of particular interest because they appear to be more bioavailable relative to inorganic Se compounds. The Se and sulfur antioxidant activity has been explained using copper-mediated DNA damage studies and UV-vis spectroscopy that have allowed identifying a copper coordination through a novel metal bond. For this reason has been described the synthesis of relevant copper selone complexes with tris(pyrazolyl)methane or tris(pyrazolyl)borate ligands (Figure 7) (Kimani et al., 2010). The determination of redox potential for Cu-Selone complexes indicated that Se coordination to copper in biological systems may prevent the reduction of Cu^{2+} by NADH required for the catalytic formation of damaging hydroxyl radical.

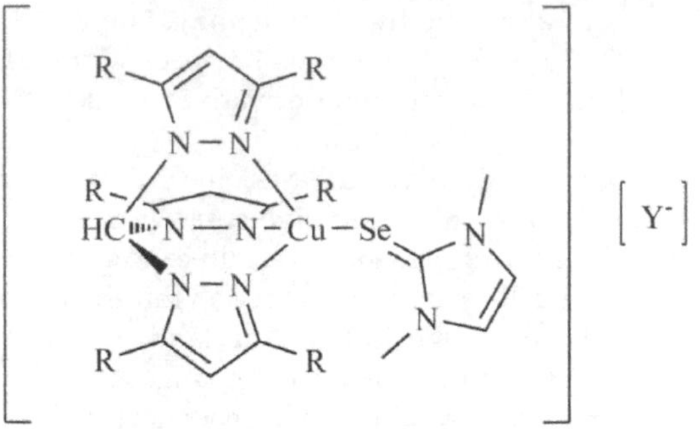

Y = BF$_4$, Cl
R = H, Me, i-Pr

Fig. 7. Chemical structure for Cu-Selone complexes. Reprinted with permission from Kimani et al., 2010. Copyright 2010 American Chemical Society.

2.7 A case study: Novel selenoderivatives as cytotoxic agents and apoptosis inducers in prostate cancer cells

In the last four years, several articles have been published by our research group related to the design, synthesis and biological evaluation of novel compounds containing Se as cytotoxic agents and apoptosis inducers. In addition, mounting evidence suggests that selenium (Se) works by inhibiting important early steps in carcinogenesis in a variety of experimental models and the anticancer activity is dependent on the chemical form of selenium. Se occurs in both organic and inorganic forms. Based on these findings we envisaged a new investigation that involves the synthesis of new compounds that incorporate the Se-containing moiety.

2.7.1 Structures and biological results

Initially, the rationale behind the design of these compounds was to maintain molecular symmetry, a structural property that is frequently present in cytotoxic and pro-apoptotic drugs (Sanmartín et al., 2006). The structures synthesised correspond to molecules with a central nucleus made up of an alkyl imidothiocarbamate (alkyl isothiourea) or alkyl imidoselenocarbamate (alkyl isoselenourea) connected by a carbonyl group on each side to two identical lateral aromatic or heteroaromatic rings mono, bi or polycyclics (Figure 8). The sulfur and selenium substituents were varied (methyl, ethyl, benzyl and isopropyl) to determine the effect of the alkyl chain length and the ramifications that this has on the activity (Plano et al., 2007, Ibáñez et al., 2011). The best results in PC-3 were obtained for the compound with X = Se, Y = C, R = CH$_3$ and R' = 4-CH$_3$. This compound was the most potent (IC$_{50}$ = 1.85 µM) and was 4.5 times more active than standard methylseleninic acid (IC$_{50}$ = 8.38 µM) and 7.3 times more active than etoposide (IC$_{50}$ = 13.6 µM), an agent used in the treatment of PC. In addition, the novel compound was less toxic than the reference and apoptotic inducer in MCF-7 and CCRF-CEM. For the heteroaromatic rings thienyl and quinolinyl were the most interesting. During the course of our work a great number of different structural classes of selenocompounds were reported (Sanmartín et al., 2008). For this reason, and in order to improve the potency of our compounds, we decided to introduce some structural modifications. Among these modifications was the preparation of new compounds with related structures based on aroyl and heteroaroyl selenylacetic acid derivatives (Figure 8). The most promising derivatives against PC-3 cancer cells were the corresponding phenyl, 3,5-dimethoxyphenyl and benzyl with TGI values of 6.8, 4.0 and 2.9 µM (Sanmartín et al., 2009). Too, there is current interest in heterocyclic compounds that contain a Se atom in the ring. Bearing this fact in mind, and as a continuation of our previous work, we proposed the synthesis 1,2,5-selenadiazolo[3,4-d]pyridines and 1,2,5-benzoselenadiazolo derivatives (Figure 8). The most promising molecule was a pyridine derivative (Plano et al., 2010b). Other explored structures were compounds with selenocyanate and diselenide moieties. Moreover, we evaluated their antioxidant-prooxidant properties so as their cytotoxic activities against PC-3 resulting eighteen of the fifty-nine compounds evaluated more potent than etoposide (Plano et al., 2010a). Taking into account that oxidation state for Se is related to antitumoral effect we have synthesized and evaluated an original series consisting of a small group of compounds which possess Se in the +4 states oxidation instead of Se +2 (Figure 8) (Plano et al., 2010a).

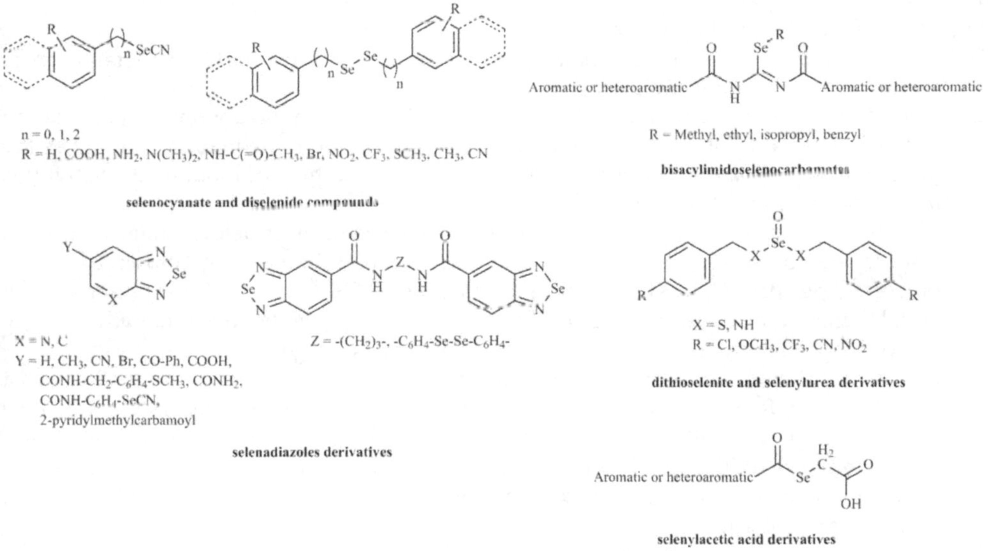

n = 0, 1, 2
R = H, COOH, NH$_2$, N(CH$_3$)$_2$, NH-C(=O)-CH$_3$, Br, NO$_2$, CF$_3$, SCH$_3$, CH$_3$, CN

selenocyanate and diselenide compounds

R = Methyl, ethyl, isopropyl, benzyl

bisacylimidoselenocarbamates

X = N, C
Y = H, CH$_3$, CN, Br, CO-Ph, COOH, CONH-CH$_2$-C$_6$H$_4$-SCH$_3$, CONH$_2$, CONH-C$_6$H$_4$-SeCN, 2-pyridylmethylcarbamoyl

Z = -(CH$_2$)$_3$-, -C$_6$H$_4$-Se-Se-C$_6$H$_4$-

selenadiazoles derivatives

X = S, NH
R = Cl, OCH$_3$, CF$_3$, CN, NO$_2$

dithioselenite and selenylurea derivatives

selenylacetic acid derivatives

Fig. 8. Selenoderivatives obtained and evaluated by our research group.

Considering that Se has been associated with an anticancer effect via the modulation of some kinase such as Akt (J.H. Lee et al., 2008) some of these compounds have been studied as kinase modulators. Some of them modulate CK1A and GS3Ka expression and a weak modification in ErB4, GS3Ka and PKCA was detected (unpublished results).

The preliminary results from the biological screening of these novel compounds are very encouraging and these systems could offer an excellent framework in this field and may ultimately lead to discovery of potent antitumour agent. Thus, the search for new drugs with Se continues to be a great challenge in medical science.

3. Conclusion

It is clear from the studies discussed above that Se compounds do have effects on growth, cell cycle and apoptosis and that such compounds offer great promise as anticancer and apoptotic agents in many tumoral processes, mainly for PC. In this chapter we have summarized information on more than twenty eight structures that contain Se – most of which were published in the last three years – and possess cytotoxic activity against PC. This list of compounds and references is by no means exhaustive and merely hints at the hundreds of other citations due to the ever increasing amount of work carried out in this field. As a result of these studies, Se derivatives are rapidly emerging as valid chemotherapeutic agents. However, various organic and inorganic selenium compounds used in some studies have produced variable results when they are tested in animal models and human subjects and more investigations are urgently needed in order to ascertain the safety in their use. We have included some structures that have not yet been evaluated in prostate cancer cells because we believe that the study of these compounds would be of interest. Although several possible mechanisms have been proposed to explain the anticancer and apoptotic properties of selenium compounds, the results described here suggest the following preliminary considerations:

1. The chemical form is a determinant factor for the activity and the metabolism is required for anticarcinogenic activity.
2. The effect of some selenium compounds mainly depends on the dose and the oxidation state of selenium. For inorganic selenium compounds the +4 oxidation state gives the highest anticarcinogenic properties and for organic selenium compounds the activity is mainly observed for the +2 oxidation state.
3. The existence of diverse responses for the same chemical structure suggests several mechanisms of action. For example, sodium selenite induced apoptosis by redox processes, decreased HDAC activity, increased of PTEN activity. The expectation of a broad therapeutic benefit from agents that target only one member of either pathway may be overly simplistic due to the complex interrelated network governing apoptosis.
4. Experimental evidence shows that molecular symmetry, as a broad concept, could be a positive factor for cancer prevention and apoptosis (sodium selenite, methylseleninic acid, p-XSC, p-XMS, BBSKE). The importance of molecular symmetry in cytotoxic and pro-apoptotic activities was reported by us in 2006. Recently, we described a new series of symmetrical organoselenium compounds that are potent as cytotoxic agents in prostate cancer cells.

This class of compound offers a great deal of promise to broaden significantly the horizons of modern apoptosis and anticancer drug discovery for the potential treatment of prostate cancer. Animal data, epidemiological data, and intervention trials have shown a clear role for selenium derivatives in both the prevention of specific cancers and antitumourigenic effects in postinitiation phases of cancer through apoptosis induction. Accordingly, in recent years there has been substantial interest directed toward the synthesis of selenium-containing derivatives that could be used as cytotoxic, cancer chemopreventive and apoptotic agents. However, a great deal of further research is needed to unravel the precise manner in which selenium compounds act.

4. Acknowledgment

The authors wish to express their gratitude to the Ministerio de Educación y Ciencia, Spain (SAF 2009-07744) for financial support.

5. References

Abdulah R, et al. (2011) Molecular targets of selenium in prostate cancer prevention (Review). *International Journal of Oncology*, Vol.39, No.2, (August 2011), pp. 301-309, ISSN 1019-6439.

Algotar AM, et al. (2011) Dose-dependent effects of selenized yeast on total selenium levels in prostatic tissue of men with prostate cancer. *Nutrition and Cancer*, Vol.63, No.1, (December 2010), pp. 1-5, ISSN 0163-5581.

Aly M, Wiklund F, & Grönberg H (2011) Early detection of prostate cancer with emphasis on genetic markers. *Acta Oncologica*, Vol.50, No.S1, (June 2011), pp. 18-23, ISSN 0284-186X.

Araldi EMV, et al. (2008) Natural and synthetic agents targeting inflammation and angiogenesis for chemoprevention of prostate cancer. *Current Cancer Drug Targets*, Vol.8, No.2, (March 2008), pp. 146-155, ISSN 1568-0096.

Arantes FFP, et al. (2010) Synthesis of novel alpha-santonin derivatives as potential cytotoxic agents. *European Journal of Medicinal Chemistry*, Vol.45, No.12, (December 2010), pp. 6045-6051, ISSN 0223-5234.

Arantes FFP, et al. (2009) Synthesis and cytotoxic activity of alpha-santonin derivatives. *European Journal of Medicinal Chemistry*, Vol.44, No.9, (September 2009), pp. 3739-3745, ISSN 0223-5234.

Berggren M, et al. (2009) Sodium selenite increases the activity of the tumor suppressor protein, PTEN, in DU-145 prostate cancer cells. *Nutrition and Cancer*, Vol.61, No.3, (May-June 2009), pp. 322-331, ISSN 0163-5581.

Choi HS, et al. (2010) Design considerations for tumour-targeted nanoparticles. *Nature Nanotechnology*, Vol.5, No.1, (January 2010), pp. 42-47, ISSN 1748-3387.

Colloca G & Venturino A (2011) The evolving role of familial history for prostate cancer. *Acta Oncologica*, Vol.50, No.1, (January 2011), pp. 14-24, ISSN 0284-186X.

Corcoran NM, et al. (2010) Open-label, phase I dose-escalation study of sodium selenate, a novel activator of PP2A, in patients with castration-resistant prostate cancer. *British Journal of Cancer*, Vol.103, No.4, (August 2010), pp. 462-468, ISSN 0007-0920.

Dennert G, et al. (2011) Selenium for preventing cancer. *Cochrane Database of Systematic Reviews*, Vol.5, Article Number.CD005195, ISSN 1469-493X.

Desai D, et al. (2010a) Synthesis and antitumor properties of selenocoxib-1 against rat prostate adenocarcinoma cells. *International Journal of Cancer*, Vol.127, No.1, (July 2010), pp. 230-238, ISSN 1097-0215.

Desai D, et al. (2010b) Synthesis and evaluation of the anti-inflammatory properties of selenium-derivatives of celecoxib. *Chemico-Biological Interactions*, Vol.188, No.3, (December 2010), pp. 446-456, ISSN 0009-2797.

El-Sayed WM, Hussin WA, & Franklin MR (2007) The antimutagenicity of 2-substituted selenazolidine-4-(R)-carboxylic acids. *Mutation Research/Genetic Toxicology and Environmental Mutagenesis*, Vol.627, No.2, (March 2007), pp. 136-145, ISSN 1383-5718.

Erkekoglu P, *et al.* (2011) Induction of ROS, p53, p21 in DEHP- and MEHP-exposed LNCaP cells-protection by selenium compounds. *Food and Chemical Toxicology,* Vol.49, No.7, (July 2011), pp. 1565-1571, ISSN 0278-6915.

Facompre ND, *et al.* (2010) 1,4-Phenylenebis(methylene)selenocyanate, but not selenomethionine, inhibits androgen receptor and Akt signaling in human prostate cancer cells. *Cancer Prevention Research,* Vol.3, No.8, (August 2010), pp. 975-984, ISSN 1940-6207.

Fairweather-Tait SJ, *et al.* (2011) Selenium in human health and disease. *Antioxidants & Redox Signaling,* Vol.14, No.7, (April 2011), pp. 1337-1383, ISSN 1523-0864.

Ferlay J, Parkin DM, & Steliarova-Foucher E (2010) Estimates of cancer incidence and mortality in Europe in 2008. *European Journal of Cancer,* Vol.46, No.4, (March 2010), pp. 765-781, ISSN 0959-8049.

Ferris-i-Tortajada J, *et al.* (2011) Constitutional risk factors in prostate cancer. *Actas Urologicas Españolas,* Vol.35, No.5, (May 2011), pp. 282-288, ISSN 0210-4806.

Freitas M, *et al.* (2011) Combined effect of sodium selenite and docetaxel on PC3 metastatic prostate cancer cell line. *Biochemical and Biophysical Research Communications,* Vol.408, No.4, (May 2011), pp. 713-719, ISSN 0006-291X.

Fu JN, *et al.* (2011) Thioredxin reductase inhibitor ethaselen increases the drug sensitivity of the colon cancer cell line LoVo towards cisplatin via regulation of G1 phase and reversal of G2/M phase arrest. *Investigational New Drugs,* Vol.29, No.4, (August 2011), pp. 627-636, ISSN 0167-6997.

Gazi MH, *et al.* (2007) Sodium selenite inhibits interleukin-6-mediated androgen receptor activation in prostate cancer cells via upregulation of c-Jun. *Clinica Chimica Acta,* Vol.380, No.1-2, (May 2007), pp. 145-150, ISSN 0009-8981.

Gjertson CK & Albertsen PC (2011) Use and assessment of PSA in prostate cancer. *Medical Clinics of North America,* Vol.95, No.1, (January 2011), pp. 191-200, ISSN 0025-7125.

Gundimeda U, *et al.* (2008) Locally generated methylseleninic acid induces specific inactivation of protein kinase C isoenzymes relevance to selenium-induced apoptosis in prostate cancer cells. *Journal of Biological Chemistry,* Vol.283, No.50, (December 2008), pp. 34519-34531, ISSN 0021-9258.

Hilchie AL, *et al.* (2010) Curcumin-induced apoptosis in PC3 prostate carcinoma cells is caspase-independent and involves cellular ceramide accumulation and damage to mitochondria. *Nutrition and Cancer,* Vol.62, No.3, pp. 379-389, ISSN 0163-5581.

Hurst R, *et al.* (2008) Se-methylselenocysteine alters collagen gene and protein expression in human prostate cells. *Cancer Letters,* Vol.269, No.1, (September 2008), pp. 117-126, ISSN 0304-3835.

Husbeck B, *et al.* (2006) Inhibition of androgen receptor signaling by selenite and methylseleninic acid in prostate cancer cells: two distinct mechanisms of action. *Molecular Cancer Therapeutics,* Vol.5, No.8, (August 2006), pp. 2078-2085, ISSN 1535-7163.

Ibáñez E, *et al.* (2011) Synthesis and antiproliferative activity of novel symmetrical alkylthio- and alkylseleno-imidocarbamates. *European Journal of Medicinal Chemistry,* Vol.46, No.1, (January 2011), pp. 265-274, ISSN 0223-5234.

Jamier V, Ba LA, & Jacob C (2010) Selenium- and tellurium-containing multifunctional redox agents as biochemical redox modulators with selective cytotoxicity. *Chemistry-a European Journal,* Vol.16, No.36, (September 2010), pp. 10920-10928, ISSN 0947-6539.

Juang S-H, et al. (2007) D-501036, a novel selenophene-based triheterocycle derivative, exhibits potent in vitro and in vivo antitumoral activity which involves DNA damage and ataxia telangiectasia–mutated nuclear protein kinase activation. *Molecular Cancer Therapeutics*, Vol.6, No.1, (January 2007), pp. 193-202, ISSN 1535-7163.

Kassam S, et al. (2011) Methylseleninic acid inhibits HDAC activity in diffuse large B-cell lymphoma cell lines. *Cancer Chemotherapy and Pharmacology*, (In press), DOI 10.1007/s00280-011-1649-1, ISSN 0344-5704.

Kimani MM, Brumaghim JL, & VanDerveer D (2010) Probing the antioxidant action of selenium and sulfur using Cu(I)-chalcogenone tris(pyrazolyl)methane and -borate complexes. *Inorganic Chemistry*, Vol.49, No.20, (October 2010), pp. 9200-9211, ISSN 0020-1669.

Knudsen BS & Vasioukhin V (2010) Mechanisms of prostate cancer initiation and progression. *Advances in Cancer Research*, Vol. 109, pp. 1-50, ISSN 0065-230X.

Kong L, et al. (2011) The suppression of prostate LNCaP cancer cells growth by Selenium nanoparticles through Akt/Mdm2/AR controlled apoptosis. *Biomaterials*, (In press), DOI 10.1016/j.biomaterials.2011.05.032, ISSN 0142-9612.

Kumi-Diaka J, et al. (2010) Genistein-selenium combination induces growth arrest in prostate cancer cells. *Journal of Medicinal Food*, Vol.13, No.4, (August 2010), pp. 842-850, ISSN 1096-620X.

Lee JH, et al. (2008) A novel activation-induced suicidal degradation mechanism for Akt by selenium. *International Journal of Molecular Medicine*, Vol.21, No.1, (January 2008), pp. 91-97, ISSN 1107-3756.

Lee JI, et al. (2009) Alpha-keto acid metabolites of naturally occurring organoselenium compounds as inhibitors of histone deacetylase in human prostate cancer cells. *Cancer Prevention Research*, Vol.2, No.7, (July 2009), pp 683-693, ISSN 1940-6207.

Li GX, et al. (2008) Superior in vivo inhibitory efficacy of methylseleninic acid against human prostate cancer over selenomethionine or selenite. *Carcinogenesis*, Vol.29, No.5, (May 2008), pp. 1005-1012, ISSN 0143-3334.

Lin L, et al. (2009) Facile synthesis and anti-tumor cell activity of Se-containing nucleosides. *Nucleosides Nucleotides & Nucleic Acids*, Vol.28, No.1, (January 2009), pp. 56-66, ISSN 1525-7770.

Liu M, et al. (2010) Preparation of tri-block copolymer micelles loading novel organoselenium anticancer drug BBSKE and study of tissue distribution of copolymer micelles by imaging in vivo method. *International Journal of Pharmaceutics*, Vol.391, No.1-2, (May 2010), pp. 292-304, ISSN 0378-5173.

Liu SA, et al. (2010) Telomerase as an important target of androgen signaling blockade for prostate cancer treatment. *Molecular Cancer Therapeutics*, Vol.9, No.7, (July 2010), pp. 2016-2025, ISSN 1535-7163.

Lunoe K, et al. (2011) Investigation of the selenium metabolism in cancer cell lines. *Metallomics*, Vol.3, No.2, (February 2010), pp. 162-168, ISSN 1756-5901.

Nadiminty N & Gao AC (2008) Mechanisms of selenium chemoprevention and therapy in prostate cancer. *Molecular Nutrition & Food Research*, Vol.52, No.11, (November 2008), pp. 1247-1260, ISSN 1613-4125.

Ozten N, *et al.* (2010) Selenomethionine and alpha-tocopherol do not inhibit prostate carcinogenesis in the testosterone plus estradiol-treated NBL rat model. *Cancer Prevention Research*, Vol.3, No.3, (March 2010), pp. 371-380, ISSN 1940-6207.

Pei ZY, *et al.* (2010) Sodium selenite inhibits the expression of VEGF, TGF beta(1) and IL-6 induced by LPS in human PC3 cells via TLR4-NF-(K)B signaling blockage. *International Immunopharmacology*, Vol.10, No.1, (January 2010), pp. 50-56, ISSN 1567-5769.

Penney KL, *et al.* (2010) A large prospective study of SEP15 genetic variation, interaction with plasma selenium levels, and prostate cancer risk and survival. *Cancer Prevention Research*, Vol.3, No.5, (May 2010), pp. 604-610, ISSN 1940-6207.

Pinto JT, *et al.* (2011) Chemopreventive mechanisms of alpha-keto acid metabolites of naturally occurring organoselenium compounds. *Amino Acids*, Vol.41, No.1, (June 2011), pp. 29-41, ISSN 0939-4451.

Pinto JT, *et al.* (2007) Differential effects of naturally occurring and synthetic organoselenium compounds on biomarkers in androgen responsive and androgen independent human prostate carcinoma cells. *International Journal of Cancer*, Vol.120, No.7, (April 2007), pp. 1410-1417, ISSN 0020-7136.

Plano D, *et al.* (2010a) Antioxidant-prooxidant properties of a new organoselenium compound library. *Molecules*, Vol.15, No.10, (October 2010), pp. 7292-7312, ISSN 1420-3049.

Plano D, *et al.* (2010b) Synthesis and in vitro anticancer activities of some selenadiazole derivatives. *Archiv der Pharmazie*, Vol.343, No.11-12, (November-December 2010), pp. 680-691, ISSN 1521-4184.

Plano D, *et al.* (2007) Novel potent organoselenium compounds as cytotoxic agents in prostate cancer cells. *Bioorganic & Medicinal Chemistry Letters*, Vol.17, No.24, (December 2007), pp. 6853-6859, ISSN 0960-894X.

Poerschke RL & Moos PJ (2011) Thioredoxin reductase 1 knockdown enhances selenazolidine cytotoxicity in human lung cancer cells via mitochondrial dysfunction. *Biochemical Pharmacology*, Vol.81, No.2, (January 2011), pp. 211-221, ISSN 0006-2952.

Rebsch CM, Penna FJ, & Copeland PR (2006) Selenoprotein expression is regulated at multiple levels in prostate cells. *Cell Research*, Vol.16, No.12, (December 2006), pp. 940-948, ISSN 1001-0602.

Roy SS, *et al.* (2010) Naphthalimide based novel organoselenocyanates: Finding less toxic forms of selenium that would retain protective efficacy. *Bioorganic & Medicinal Chemistry Letters*, Vol.20, No.23, (December 2010), pp. 6951-6955, ISSN 0960-894X.

Sanmartin C, *et al.* (2009) Synthesis and Pharmacological Screening of Several Aroyl and Heteroaroyl Selenylacetic Acid Derivatives as Cytotoxic and Antiproliferative Agents. *Molecules*, Vol.14, No.9, (September 2009), pp. 3313-3338, ISSN 1420-3049.

Sanmartin C, Plano D, & Palop JA (2008) Selenium compounds and apoptotic modulation: A new perspective in cancer therapy. *Mini-Reviews in Medicinal Chemistry*, Vol.8, No.10, (September 2008), pp. 1020-1031, ISSN 1389-5575.

Sanmartin C, Font M, & Palop JA (2006) Molecular symmetry: A structural property frequently present in new cytotoxic and proapoptotic drugs. *Mini-Reviews in Medicinal Chemistry*, Vol.6, No.6, (January 2006), pp. 639-650, ISSN 1389-5575.

Schmid H-P, *et al.* (2011) Nutritional aspects of primary prostate cancer prevention, In: *Clinical Cancer Prevention,* H-J Senn & F Otto (Eds.), pp. 101-107, Springer-Verlag Berlin Heidelberg, ISSN 978-3-642-10858-7.

Schröder FH (2010) Prostate cancer around the world. An overview. *Urologic Oncology-Seminars and Original Investigations,* Vol.28, No.6, (November-December 2010), pp. 663-667, ISSN 1078-1439.

Sharma AK, *et al.* (2011) The Akt inhibitor ISC-4 activates prostate apoptosis response protein-4 and reduces colon tumor growth in a nude mouse model. *Clinical Cancer Research,* (In press), DOI 10.1158/1078-0432, ISSN 1078-0432.

Sharma AK, *et al.* (2008) Synthesis and anticancer activity comparison of phenylalkyl isoselenocyanates with corresponding naturally occurring and synthetic isothiocyanates. *Journal of Medicinal Chemistry,* Vol.51, No.24, (December 2008), pp. 7820-7826, ISSN 0022-2623.

Shi CJ, *et al.* (2003a) A novel organoselenium compound induces cell cycle arrest and apoptosis in prostate cancer cell lines. *Biochemical and Biophysical Research Communications,* Vol.309, No.3, (September 2003), pp. 578-583, ISSN 0006-291X.

Shi CJ, *et al.* (2003b) Induction of apoptosis in prostate cancer cell line PC-3 by BBSKE, a novel organoselenium compound, and its effect in vivo. *Zhonghua Yi Xue Za Zhi,* Vol.83, No.22, (November 2003), pp. 1984-1988, ISSN 0253-9624.

Silberstein JL & Parsons JK (2010) Prostate cancer prevention: concepts and clinical recommendations. *Prostate Cancer and Prostatic Diseases,* Vol.13, No.4, (December 2010), pp. 300-306, ISSN 1365-7852.

Sinha I, *et al.* (2011) Methylseleninic acid down regulates hypoxia inducible factor-1α in invasive prostate cancer. *International Journal of Cancer,* (In press), DOI 10.1002/ijc.26141, ISSN 1097-0215.

Sinha R, *et al.* (2008) Effects of naturally occurring and synthetic organoselenium compounds on protein profiling in androgen responsive and androgen independent human prostate cancer cells. *Nutrition and Cancer,* Vol.60, No.2, (March-April 2008), pp. 267-275, ISSN 0163-5581.

Strope SA & Andriole GL (2010) Update on chemoprevention for prostate cancer. *Current Opinion in Urology,* Vol.20, No.3, (May 2010), pp. 194-197, ISSN 0963-0643.

Sung SY, *et al.* (2006) Oxidative stress induces ADAM9 protein expression in human prostate cancer cells. *Cancer Research,* Vol.66, No.19, (October 2006), pp. 9519-9526, ISSN 0008-5472.

Tabassum A, Bristow RG, & Venkateswaran V (2010) Ingestion of selenium and other antioxidants during prostate cancer radiotherapy: A good thing? *Cancer Treatment Reviews,* Vol.36, No.3, (May 2010), pp. 230-234, ISSN 0305-7372.

Terazawa R, *et al.* (2010) Identification of organoselenium compounds that possess chemopreventive properties in human prostate cancer LNCaP cells. *Bioorganic & Medicinal Chemistry,* Vol.18, No.19, (October 2010), pp. 7001-7008, ISSN 0968-0896.

Tian JQ, Ning SC, & Knox SJ (2010) Sodium selenite radiosensitizes hormone-refractory prostate cancer xenograft tumors buy not intestinal crypt cells in vivo. *International Journal of Radiation Oncology Biology Physics,* Vol.78, No.1, (September 2010), pp. 230-236, ISSN 0360-3016.

Vidlar A, *et al.* (2010) The safety and efficacy of a silymarin and selenium combination in men after radical prostatectomy – a six month placebo-controlled double-blind clinical trial. *Biomedical Papers-Olomouc,* Vol.154, No.3, (September 2010), pp. 239-244, ISSN 1213-8118.

Wang L, *et al.* (2009) Methyl-selenium compounds inhibit prostate carcinogenesis in the transgenic adenocarcinoma of mouse prostate model with survival benefit. *Cancer Prevention Research,* Vol.2, No.5, (May 2009), pp. 484-495, ISSN 1940-6207.

Wang Z, *et al.* (2010) Persistent P21Cip1 induction mediates G(1) cell cycle arrest by methylseleninic acid in DU145 prostate cancer cells. *Current Cancer Drug Targets,* Vol.10, No.3, (May 2010), pp. 307-318, ISSN 1568-0096.

Wartenberg M, *et al.* (2010) Glycolytic pyruvate regulates P-glycoprotein expression in multicellular tumor spheroids via modulation of the intracellular redox state. *Journal of Cellular Biochemistry,* Vol.109, No.2, (February 2010), pp. 434-446, ISSN 0730-2312.

Wilson BAP, *et al.* (2011) High-throughput screen identifies novel inhibitors of cancer biomarker α-methylacyl coenzyme A racemase (AMACR/P504S). *Molecular Cancer Therapeutics,* Vol.10, No.5, (May 2011), pp. 825-838, ISSN 1535-7163.

Xiang N, Zhao R, & Zhong WX (2009) Sodium selenite induces apoptosis by generation of superoxide via the mitochondrial-dependent pathway in human prostate cancer cells. *Cancer Chemotherapy and Pharmacology,* Vol.63, No.2, (January 2009), pp. 351-362, ISSN 0344-5704.

Xiang N, *et al.* (2008) Selenite reactivates silenced genes by modifying DNA methylation and histones in prostate cancer cells. *Carcinogenesis,* Vol.29, No.11, (November 2008), pp. 2175-2181, ISSN 0143-3334.

Zhang HT, *et al.* (2010) Activation of FOXO1 is critical for the anticancer effect of methylseleninic acid in prostate cancer cells. *Prostate,* Vol.70, No.12, (September 2010), pp. 1265-1273, ISSN 0270-4137.

Zhang J, *et al.* (2011) Mouse prostate proteomes are differentially altered by supranutritional intake of four selenium compounds. *Nutrition and Cancer,* (In press) DOI 10.1080/01635581.2011.563029, ISSN 0163-5581.

Zhang J, *et al.* (2010) Proteomic profiling of potential molecular targets of methyl-selenium compounds in the transgenic adenocarcinoma of mouse prostate model. *Cancer Prevention Research,* Vol.3, No.8, (August 2010), pp. 994-1006, ISSN 1940-6207.

Zhou H-y, *et al.* (2010) LC-MSn analysis of metabolites of 1, 2- bis (1, 2-benzisoselenazolone-3(2H)-ketone) -ethane, a novel anti-cancer agent in rat. *Yaoxue Xuebao,* Vol.45, No.5, (May 2010), pp. 627-631, ISSN 0513-4870.

11

Injection Site Granulomas Resulting from Administration of Leuprorelin Acetate

Taku Suzuki and Hideki Mukai

Toho University, Medical Center, Ohashi Hospital, Department of Dermatology

Japan

1. Introduction

Leuprorelin acetate is a luteinizing hormone releasing hormone (LHRH) agonist and was launched in 1997. It has been used for sex hormone-dependent diseases such as prostate cancer, endometriosis, premenopausal breast cancer, and central precocious puberty. In Japan, a preparation for administration at monthly intervals (Leuprin®) has been available since 1999, and a continuous sustained release preparation for administration every 3 months (Leuprin SR®) since 2002. In recent years, there has been a considerable increase in the frequency of foreign body granulomas, particularly in patients in whom a 1-monthly preparation was changed to a 3-monthly continuous sustained release preparation. We report two such cases that we encountered and present a literature review.

2. Case

Case 1: A 77-year-old Japanese male had been treated for prostate cancer with monthly subcutaneous `injections of depot leuprorelin acetate since August 2005. In December 2005, his treatment was changed to the 3-monthly leuprorelin acetate preparation. One month later, he presented with a nodule at the injection site. The nodule was 15 mm in diameter, firm and tethered to the overlying skin **(Photograph 1)**. Skin biopsy revealed a granuloma with epithelioid cells, and multinucleated giant cells were observed in the subcutaneous tissue by hematoxylin–eosin staining. The granuloma contained vacuoles of various sizes, and portions of it were phagocytosed **(Photograph 3)**. In addition, inflammatory cell infiltration was observed, mainly of lymphocytes and neutrophils, along with eosinophils **(Photograph 4)**.

His treatment was then changed to goserelin acetate (Zoladex®) for subsequent injections,no problems occurred thereafter.

Case 2: A 78-year-old Japanese male had been treated for prostate cancer with monthly subcutaneous injections of depot leuprorelin acetate since October 2002. In February 2003, his treatment was changed to the 3-monthly preparation. After the sixth administration, he presented with a nodule at the injection site.

Laboratory tests showed no abnormalities in blood count, blood biochemistry, and urine. Serum PSA was high at 5.14 ng/ mL, while γ-SM was within normal limits (0.4 ng/ mL). The nodule was 30 × 35 mm in diameter, painless, firm, and tethered to the overlying skin **(Photograph 2)**.

Skin biopsy showed a granuloma with epithelioid cells and multinucleated giant cells, and lymphocytes were observed from the subdermal layer to the subcutaneous tissue **(Photograph 5)**. His treatment was changed to goserelin acetate (Zoladex®) for subsequent injections, and no problems occurred thereafter.

Intradermal and patch tests were not performed in either patient because we were unable to obtain consent from them.

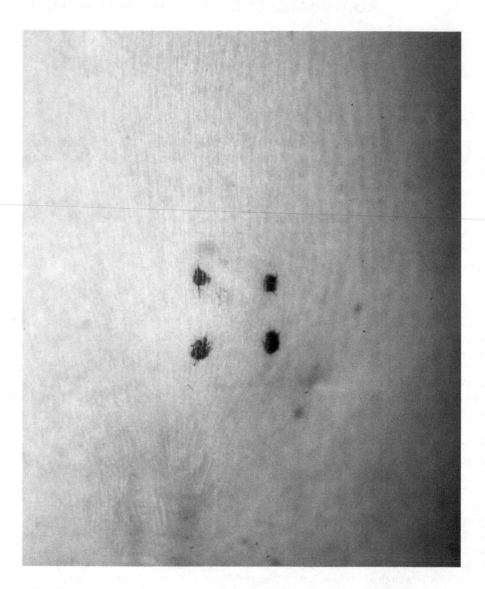

Fig. 1. Case 1 presented with a subcutaneous nodule (dotted area) in the right navel area. The solitary nodule was 15 mm in diameter, slightly firm, and only slightly mobile.

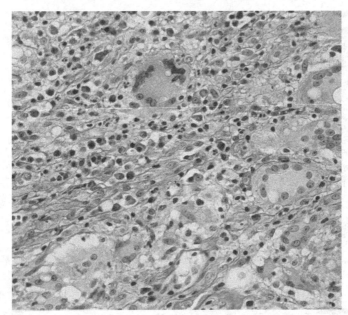

Fig. 2. Case 2 presented with a subcutaneous nodule with an injection scar on the right upper arm. The solitary nodule was 30 × 35 mm in size, slightly firm, and mobile.

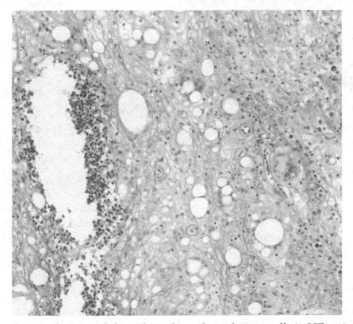

Fig. 3. It showed several eosinophils with multinucleated giant cells in HE staining (original magnification ×400).

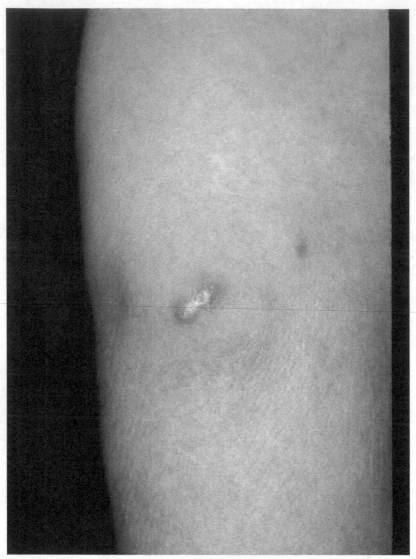

Fig. 4. It showed an epithelial granuloma with foreign body multinucleated giant cells containing microspheres and scattered eosinophils. The granuloma with multinucleated giant cells, eosinophils, and numerous vacuoles was located in the subcutaneous tissue (hematoxylin–eosin staining; original magnification ×200).

3. Discussion

Treatments for prostate cancer include hormone therapy, surgical treatment, radiation therapy, and chemotherapy. Although treatment plans differ according to the stage of disease, endocrine therapy is used for clinically localized cancer, locally invasive cancer, and distant metastasis such as to the bone. Among the endocrine therapies, the first choice for treatment in the initial stage is an LHRH agonist or a combination of an LHRH agonist and an anti-androgen.

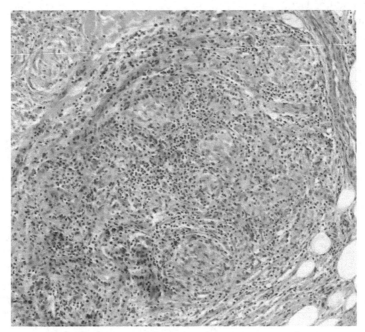

Fig. 5. In the subdermal layer beneath the subcutaneous fat tissue, there was a granuloma, part of which contained multinucleated giant cells (hematoxylin–eosin staining; original magnification ×100).

Leuprorelin acetate is a derivative of LHRH with a substituted amino acid sequence; it is a superagonist with an activity approximately 100-fold higher than the natural form. Continuous administration of leuprorelin acetate causes downregulation of the LHRH receptor, has an antagonist-like action, and depresses gonadal function. Therefore, it is used for treating sex hormone-dependent diseases. At present, a preparation of leuprorelin acetate designed for administration at intervals of 3 months is indicated for prostate cancer and premenopausal breast cancer.

The side effect profile of systemic LHRH agonist injections is below

- fast and irregular heart beat
- bone, muscles, and joint pain
- fainting and fast and irregular breathing and shortness of breath
- numbness and tingling in the hands and feet
- swelling of the eyes and the eyelids
- skin rash or hives and itching
- pains in the chest or tightness of chest and wheezing
- pain in the groin or the legs, especially the calves

If these symptoms are severe, they may require consultation with a physician. Other more common symptoms that are less severe include:

- hot flashes
- burning, itching, redness, and swelling at the injection site
- blurred vision
- dizziness and headaches
- nausea and vomiting and constipation
- gynecomastia (swelling or tenderness and pain of the breasts)
- swelling or feet and lower legs
- trouble sleeping
- decreased size of testicles
- inability to maintain an erection satisfactory for intercourse
- decrease in interest in sex

The side effect profile of local LHRH agonist injections is below[2]

- erythema
- nodule
- induration
- dermatitis

Previous reports of foreign body granuloma formation resulting from the use of leuprorelin acetate are summarized in Table 1. Sixty-six cases have been reported globally, and most of these reports (58 cases, 87.9%) are from Japan. As mentioned below, the difference in the number of reports between Japan and other countries is believed to be related to the depth

country	Japan: 58 cases Others: 8 cases
disease	prostate cancer: 62 cases central precocious puberty: 4 cases
age	1~89(average: 76.3)
lesion	Upper arm: 30cases Abdomen: 15cases Buttock: 1case Unknown: 20cases
Kind and the number of times of drugs (except for 18 cases of unknown)	1-month depot preparation:12cases 1 ~about60times(average:27.8times)
	3-months depot preparation :36cases 2~7times(average:2.6times)
	<past history of LH-RH agonist:24cases> month depot preparation: 19cases (once~five years; average12.8times) bicalutamide：3cases(unspecified) goserelin acetate：2cases(unspecified)

Table 1. Summary of 66 cases

of insertion of the injection needle. All caese were single .The underlying disease was prostate cancer in all cases except four with central precocious puberty. Regarding the cases of prostate cancer, we found that the range of patient ages was 60–89 years, with a mean of 76.3 years, which is consistent with the mean age of prostate cancer onset. The 1-monthly preparation was used in 12 patients, the 3-monthly preparation in 36 patients, and the preparation type was unknown in 18 patients. Among the patients who received the 3-monthly preparation, 24 had a treatment history with LHRH agonists including leuprorelin acetate. Most of these patients (19 of them) had previously received the 1-monthly preparation. The injection site was the upper arm in 30 patients, the abdomen in 15 patients, the buttock in 1 patient, and unknown in 20 patients. Among those whose injection sites were known, either the injection sites were changed or the dermatological symptoms were observed at another site in 16 patients. Histologically, all cases had foreign-body granulomatous tissue reaction.

Various opinions on the cause of local reactions to depot leuprorelin acetate have been suggested, including the base used and the nature of the preparation itself. Manasco et al. stated that an identical reaction was observed when base alone was injected, and that natural LHRH did not cause a similar reaction. However, Neely et al. administered an alternative drug without the base and observed erythema. In an animal experiment, they also observed a strong reaction when a high concentration of leuprorelin acetate was combined with the base. Therefore, the local reaction was thought to be associated not only with the base, but also with the preparation itself.

The leuprorelin acetate preparation contained controlled release solid dispersion microspheres comprising lactic acid–glycolic acid copolymers, which slowly disseminated throughout the body. Subsequently, there was a continuous inflammatory response to the leuprorelin acetate, and multinucleated giant cells appeared as a result of the recognition of foreign bodies because of the long-term presence of the microspheres themselves. Therefore, histologically, a foreign-body granuloma was formed. The injection dose and needle insertion depth could have also contributed to this finding. There was a 3-fold difference in the leuprorelin acetate content between the 1-monthly and 3-monthly preparations. Therefore, the 3-monthly preparation was more likely to cause an inflammatory response. Regarding the needle insertion depth, injections are administered intramuscularly in Europe and the USA, and subcutaneously in Japan. The difference in the number of reported cases between Europe and the USA on one hand and Japan on the other hand may be related to this difference in needle insertion depth.

The number of prostate cancer cases is increasing in Japan with a concomitant increase in the frequency of use of leuprorelin acetate. The number of reported cases with granuloma may increase in the future. If a granuloma develops as a result of the use of this preparation, we believe that dermatologists should be obliged to provide appropriate advice to other physicians, such as a change of drug. And physician should pay attention to perform the injection of LA in enough subcutaneous depth and exchange injection sites everytimes.

4. References

Adachi H, Hashimoto J,Hota H.Two cases of granuloma due to leuprorelin acetate subcutaneous injection. Jpn J Urology ; 106: 456, 2006(in Japanese)

Arai Y, Ebihara K,Okubo Y.et al A case of granuloma leuprorelin acetate subcutaneous injection. Jpn J Dermatol; 116: 963, 2006(in Japanese)

Egi M, Maeda M.Furuya K.Skin disorder by leuprorelin acetate.Nishinihon Journal of Dermatology ;66:206,2004(in Japanese)

Ferran M,Baena V,Pujol RM.et al Depot Leuprorelin Acetate-induced Granulomatous Manifested as Persistent Suppurative Nodules. Acta Derm Venerol ; 86: 453-455, 2006

Fujita R, Sakuma S,Komiya H. A case of subcutaneous tumor due to leuprorelin acetate one-month preparation.Nishinihon Journal of Urology ;68:159-161,2006(in Japanese)

Goto N, Mori R.Kudo H.Three cases due to leuprorelin acetate. Skin Research; 4: 507, 2005(in Japanese)

Hatcho Y,Ide Y,Masuda M.et al Two cases of granuloma due to leuprorelin acetate subcutaneous injection. Rinsho hihuka;48:1055-1057,2006(in Japanese)

Hirashima N, Shinogi T,Narisawa H.et al A case of cutaneous injury induced by subcutaneous injection of leuprolide acetate. Nishinihon Journal of Dermatology ;63:384-386,2001(in Japanese)

Ishigami T, Urano,Hujii Y.Four cases of skin disorder due to leuprorelin acetate. Nishinihon Journal of Dermatology;68:223,2006(in Japanese)

Kato A,Noro S,Kawana S.et al A case of granuloma due to leuprorelin acetate. rinsho derma ;60:1013-1016,2006(in Japanese)

Kawase A,Mizoguchi M,Iwamoto T,et al.A case of foreign body granuloma induced by injecton of leuprorelin acetate. Jpn J Dermatol;114:574,2004(in Japanese)

Koura S, Watanabe T.A suspected case of granuloma due to leuprorelin acetate. Nishinihon Journal of Dermatology ; 68: 220, 2006(in Japanese)

Liu XS, Folia C, Gomella LG. Pharmacology for common urologic diseases: 2011 review for the primary care physician. Can J Urol. 2011 ;18 Suppl:24-38

Manasco PK,Pescovitz OH, Blizzard RM.Local reactions to depot leuprolide therapy for central precocious puberty.et al. J Pediatr ; 123: 334-335, 1993

Marumo K, Baba S, Murai M. Erectile function and nocturnal penile tumescence in patients with prostate cancer undergoing luteinizing hormone-releasing hormone agonist therapy. Int J Urol. 1999;6:19

Mizoguchi K, Hamasaki Y,Igawa H.et al A case of drug induced granulomatous reaction by leuprorelin acetate for prostate cancer. Jpn J Dermatol; 114: 163-167, 2004(in Japanese)

Muya M, Takijiri C,Shirahara S.Two cases of granuloma caused by subcutaneous injection of leuprorelin acetate. Rinsho Hifuka;53:801-803,1999(in Japanese)

Nagata K,Shinoda S,Yonehara S.et al Two cases of granuloma due to leuprorelin acetate. Rinsho Hihuka ; 47: 784-787, 2005(in Japanese)

Navon L, Morag A. Advanced prostate cancer patients' ways of coping with the hormonal therapy's effect on body, sexuality, and spousal ties. Qual Health Res. 2003;13:1378

Neely EK, Hintz RL, Parker B et al.Two-year results of treatment with depot leuprolide acetate for central precocious puberty. J Pediatr;121:634-640,1992

Nomoto H, Ishida K,Kitagawa T.et al Granuloma due to leuprorelin acetate subcutaneous injection. Jpn J Dermatol; 116: 1089, 2006(in Japanese)

Ohara N, Mihara S,Usui T.et al A case of granuloma due to leuprorelin acetate . rinsho derma ;48:781-783,2006(in Japanese)

Ota K,Terao A,et al.Subcutaneous granuloma with formation caused by a slow-release leuprorelin acetate preparation. Nishinihon Journal of Urology;68: 267-269,2006(in Japanese)

Ouchi T, Naho MIYATA,Makoto S.et al Granuloma caused by subcutaneous injection of leuprorelin acetate product:Case report and histopathological findings; J Dermatol;33:719-721,2006

Quella S, Loprinzi CL, Dose M. A qualitative approach to defining "hot flashes" in men. Urol Nurs. 1994; 14: 155-158

Role of Estrogen in Normal Male Function: Clinical Implications for Patients with Prostate Cancer on Androgen Deprivation Therapy. The Journal of Urology 185, 17-23, 2011

Sadahira C,Yoneda K.Kubota Y. et al. A cases of granuloma due to leuprorelin acetate. Japanese Journal of Dermatoallergology; 13:138-143, 2005(in Japanese)

Saimoto H,Horikawa S,Nagai N.et al A case of subcutaneous allergy granuloma due to leuprorelin acetate. Acta Urologica Japonica;50:834,2004(in Japanese)

Sakamoto R,Kanekura T,Kanzaki T.et al Granulomas induced by subcutaneous injection of leuprorelin acetate, J Dermatol;33:43-45,2006

Shimizu H,Shimoura S,Sarayama Y.et al Granuloma The granuloma by the acetic acid Lew professional re phosphorous pharmaceutical administration is formed by a base remaining in subcutis for a long term. Jpn J Dermatol ; 116: 781,2006(in Japanese)

Sugano Y, Fujii K,Ogou N.A case of lipogranukoma induced by subcutaneous injection of the drug for prostate carcinoma. Jpn J Dermato;107:899,1997(in Japanese)

Tachibana M,Yamano Z,Chimogaki H,Hamami G.et al Cutaneous epitheloid granulomas caused by subcutaneous infusion of leuprorelin acetate:a case report.Hinyokika Kiyo;50:199-202,2004(in Japanese)

Taguchi S,Ishi Y.Granuloma due to leuprorelin acetate. Jpn J Dermatol;114:1440,2004(in Japanese)

Takahashi G,Hashimoto Y.Iizuka H.et al A case of granuloma due to leuprorelin acetate injection. Rinsho hihuka ; 47: 782-783, 2005(in Japanese)

Takakura Y. DDS type injecton.Journal of Practical Pharmacy;56:2437-2440,2005(in Japanese)

Tanaka E, Tanaka A.Hori K. Granuloma due to leuprorelin acetate subcutaneous injection. Rinsho hihuka ; 48: 411-415, 2006(in Japanese)

Tanaka S. Tamura M.Three cases of granuloma due to leuprorclin acetate. rinsho derma;47:788-792,2005(in Japanese)

Taneda T,Kanno T,Kanamaru H.et al Surgical manegement of inflammatory granuloma which developed following subcutaneous injection of leuprorelin acetate. Acta Urologica Japonica;51:487-489,2005(in Japanese)

Tonini G,Forleo V,Rustico M.et al Local reactions to lutenizing hormone releasing hormone analog therapy. J Pediatr ; 126: 159-160, 1995

Watanabe T, Yamada N.Yamamoto O.Histopathological Examination of the histopathology of six granuloma that resulted from acetic acid Lew professional re phosphorous hypodermic injection Jpn J Dermatol;116:803,2006(in Japanese)

Yasukawa K,Sugawara H,Kato N.et al Leuprorelin acetate granulomas:case reports and review of the literture. Br J Dermatol; 152: 1045-1047,2005

Yamashita F.,Hirai S,Ikeda S.et al A case of foreign granuloma due to leuprorelin acetate 3-month preparations. Hifubyo Shinryo; 27: 1277-1280,2005 (in Japanese)

Yamashita F.,Hirai S,Ikeda S.et al A case of foreign granuloma due to leuprorelin acetate 3-month preparations. Hifubyo Shinryo;27:1277-1280,2005(in Japanese)

Yasukawa K,Sugawara H,Kato N.et al Leuprorelin acetate granulomas:case reports and review of the literture. Br J Dermatol; 152: 1045-1047, 2005

Zippe CD, Raina R, Thukral M, et al. Management of erectile dysfunction following radical prostatectomy. Curr Urol Rep. 2001;2:495–503

12

Stem Like Cells and Androgen Deprivation in Prostate Cancer

Yao Tang, Mohammad A. Khan, Bin Zhang and Arif Hussain
University of Maryland School of Medicine and Baltimore VA Medical Center
USA

1. Introduction

Cancer stem cells (CSC) have been hypothesized to contribute to tumor initiation and recurrence, but the very existence of CSC is currently under debate. Increased expression of stem cell markers in cancer tissues after various treatments has been observed in both experimental animal models and patients for a number of cancer types. Cancer cells that express stem cell markers are generally called stem-like cells (SLC) since the exact origin of these cells is often not clear.

Using human LNCaP prostate cancer cell-based mouse xenografts as well as a transgenic model of prostate cancer (TRAMP), we studied the possible origin of SLC and their potential role in cancer recurrence after androgen deprivation therapy (ADT). We found that the proportion of SLC within a tumor can change over time, particularly after anti-cancer therapy (Tang et al., 2010). A significant increase in the SLC population occurred in tumors soon after ADT (surgical castration), but then returned to basal levels when the tumors resumed growth after the initial response to ADT. Several stem cell markers were found to be elevated during this period. This phenomenon was observed in both LNCaP xenografts and in TRAMP mice. These observations suggest that ADT may induce a 'stemness' stage in tumors which, although transient, could allow tumor cells to adapt to the anti-tumor effects of ADT and enhance their survival. A similar phenomenon was observed in LNCaP xenografts after docetaxel treatment. We believe stemness may have a biological function in self protection; it may be one pathway by which tumor cells can survive and recur after anti-cancer treatment.

2. Cancer stem cell or cancer cell stemness

The concept of cancer stem cells (CSC) is built upon the hypothesis that tumor tissues harbor a very small population of cells that is responsible for tumor initiation and recurrence due to its capacity for self-renewal and multilineage differentiation, as well as relative drug resistance. However, the frequency of CSC can be highly variable among different tumor types, and even among tumors of the same type (Visvader & Lindeman, 2008). For instance, in clinical samples, the CSC population in melanomas (ABCB5+) ranges between 1.6 - 20% (Schatton et al., 2008), and in colorectal carcinomas (CD133+) between 1.8 - 24.5% (O'Brien et al., 2007). The factors governing the different frequencies of CSC within tumors are not clearly delineated, although communication with surrounding cells and stroma, alterations in pH, chemokines/cytokines in the microenvironment, locoregional angiogenesis, and host response to local tissue damage could all potentially affect the CSC population to varying degrees.

A number of cell surface markers have been used to identify CSC in human cell cultures and *in vivo* experiments, including CD44, CD133, and c-Kit, among others. The relevance of some of the common stem cell markers such as CD44 with respect to stem-cell like properties and growth characteristics, however, is not altogether clear, particularly in established long term cell culture lines. For instance, in human prostate cancer cell lines, CD44 has been used to identify CSC; isolated CD44+ cells from prostate cancer cell lines and xenograft tumors show stem-like functions in terms of self-renewal, clonogenicity, tumorigenicity, as well as tumor metastasis (Patrawala et al., 2006; H. Li et al., 2008). However, significant differences in CD44 expression can exist between various prostate cancer cell lines in culture. For instance, by flowcytometry, CD44+ cells can represent 80-90% of the population in PC3 and DU145 cell lines (Patrawala et al., 2006; H. Li et al., 2008), but in LNCaP they are undetectable. The side population (SP) assay, which is based on exclusion of vital dyes, has also been used to identify a small subpopulation of cells enriched in self-renewal function particularly that derived from the bone marrow (Goodell et al., 1996). No difference in SP fractions is observed among PC3, DU145 and LNCaP cell lines, and their relevance to the overall biology of these cancer cells is not clear.

A recent comprehensive analysis of stem cell makers in the NCI60 Tumor Cell Line Panel demonstrates the presence of these various markers, but they are expressed in rather complex combinatorial patterns in cancer cell lines of different lineages (Stuelten et al., 2010). This and other studies suggest that established immortal cancer cell lines harbor SLC subpopulations, but also underscore the complexity of stem cell biology. Although mounting evidence supports the existence of CSC in various types of tumors (Baker, 2008; Dalerba et al., 2007; Lobo et al., 2007; C. Tang et al., 2007; Huntly & Gilliland, 2005), how cells with stem cell like-properties affect the growth characteristics and/or metastatic potential of tumors still remains an open question (Dalerba et al., 2007; Fabian et al., 2009; Jordan, 2009; Marotta & Polyak 2009; Clevers, 2011).

Another term, stemness, is frequently used in stem cell studies, but its exact definition has not been universally accepted (Leychkis et al., 2009; Hoffmann & Tsonis, 2011). Epithelial-mesenchymal and mesenchymal-epithelial transition states are also relevant not only to embryogenesis but to tumorigenesis; how these may relate to stemness is an area of active investigation ((Yang & Weinberg, 2008). In general, stemness represents a *state* in which cells are characterized by self-renewal and plasticity. In cancer tissue, the stemness state may be a transiently acquired property by a subpopulation of tumor cells that likely also involves input from surrounding cells. Biological or pharmacological stress, or changes in the tumor microenvironment, could serve as potential triggers for inducing this state, which may then allow for adaptation, survival and eventual disease progression.

3. Anti-tumor therapy and stem like cells in prostate cancer

Over the last several years we have utilized an LNCaP-based xenograft model and a genetically engineered transgenic mouse model, TRAMP, to study the effects of androgen deprivation and chemotherapy on prostate cancer (Y. Tang et al., 2006, 2008, 2009, 2010). Tumor tissues were collected at different time points before and after various treatments, and the expression patterns of several stem cell markers were evaluated in an effort to better understand treatment response and potential mechanisms of tumor recurrence.

3.1 LNCaP xenograft based studies

LNCaP is a hormone-sensitive human prostate cancer cell line. Withdrawal of androgens *in vitro* interrupts its growth and induces apoptosis. *In vivo*, LNCaP tumors in male SCID mice cease growth for up to 2-3 weeks after surgical castration (bilateral orchiectomy), which is invariably followed by accelerated tumor growth (Figure 1A). Immunohistochemical (IHC) analysis of proliferation-related (Ki67) and angiogenesis-related (CD105) markers in castrated and non-castrated mice is shown in Figures 1B and 1C. It is apparent that a significant decrease in overall proliferation occurs only in the castrated mice between one and two weeks after castration, followed then by recovery of proliferative potential. This recovery of cell proliferation appears to parallel increased angiogenesis, which is observed at the IHC level between two and three weeks post castration. In non-castrated mice, on the other hand, tumors continue to grow unabated over time, with no observable changes in cell proliferation or overall angiogenesis noted over this period of continued growth (Figures 1A-C).

To determine whether SLC play any role in the above model, we also studied several stem cell markers. Recent studies suggest that SLC are a heterogeneous population with diverse biological properties, and that multiple subpopulations with stem cell-like characteristics can coexist in the same tumor (Hermann et al., 2007; Ma et al., 2008; Hope et al., 2004). Since there is no single specific 'standard' marker for identifying cancer stem cells, we selected several antigens that have been implicated in one way or the other in stem cell biology; specifically, CD44, CD133, and c-Kit (CD117) for IHC studies, and human ALDH (aldehyde dehydrogenase), Shh (sonic hedgehog), p63, BCRP (breast cancer resistant protein), Notch1 and bcl-2 for western blot analyses. Tumor samples were collected at days 5, 10, 15, 20, 25, and 30 post castration, and tumors from non-castrated mice collected at similar time points served as controls.

By IHC, expressions of c-Kit (Figure 1D) and CD44 (Figure 1E), but not CD133, were significantly increased in LNCaP xenograft tumors at the day 15 time point after castration but not at other time points in either castrated or control mice. Representative images of c-Kit and CD44 at day-15 (Cas-15) and day 30 (Cas-30) are shown in Figure 1E. Interestingly, we noted that the distribution of CD44+ and c-Kit+ cells in tumor tissues was different. Most of the CD44+ cells were found in the periphery of tumor islands, whereas c-Kit+ cells were present within the tumor mass (Figure 1E). This suggests that these two proteins can be expressed in different cells within the LNCaP tumors, and may potentially signify the presence of different subtypes of SLC in these tumors. In untreated control mice, on the other hand, SLC markers do not change significantly over time despite continued tumor growth, as shown in Figure 1D.

Data for several proteins evaluated by western blots are summarized in Table 1. It is apparent from these initial studies that there is a trend for Shh, Notch, ALDH, BCRP and p63 to be over expressed at least 2-fold at day 15 compared to the other time points post castration in most or all the tumor samples tested, while Bcl2 is over expressed in 2 of the 4 tumors evaluated at this time point.

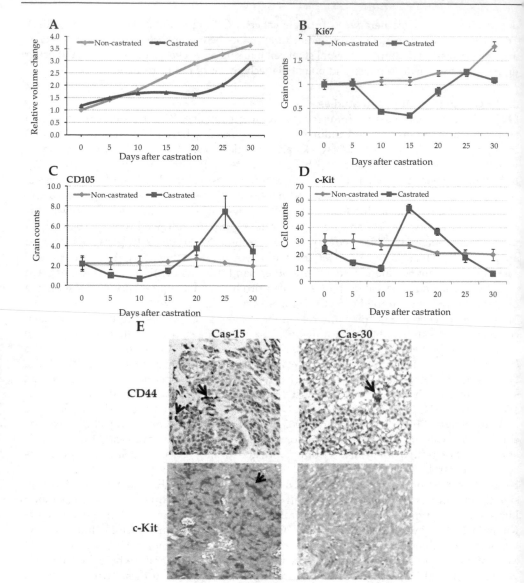

A. *Relative tumor volumes at different time points. Male SCID mice (6-8 wks of age), were inoculated sq with 5 x 10⁶ LNCaP cells per flank. The tumor volumes are shown as the average tumor volume at each time point (5-10 mice) divided by the average tumor volume at day 0.* **B-D**. *Protein expression patterns are summarized as histographs based on IHC data. Cryosections or FFPE (formalin-fixed paraffin-embedded) tissue sections of tumors from each time point (n=4-5) were analyzed for the expression of Ki67 (**B**), CD105 (**C**), and c-Kit (**D**). Five to ten images per section were taken randomly and digitized using the autoscan function of MCID 7.0 software which was set with respect to grain counts (CD105, Ki67) or positively staining cells (c-Kit). Data were analyzed using SigmaPlot. E. Representative images demonstrating expressions of CD44 and c-Kit in tumors at days 15 (Cas-15) and 30 (Cas-30) post castration. (Amplification: 200x).*

Fig. 1. Evaluation of LNCaP tumors in castrated and non-castrated mice.

We also carried out pilot studies with docetaxel chemotherapy in the LNCaP xenografts (Figure 2). Specifically, LNCaP-bearing SCID mice were treated with docetaxel when tumour volumes reached approximately 300 cc (docetaxel was given IP at 8 mg/kg every 3 to 4 days X 4 doses over a two week period). Tumors were harvested from the mice at

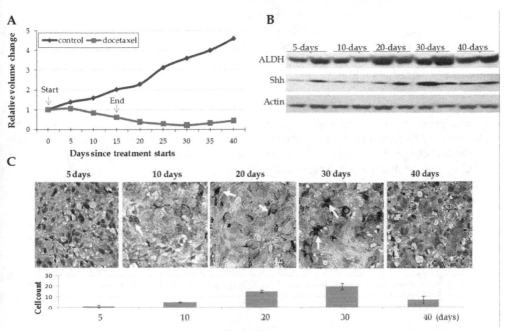

A. *Tumor volumes at different time points. Arrows indicate start and end of docetaxel treatments.* B. *Representative western blot. Expressions of ALDH and Shh at different time points from start of treatment were determined in tumor samples (n=5 per time point).* C. *IHC. c-Kit expression in various tumor tissues. The selected images are representative of 3-5 tumors per time point. Five to 10 images per slide were taken and digitized using MCID 7.0 software. Data were analyzed with SigmaPlot and plotted using Microsoft Excel.*

Fig. 2. Evaluation of LNCaP tumors in docetaxel-treated mice.

	Day-5	Day-10	Day-15	Day-20	Day-25	Day 30
ALDH	0/6	0/6	6/6	3/6	0/6	0/6
Shh	0/6	0/6	6/6	0/6	0/6	0/6
Notch	0/6	0/6	4/6	0/6	0/6	0/6
p63	0/4	ND	4/4	ND	ND	0/4
BCRP	0/4	ND	4/4	ND	ND	0/4
bcl-2	0/4	ND	2/4	ND	ND	0/4

Equal amounts of protein from 3-5 tumors at each time point were analyzed with western blots. After normalization to β–actin, at least double the mean of the band intensities with respect to the non-castrated control samples in each reaction was considered to be overexpressed. ND: not done.

Table 1. The expression of stem cell markers in LNCaP xenografts post castration.

different time points post docetaxel treatment as shown in Figure 2A, and evaluated for ALDH and Shh expression by western blots and for c-Kit expression by IHC (Figures 2B and 2C). Although our analysis is limited, interestingly, as is the case with castrated mice, increased levels of ALDH, Shh and c-Kit were observed in the docetaxel treated mice at points of maximal anti-tumor response (Figures 2A-C). These initial studies suggest that docetaxel treatment can also induce enhanced expression of some of the proteins associated with SLC, although the kinetics of this response are somewhat different than observed in tumors from castrated mice. Thus, there is a trend towards enhanced expression of SLC-related proteins in both castrated mice and docetaxel treated mice at points of maximal anti-tumor response (i.e. when tumors are at their smallest sizes).

3.2 TRAMP based studies

A similar phenomena of enhanced SLC expression post castration was also observed in the TRAMP model in which probasin promoter-driven T antigen expression in mouse prostatic epithelia induces prostate cancers in male mice as they mature sexually (by 8 to 12 weeks of age)(Greenberg et al., 1995; Y. Tang et al. 2008).

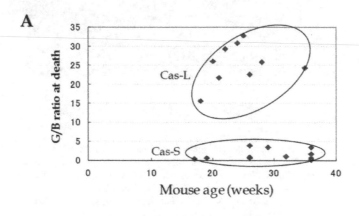

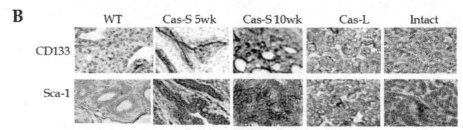

A. *Effects of castration on genitourinary (GU) organs. Based on G/B ratios (GU organs versus mouse body weight), TRAMP mice were divided into two groups after castration – those with G/B ratios ≤ 3.0 (Cas-S) and others with G/B ratios > 20 (Cas-L).* **B**. *IHC. Expressions of CD133 and Sca-1 in TRAMP mouse prostates. These proteins are highly expressed in Cas-S tumors around 5 (Cas-S 5wk; n=3) and 10 wks (Cas-S 10wk; n=3) post castration, but not in Cas-L tumors (n=3). Prostate tumors from non-castrated mice (intact; n=3) and normal prostate tissues from wild-type siblings (n=3) served as controls.*

Fig. 3. Evaluation of tumors in TRAMP mice.

We previously reported that castration of these mice at 12 weeks of age resulted in two different outcomes with respect to anti-tumor response (Y. Tang et al., 2008). In one group of mice, significant locoregional disease progression occurred subsequent to the castration without any evidence of tumor shrinkage such that the mice ended up with large prostatic tumors (designated Castration-Large or Cas-L); in these mice, the average genitourinary (GU) organ weight (which included prostate gland and seminal vesicles) to total body weight (G/B) ratios were 25.43 ± 5.25 (Figure 3A) (Y. Tang et al., 2008). Other mice (designated Castration-Small or Cas-S) had a positive response to castration in that prominent shrinkage of the prostate gland and other GU organs occurred so that the average G/B ratios were around 1.41 ± 1.31 (Figure 3A); despite a positive response to castration the prostate glands still harbored cancer cells. Analysis of two SLC markers, Sca1 (which is mouse-specific) and CD133, in mice responding positively to castration (i.e. small G/B ratios) revealed significant increase of both markers at weeks 5 (Cas-S 5wk) and 10 (Cas-S 10wk) (Figure 3B). By contrast, in Cas-L tumors and in tumors from non-castrated mice, Sca1 and CD133 levels remained low (Figure 3B).

4. Discussion

The above studies indicate that enhanced expression of SLC-related proteins can occur in prostate tumors in response to anti-proliferative/cytotoxic treatments such as androgen deprivation or chemotherapy. Further, this SLC response appears to be transient in nature in that it is generally limited to the time period of maximal anti-tumor response to treatment.

The increased expression of these SLC-related proteins observed in our tumor samples could be due to more proteins being expressed per cell but within a limited number of the cells, or alternatively more cells that express these proteins (but not necessarily at significantly higher levels than baseline) may be recruited, or it could be a combination of these two processes. Regardless of the specifics of the underlying processes associated with each individual protein in terms of patterns and mechanisms of expression, our results indicate that the *overall* expressions of several SLC markers in tumors change as a function of time post treatment. These transient elevations of a relatively broad range of stem cell markers indicate a complex tissue response in which not only tumor cells but other surrounding cells could be involved. We hypothesize that this transient period represents a stemness stage during which cancer cells and surrounding cells can adapt to a changed microenvironment.

Elevations of stem cell related proteins have also been observed by others. For instance, CD44 over expression in breast cancer patients after chemotherapy (X. Li et al., 2008), CD133 over expression in human glioblastoma after radiation (Bao et al., 2006), and ALDH1 over expression and increased enzyme activity in human colorectal xenograft tumors after chemotherapy (Dylla et al., 2008) have been reported. Other forms of stress such as hypoxia and products of metabolism, including lactate and ketones, have also recently been shown to induce stemness in tumor tissues (Kim et al., 2009; Martinez-Outschoorn et al., 2011). Thus, emerging data suggest a correlation between SLC and anti-cancer therapy or other forms of cellular stress, although the exact role of the SLC population in tumor recurrence remains unclear.

Xin et al have shown that prostate glands in C57BL6 wild type mice undergoing castration are enriched in Sca1+ cells, and which are found primarily in the relatively treatment-resistant G0 phase of the cell cycle (Xin et al., 2005). These cells are capable of regenerating tubular structures containing basal cells and luminal cells in a dissociated prostate regeneration system, demonstrating their plasticity and role in prostate regeneration. Moreover, enriched SLC populations have been reported in several tumor-free tissues following local damage (Beltrami et al., 2003; Amcheslavsky et al., 2009). Thus, stemness may represent a protective response by tissue cells, including cancerous cells, to damage or environmental change. This stemness state may in turn allow cells to survive, adapt and grow. Stemness is not an unusual characteristic; many cells possess this ability. As indicated by Zipori et al, all cells possess the molecular machinery that enables them to return to a relatively undifferentiated stem cell-like state when appropriately challenged (Zipori, 2009). Several recent studies have also documented de-differentiation in mature cells (Brawley & Matunis, 2004; Monje et al., 2010; Red-Horse et al., 2010; Shoshani & Zipori, 2011) During tumor recurrence/progression, the de-differentiated SLC can re-differentiate back into the original tumor, or under other conditions, they could trans-differentiate to a different phenotype. Our TRAMP mice castrated at 12 weeks of age all eventually developed prostate cancer, including distant metastasis in over 70% of the animals (Y. Tang et al., 2008, 2009). In several of these mice, neuroendocrine carcinoma (NEC) partially or completely replaced the original adenocarcinomas in the prostate gland and/or distant metastatic sites (Y. Tang et al., 2009); this was rarely observed in the non-castrated mice. Thus, in TRAMP mice regrowth after castration can lead to 'differentiation' along the same original adenocarcinoma pathway or trans-differentiation along the NEC pathway.

A recent study showed that certain differentiated cells in breast tissue *spontaneously* converted to a stem cell-like state (Chaffer et al., 2011). This challenges the scientific dogma that differentiation is a one way path, i.e. once cells specialize they cannot return to a SLC state on their own. Thus, a considerable degree of plasticity exists among cells in their ability to reprogram themselves to a more permissive state not only when appropriately challenged, but under certain conditions this seems to occur spontaneously. The state of 'stemness' that occurs in response to androgen deprivation in our xenograft and transgenic prostate cancer models appears to be transient. Interestingly, recent work has shown that cancer cells in culture exposed to various drugs can undergo histone deacetylation mediated chromatin changes that result in transient reversible drug tolerant states (Sharma et al., 2010).

5. Conclusion

The transient nature of various adaptive responses noted above suggests that to maximize anti-cancer treatments, not only more effective agents need to be developed, but also the relative timing of these treatments with respect to the transient cellular states need to be taken into account. Thus, given that various adaptive cellular processes are dynamic, real time detection and targeting of cancer cells undergoing de-differentiation may improve the efficacy of anti-cancer therapies.

6. Acknowledgment

This work was supported by a Merit Review Award, Department of Veterans Affairs (A. H.).

7. References

Amcheslavsky, A., Jiang, J. and Ip, Y.T., 2009. Tissue damage-induced intestinal stem cell division in Drosophila. Cell Stem Cell, Vol.4, No.1, (January 9, 2009), pp. 49-61, ISSN 1875-9777

Baker, M., 2008. Cancer stem cells, becoming common. In: Nature Report Stem Cell, Vol.153, December 2008, Available from: http://www.natuture.com/stemcells/2008/0812/081203/full/stemcells.2008.153.html

Bao, S., Wu, Q., McLendon, R.E., Hao, Y., Shi, Q., Hjelmenland, A.B., Dewhirst, M.W., Bigner, D.D. and Rich, J.N., 2006. Glioma stem cells promote radioresistance by preferential activation of the DNA damage response. Nature,Vol.444, (December 7, 2006), pp. 756-760, ISSN 1475-4687

Beltrami, A.P., Barlucchi, L., Torella, D., Baker, M., Limana, F., Chimenti, S., Kasahara, H., Rota, M., Musso, E., Urbanek, K., Leri, A., Kajstura, J., Nadal-Ginard, B. and Anversa, P., 2003. Adult cardiac stem cells are multipotent and support myocardial regeneration. Cell, Vol.114, No.6, (September 19, 2003), pp. 763-776, ISSN 1097-4172; 0092-8674

Brawley, C. and Matunis, E., 2004. Regeneration of male germline stem cells by spermatogonial dedifferentiation in vivo. Science (New York, N.Y.), Vol.304, (May 28, 2008), pp. 1331-1334, ISSN 1095-9203; 0036-8075

Chaffer, C.L., Brueckmann, I., Scheel, C., Kaestli, A.J., Wiggins, P.A., Rodrigues, L.O., Brooks, M., Reinhardt, F., Su, Y., Polyak, K., Arendt, L.M., Kuperwasser, C., Bierie, B. and Weinberg, R.A., 2011. Normal and neoplastic nonstem cells can spontaneously convert to a stem-like state. Proceedings of the National Academy of Sciences of the United States of America, Vol.108, No.19, (May 10, 2011), pp. 7950-7955, ISSN 1091-6490; 0027-8424

Clevers, H., 2011. The cancer stem cell: premises, promises and challenges. Nature Medicine, Vol.17, No.3, (March 2011) pp. 313-319, ISSN 1546-170x; 1078-8956

Dalerba, P., Cho, R.W. and Clarke, M.F., 2007. Cancer stem cells: models and concepts. Annual Review of Medicine, Vol.58, (February 2007), pp. 267-284, ISSN 0066-4219

Dylla, S.J., Beviglla, L., Park, I.K., Chartier, C., Raval, J., Ngon, L., Pickell, K., Aguilar, J., Lazetic, S., Smith-Berdan, S., Clarke, M.F., Hoey, T., Lewicki, J. and Gurney, A.L., 2008. Colorectal cancer stem cells are enriched in xenogeneic tumors following chemotherapy. PloS One, Vol.3, No.6, (June 13, 2008) pp. e2428, ISSN 1932-6203

Fabian, A., Barok, M., Vereb, G. and Szollosi, J., 2009. Die hard: are cancer stem cells the Bruce Willises of tumor biology? Cytometry.Part A : The Journal of the International Society for Analytical Cytology, Vol.75, No.1, (January 2009), pp. 67-74, ISSN 1552-4930

Goodell, M.A., Brose, K., Paradis, G., Conner, A.S. and Mulligan, R.C., 1996. Isolation and functional properties of murine hematopoietic stem cells that are replicating in vivo. The Journal of Experimental Medicine, Vol.183, No.4, (April 1, 1996), pp. 1797-1806, ISSN 0022-1007

Greenberg, N.M., Demayo, F., Finegold, M.J., Medina, D., Tilley, W.D., Aspinall, J.O., Cunha, G.R., Donjacour, A.A., Matusik, R.J. and Rosen, J.M., 1995. Prostate cancer in a transgenic mouse. Proceedings of the National Academy of Sciences of the United States of America, Vol.92, No.8, (April 11, 1995), pp. 3439-3443, ISSN 0027-8424

Hermann, P.C., Huber, S.L., Herrler, T., Aicher, A., Ellwart, J.W., Guba, M., Bruns, C.J. and Heeschen, C., 2007. Distinct populations of cancer stem cells determine tumor growth and metastatic activity in human pancreatic cancer. Cell Stem Cell, Vol.1, No.3, (September 13, 2007), pp. 313-323, ISSN 1875-9777

Hoffmann, A. and Tsonis, P.A., 2011. Traveling backward: de-differentiation to stemness. Molecular Interventions, Vol.11, No.1, (February 2011), pp. 15-17, ISSN 1543-2548; 1534-0384

Hope, K.J., Jin, L. and Dick, J.E., 2004. Acute myeloid leukemia originates from a hierarchy of leukemic stem cell classes that differ in self-renewal capacity. Nature Immunology, Vol.5, No.7, (July 2004), pp. 738-743, ISSN 1529-2908

Huntly, B.J. and Gilliland, D.G., 2005. Cancer biology: summing up cancer stem cells. Nature, Vol.435, (June 30, 2005), pp. 1169-1170, ISSN 1476-4687

Jordan, C.T., 2009. Cancer stem cells: controversial or just misunderstood? Cell Stem Cell, Vol.4, No.3, (March 6, 2009), pp. 203-205, 1875-9777

Kim, Y., Lin, Q., Zelterman, D. and Yun, Z., 2009. Hypoxia-regulated delta-like 1 homologue enhances cancer cell stemness and tumorigenicity. Cancer Research, Vol.69, No.24, (December 15, 2009), pp. 9271-9280, ISSN 1538-7445; 0008-5472

Leychkis, Y., Munzer, S.R. and Richardson, J.L., 2009. What is stemness? Studies in History and Philosophy of Science Part C: Studies in History and Philosophy of Biological and Biomedical Sciences, Vol.40, No.4, (December 2009), pp. 312-320, ISSN 1369-8486

Li, H., Chen, X., Calhoun-Davis, T., Claypool, K. and Tang, D.G., 2008. PC3 human prostate carcinoma cell holoclones contain self-renewing tumor-initiating cells. Cancer Research, Vol.68, No.6, (May 15, 2008), pp. 1820-1825, ISSN 1538-7445; 0008-5472

Li, X., Lewis, M.T., Huang, J., Gutierrez, C., Osborne, C.K., Wu, M., Hilsenbeck, S.G., Pavlick, A., Zhang, X., Chamness, G.C., Wong, H., Rosen, J. and Chang, J.C., 2008. Intrinsic Resistance of Tumorigenic Breast Cancer Cells to Chemotherapy. JNCI Journal of the National Cancer Institute, Vol.100, No.9, (May 7, 2008), pp. 672-679, ISSN 1460-2105

Lobo, N.A., Shimono, Y., Qian, D. and Clarke, M.F., 2007. The biology of cancer stem cells. Annual Review of Cell and Developmental Biology, Vol.23, pp. 675-699, ISSN 1081-0706

Ma, S., Chan, K.W., Lee, T.K., Tand, K.H., Wo, J.Y., Zheng, B.J. and Guan, X.Y., 2008. Aldehyde dehydrogenase discriminates the CD133 liver cancer stem cell populations. Molecular Cancer Research, Vol.6, No.7, (July 2008), pp. 1146-1153, ISSN 1541-7786

Marotta, L.L. and Polyak, K., 2009. Cancer stem cells: a model in the making. Current Opinion in Genetics & Development, Vol.19, No.1, (February 2009), pp. 44-50, ISSN 1879-0380

Martinez-outschoorn, U.E., Prisco, M., Ertel, A., Tsirigos, A., Lin, Z., Pavlides, S., Wang, C., Flomenberg, N., Knudsen, E.S., Howell, A., Pestell, R.G., Sotgia, F. and Lisanti, M.P., 2011. Ketones and lactate increase cancer cell "stemness," driving recurrence, metastasis and poor clinical outcome in breast cancer: Achieving personalized medicine via Metabolo-Genomics. Cell Cycle (Georgetown, Tex.), Vol.10, No.8, (April 15, 2011), pp. 1271-1286, ISSN 1551-4005

Monje, P.V., Soto, J., Bacallao, K. and Wood, P.M., 2010. Schwann cell dedifferentiation is independent of mitogenic signaling and uncoupled to proliferation: role of cAMP and JNK in the maintenance of the differentiated state. The Journal of Biological Chemistry, Vol.285, No.40, (October 1, 2010), pp. 31024-31036, ISSN 1083-351x; 0021-9258

O'Brien, C.A., Pollett, A., Gallianger, S. and Dick, J.E., 2007. A human colon cancer cell capable of initiating tumour growth in immunodeficient mice. Nature, Vol.445, No.7123, (January 4, 2007), pp. 106-110, ISSN 1476-4687; 0028-0836

Patrawala, L., Calhoun, T., Schneider-Broussard, R., Li, H., Bhatia, B., Tand, S., Reilly, J.G., Chandra, D., Zhou, J., Claypool, K., Coghlan, L. and Tang, D.G., 2006. Highly purified CD44+ prostate cancer cells from xenograft human tumors are enriched in tumorigenic and metastatic progenitor cells. Oncogene, Vol.25, No.12, (March 16, 2006), pp. 1696-1708, ISSN 0950-9232

Red-Horse, K., Ueno, H., Weissman, I.L. and Krasnow, M.A., 2010. Coronary arteries form by developmental reprogramming of venous cells. Nature, Vol.464, No.7288, (March 25, 2010), pp. 549-553, ISSN 1476-4687; 0028-0836

Schatton, T., Murphy, G.F., Frank, N.Y., Yamaura, K., Waaga-Gasser, A.M., Gasser, M., Zhan, Q., Jordan, S., Duncan, L.M., Weishaupt, C., Fuhlbrigge, R.C., Kupper, T.S., Sayegh, M.H. and Frank, M.H., 2008. Identification of cells initiating human melanomas. Nature, Vol.451, No.7176, (January 17, 2008), pp. 345-349, ISSN 1476-4687; 0028-0836

Sharma, S.V., Lee, D.Y., Li, B., Quinlan, M.P., Takahashi, F., Maheswaran, S., McDermott, U., Azizian, N., Zou, L., Fischbach, M.A., Wong, K.K., Brandstetter, K., Wittner, B., Ramaswamy, S., Classon, M. and Settleman, J., 2010. A chromatin-mediated reversible drug-tolerant state in cancer cell subpopulations. Cell, Vol.141, No.1, (April 2, 2010), pp. 69-80, ISSN 1097-4172; 0092-8674

Shoshani, O. and Zipori, D., 2011. Mammalian Cell Dedifferentiation as a Possible Outcome of Stress. Stem Cell Reviews, http://www.springerlink.com/content/tw8756x14w 1118kn/, (January 29, 2011), ISSN 1558-6804; 1550-8943

Stuelten, C.H., Mertins, S.D., Busch, J.I., Gowens, M., Scudiero, D.A., Burkett, M.W., Hite, K.M., Alley, M., Hollingshead, M., Shoemaker, R.H. and Niederhuber, J.E., 2010. Complex display of putative tumor stem cell markers in the NCI60 tumor cell line panel. Stem Cells (Dayton, Ohio), Vol.28, No.4, (April 2010), pp. 649-660, ISSN 1549-4918; 1066-5099

Tang, C., Ang, B.T. and Pervaiz, S., 2007. Cancer stem cell: target for anti-cancer therapy. Journal of the Federation of American Societies for Experimental Biology, Vol.21, No.14, (December 1, 2007), pp. 3777-3785, ISSN 0892-6638; 1530-6860

Tang, Y., Khan, M.A., Goloubeva, O., Lee, D.I., Jelovac, D., Brodie, A.M. and Hussain, A., 2006. Docetaxel followed by castration improves outcomes in LNCaP prostate cancer-bearing severe combined immunodeficient mice. Clinical Cancer Research, Vol.12, No.1, (January 1, 2006), pp. 169-174, ISSN 1078-0432

Tang, Y., Wang, L., Goloubeva, O., Khan, M.A., Zhang, B. and Hussain, A., 2008. Divergent Effects of Castration on Prostate Cancer in TRAMP Mice: Possible Implications for Therapy. Clinical Cancer Research, Vol.14, No.10, (May 15, 2008), pp. 2936-2943, ISSN 1078-0432

Tang, Y., Wang, L., Goloubeva, O., Khan, M.A., Lee, D. and Hussain, A., 2009. The relationship of neuroendocrine carcinomas to anti-tumor therapies in TRAMP mice. The Prostate, Vol.69, No.16, (December 1, 2009), pp. 1763-1773, ISSN 1097-0045

Tang, Y., Hamburger, A.W., Wang, L., Khan, M.A. and Hussain A., 2010. Androgen deprivation and stem cell markers in prostate cancers. International Journal of

Clinical and Experimental Pathology, Vol.3, No.2, (November 2009), ISSN 1936-2625

Visvader, J.E. and Linderman, G.J., 2008. Cancer stem cells in solid tumours: accumulating evidence and unresolved questions. Nature Reviews. Cancer, Vol.8, No.10, (October 2008), pp. 755-768, ISSN 1474-1768; 1474-175x

Xin, L., Lawson, D.A. and Witte, O.N., 2005. The Sca-1 cell surface marker enriches for a prostate-regenerating cell subpopulation that can initiate prostate tumorigenesis. Proceedings of the National Academy of Sciences of the United States of America, Vol.102, No.19, (May 10, 2005), pp. 6942-6947, ISSN 0027-8424

Yang, J. and Weinberg, R.A., 2008. Epithelial-mesenchymal transition: at the crossroads of development and tumor metastasis. Developmental Cell, Vol.14, No.6, (May 16, 2008), pp. 818-829, ISSN 1097-4172

Zipori, D., 2009. The stem state: Stemness as a state in the cell's life cycle. In: Biology of Stem Cells and the Molecular Basis of the Stem State, K. Turksen, (Ed.), pp. 200-206. Humana Press, New York

13

Inhibition of Advanced Prostate Cancer by Androgens and Liver X Receptor Agonists

Chih-Pin Chuu[1,2], Hui-Ping Lin[1,2], Ching-Yu Lin[1,2],
Chiech Huo[1,2,3] and Liang-Cheng Su[1,2]

[1]*Affiliated University, Institute of Cellular and System Medicine*
[2]*Translational Center for Glandular Malignancies, National Health Research Institutes*
[3]*Department of Life Sciences, National Central University*
Taiwan

1. Introduction

Prostate cancer is the most frequently diagnosed non-cutaneous tumor of men in western countries. National Cancer Institute estimated that more than 217,000 people were diagnosed and 32,000 people died of prostate cancer in the United States in 2010. Currently, primary therapies for prostate cancer include radical prostatectomy, radiation therapy, high-intensity focused ultrasound, chemotherapy, cryosurgery, hormonal therapy, and combination of different treatments. Approximately 20-40% of patients treated with radical prostatectomy will have tumor recurrence and elevation of serum prostate-specific antigen (PSA) (Sadar 2011). More than 80% of patients who died from prostate cancer developed bone metastases, primary metastatic sites include bones and lymph nodes (Bubendorf et al 2000, Ibrahim et al 2010, Keller et al 2001).

In 1941, Huggins and Hodges reported that androgen ablation therapy caused regression of primary and metastatic prostate cancer (Huggins C 1941). Since then, androgen ablation therapy, using luteinizing hormone-releasing hormone agonists (LH-RH) or bilateral orchiectomy, has become one of the primary treatment for prostate cancer (Seruga and Tannock 2008). More than 80% of men with these advanced prostate cancers respond to androgen ablation therapy, resulting in tumors shrinkage and reduction of serum PSA (Seruga and Tannock 2008). Anti-androgens are frequently used in conjunction with androgen ablation therapy as a combined androgen blockade to improve therapeutic outcome (Klotz et al 2004). However, 80-90% of the patients who receive androgen ablation therapy ultimately develop recurrent tumors in 12-33 months. The median overall survival of patients after tumor relapse is 1-2 years (Fowler et al 1998, Hellerstedt and Pienta 2002). In addition, androgen deprivation therapy is associated with several undesired side-effects, including sexual dysfunction, osteoporosis, hot flashes, fatigue, gynecomastia, anemia, depression, cognitive dysfunction, increased risk of diabetes, and cardiovascular diseases (Keating et al 2006, Keating et al 2010, Saigal et al 2007, Seruga and Tannock 2008). Androgen deprivation therapy using LH-RH agonists was reported to increase risk of incident diabetes, incident coronary heart disease, myocardial infarction, sudden cardiac death, and stroke (Keating et al 2006, Keating et al 2010, Saigal et al 2007). Combined androgen blockade was associated with increased risk of incident coronary heart disease (Keating et al 2010). Orchiectomy was associated with coronary heart disease and myocardial infarction (Keating et al 2010). Therefore, shortening the period of androgen ablation therapy may protect the patients.

Liver X receptors (LXRs) are ligand-activated transcriptional factors that belong to the nuclear receptor superfamily. LXRs are important regulators of cholesterol, fatty acid, and glucose homeostasis (Chuu et al 2007). There are two LXR isoforms. LXRα expression is most abundant in liver, kidney, intestine, fat tissue, macrophages, lung, and spleen, while LXRβ is ubiquitously expressed (Chuu et al 2007, Edwards et al 2002, Willy et al 1995). A specific group of oxysterols are natural ligands for LXRs (Chuu et al 2007, Forman et al 1997, Janowski et al 1996). LXR agonists are effective for treatment of murine models of atherosclerosis, diabetes, and Alzheimer's disease (Alberti et al 2001, Blaschke et al 2004, Cao et al 2003, Chuu et al 2007, Edwards et al 2002, Efanov et al 2004, Joseph et al 2002, Joseph et al 2003, Koldamova et al 2005, Peet et al 1998, Song et al 2001, Song and Liao 2001). Our and other groups' previous studies suggested that androgen and LXR agonists may suppress tumor growth of hormone-refractory prostate cancer cells (Chuu et al 2006, Chuu et al 2007, Chuu and Lin 2010, Fukuchi et al 2004b). We thus discuss the possibility of manipulating androgen/androgen receptor (AR) signaling and LXR signaling as a treatment for advanced prostate cancers.

2. Androgens and androgen receptor in prostate cancer

Androgens include testosterone, dehydroepiandrosterone, androstenedione, androstenediol, androsterone, and dihydrotestosterone (DHT). Androgens are mainly produced by testes, while the rest amount of androgens are produced from the adrenal glands. Androgens are important for growth and survival of the prostate cells. Testosterone is the main circulating androgen in human body, while DHT is the more potent androgen (Anderson and Liao 1968, Kokontis and Liao 1999, Liang and Liao 1992). 90% of the free testosterone enters prostate cells is converted to dihydrotestosterone (DHT) by the enzyme 5α-reductase (Liang and Liao 1992). The average serum testosterone level declines with age from approximately 620-670 ng/dl at age 25-44 to 470-520 ng/dl at age 65-84 (Vermeulen 1996). Low serum testosterone level was associated with an increased risk of prostate cancer (Morgentaler and Rhoden 2006), and prostate tumors arising in a low testosterone environment appeared to be more aggressive (Hoffman et al 2000, Lane et al 2008), suggesting a potential therapeutic role for androgen in advanced prostate cancer treatment.

Androgen receptor (AR) is an androgen-activated transcription factor and belongs to the steroid nuclear receptor family. AR is composed of an N-terminal domain, a central DNA-binding domain, and a C-terminal ligand-binding domain (Chang et al 1988a, Chang et al 1988b, Feldman and Feldman 2001). After binding ligand DHT, AR dissociates from heat-shock proteins, phosphorylates, dimerizes, transocates into the nucleus, and binds to androgen-response elements (ARE) in the promoter regions of its target genes under the regulation of co-activators and co-repressors (Feldman and Feldman 2001). Target genes of AR regulate growth, survival, and the production of prostate-specific antigen (PSA) in prostate cells.

Gene microarray study of seven different human prostate cancer xenograft models demonstrated that increase of AR mRNA is the only change consistently associated with the development of androgen-independency phenotype following androgen ablation therapy, and elevation of AR mRNA and protein are both necessary and sufficient progression of prostate cancer towards androgen-independency (Culig et al 1999, Joly-Pharaboz et al 1995). Elevated AR expression in androgen-independent prostate cancer cells or recurrent hormone-refractory tumors has been observed in our progression model (Chuu et al 2005, Chuu et al 2006, Kokontis et al 1994, Kokontis et al 1998, Kokontis et al 2005, Umekita et al 1996) and several other groups (Chen et al 2004a, de Vere White et al 1997, Edwards et al 2003, Ford et al 2003, Gregory et al 2001, Hara et al 2003, Holzbeierlein et al 2004, Kim et al 2002, Linja et al 2001, Shi et al 2004, Singh et al 2004, Visakorpi et al 1995, Wang et al 2001, Zhang et al 2003). Mechanisms contribute to the progression towards androgen-independency including AR gene amplification, AR mutation, bypass of androgenic activation of AR, or bypass AR signaling for cell survival and proliferation (Feldman and Feldman 2001).

3. Androgenic suppression of advanced prostate cancer cells

3.1 Androgenic suppression *in vitro*

LNCaP is one of the most commonly used cell line for prostate cancer research, which was derived from a human lymph node metastatic lesion of prostate adenocarcinoma (Chuu et al 2007, Horoszewicz et al 1980). LNCaP expressed AR and inducible PSA. Previously, we cultured androgen-sensitive LNCaP 104-S cells in androgen-depleted conditions *in vitro* to establish relapsed hormone-refractory prostate cancer cells mimic clinical situation in which prostate cancer recurs during androgen deprivation (Kokontis et al 1994a, Kokontis et al 1998b). After 3 months in medium depleted with androgens, most LNCaP 104-S cells underwent G1 cell cycle arrest and apoptosis. A few colonies of cells, named 104-I cells, evolved that proliferated very slowly in the absence of androgen (Kokontis et al 1994). After approximately 11 months, cells called 104-R1 cells emerged that grew much more rapidly in the absence of androgen. After 20 months, 104-R2 cells evolved which proliferated in the absence of androgen at a rate comparable to the proliferation rate of 104-S cells grown in androgen (Kokontis et al 1994, Kokontis et al 1998).

During the transition of 104-S cells to 104-R1 and 104-R2 cells, AR mRNA and protein level elevated several folds (Chuu et al 2005, Chuu et al 2006, Kokontis et al 1994, Kokontis et al 1998). Proliferation of 104-R1 and 104-R2 cells is androgen-independent but is unexpectedly suppressed by physiological concentrations of androgen both *in vitro* and *in vivo* (Chuu et al 2005, Chuu et al 2006, Kokontis et al 1994, Kokontis et al 1998b, Kokontis et al 2005, Umekita et al 1996). When 104-R1 cells were incubated for several weeks in a high concentration of synthetic androgen R1881 (20 nM), cells named R1Ad adapted after a period of growth arrest (Kokontis et al 1998). Growth of R1Ad cells is slow and not dependent on androgen but is stimulated by 10 nM R1881.

To further mimic the clinical situation of combined androgen deprivation and anti-androgen therapy, LNCaP 104-S cells were incubated with 5 μM Casodex (biculatimide) in androgen-deprived medium. After four weeks, Casodex-resistant colonies appeared at low frequency (1 in 1.4×10^5) as most of the cells appeared to undergo senescent cell death. The relapsed cells, called CDXR, had increased AR expression and were repressed by androgen (Kokontis et al 2005). Unlike 104-R1 cells, most CDXR cells grown in 10 nM R1881 underwent apoptosis 6 to 8 days after R1881 exposure. However, 1 in 1.9×10^3 cells relapsed as androgen-insensitive that were not repressed by R1881 or Casodex. These sublines, designated IS, showed greatly reduced AR expression (Kokontis et al 2005). Growth of IS cells was not stimulated by R1881 or suppressed by Casodex. 104-R2 cells, like CDXR cells, gave rise to androgen-insensitive cells after androgen treatment (unpublished data). Therefore, during progression from 104-R1 to 104-R2 stages, the cells appear to pass a point where cells can no longer recover responsiveness to androgen, but instead progress to androgen insensitivity (Liao et al 2005). Direct progression of 104-S cells to the CDXR stage by selection in androgen-depleted medium containing anti-androgen seems to bypass this intermediate 104-R1 stage. Androgen-suppressive phenotype and elevated AR of hormone-refractory LNCaP cells was observed by several other groups (Culig et al 1999, Joly-Pharaboz et al 1995, Joly-Pharaboz et al 2000, Shi et al 2004, Soto et al 1995). The progression model of LNCaP is shown in Figure 1.

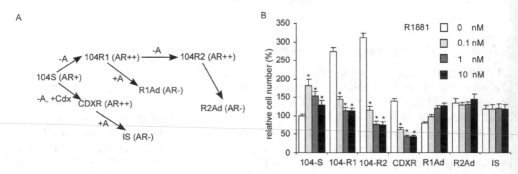

Fig. 1. The LNCaP cell line progression model. (A) AR expression level increases during the progression from androgen-dependent LNCaP 104-S cells to androgen-independent 104-R1, 104-R2, and CDXR cells. Proliferation of LNCaP 104-R1, 104-R2, CDXR cells are suppressed by androgen, but these cells can adapt to androgenic suppression and evolve as R1Ad, R2Ad, and IS cells. R1Ad, R2Ad, and IS cells express very little AR. (B) Effect of 96 h treatment of synthetic androgen (0, 0.1, 1, 10 nM) R1881 on 104-S, 104-R1, 104-R2, CDXR, R1Ad, R2Ad, IS cells was assayed by 96-well proliferation assay.

LNCaP cells express a mutant AR (T877A) that displays relaxed ligand binding specificity (Kokontis et al 1991, Veldscholte et al 1990), however, androgenic suppression is not limited to LNCaP cells. ARCaP is an AR-positive, tumorigenic, and highly metastatic cell line derived from the ascites fluid of a patient with advanced metastatic disease. Proliferation of ARCaP cells is suppressed by androgen (Zhau et al 1996). MDA PCa 2b-hr was generated *in vitro* from bone metastasis-derived, androgen-dependent MDA PCa 2b human PC cells with higher AR proteins. Proliferation of MDA PCa 2b-hr was inhibited by testosterone concentration higher than 3.5 nM or Casodex (Hara et al 2003). PC-3 is a commonly used human prostate cancer cell lines established from bone-derived metastases with no AR expression (Chuu et al 2007). Physiological concentration of DHT caused growth inhibition, G1 cell cycle arrest, and apoptosis in PC-3 cells over-expressing full length wild-type AR (Heisler et al 1997, Litvinov et al 2004, Yuan et al 1993).

3.2 Androgenic suppression *in vivo*
Castration causes regression of 104-S xenografts but tumor relapsed after 8 weeks as androgen-independent relapsed tumors 104-Rrel with elevated mRNA and protein

expression of AR (Chuu et al 2006). Low serum level of testosterone (130 ± 60 ng/dl), stop tumor growth of 104-Rrel tumors but tumor growth resumed in 4 weeks. High serum level of testosterone (2970 ± 495 ng/dl), which is approximately 5-fold higher than normal level, caused regression of 104-Rrel tumors growth. However, all 104-Rrel cells adapted to androgen and relapsed after 4 weeks as androgen-stimulated 104-Radp tumors (Chuu et al 2006) (Figure 2). Growth of the LNCaP 104-R1 tumors was also suppressed by androgen, but all tumors adapted to androgenic suppression and relapsed as androgen-stimulated R1Ad tumors in 5-6 weeks (Chuu et al 2005). Growth of R1Ad tumors was stimulated by testosterone and removal of testosterone totally stopped the tumor growth (Chuu et al 2005, Chuu et al 2006). Both 104-Radp and R1Ad tumors express very little AR and PSA mRNA and protein or serum PSA level (Figure 2), similar to R1Ad cells observed in cell culture (Chuu et al 2005, Chuu et al 2006, Kokontis et al 1998).

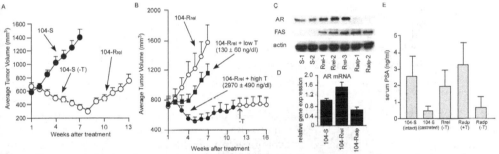

Fig. 2. Progression of androgen-dependent LNCaP 104-S tumors to androgen-independent 104-Rrel tumors, and androgenic growth suppression of 104-Rrel tumors. (A) Mice were injected subcutaneously with androgen-dependent 104-S cells. After allowing tumors to grow for 7 weeks, mice were separated into control (filled circles, 14 mice with 19 tumors) and castration groups (open circles, 24 mice with 36 tumors) and the time was designated as week 1 (Chuu et al 2006). (B) Mice in the castrated group in (A) at the 14th week were separated into 3 groups including a control group (open circles, 6 mice with 9 tumors), a low dosage testosterone treatment group that received a subcutaneous implant of a 20 mg TP/cholesterol (1:9) pellet (filled squares, 9 mice with 12 tumors), and a high-dosage testosterone treatment group that received a subcutaneous implant of a 20 mg pure TP pellet (filled circles, 10 mice with 12 tumors) (Chuu et al 2006). Tumor volumes are expressed as the mean + standard error. (C) PSA, AR, and actin protein levels in 104-S tumor (in intact mice), 104-Rrel-T tumors, 104-Radp-1+T tumors, and 104Radp-T were assayed by Western blot (Chuu et al 2005). (D) Serum PSA level of mice with 104-S tumors (in intact mice), 104-Rrel-T tumors, 104-Rrel+T tumors, Radp+T tumors, Radp-T tumors was determined by Elisa kit (Chuu et al 2005).

Both early and late treatment of androgen caused regression of CDXR3 tumors. 70% of tumors regress completely and the rest of tumors relapse after 60-90 days of treatment (Kokontis et al 2005) (Figure 3). The relapsed tumors show diminished expression of AR and no longer require androgen for growth, essentially identical to the behavior of IS3 cells that emerged after androgen exposure *in vitro* (Kokontis et al 2005). It is worthwhile to notice that 100% of 104-R1 tumor being treated with testosterone relapsed in 4-5 weeks, while only 30% of CDXR tumors relapsed after 9-13 weeks after testosterone treatment (Chuu et al

2005, Kokontis et al 2005). This is probably due to the apoptosis induced in CDXR cells but not in 104-R1 cells by androgen (Kokontis et al 1998, Kokontis et al 2005). Regression and relapse after androgen treatment of LNCaP xenograft was also observed by other group (Joly-Pharaboz et al 2000) and ARCaP xenograft (Zhau et al 1996).

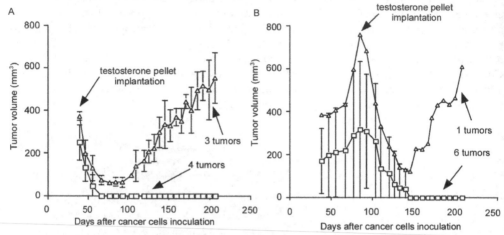

Fig. 3. Regression and relapse of LNCaP CDXR-3 tumor xenografts in nude mice treated with testosterone (A) LNCaP CDXR-3 tumor xenografts in castrated male nude mice were allowed to grow until they reached an average volume of 400 mm³ on the 38th day. All mice carrying tumors received a subcutaneous implant of a 20mg testosterone. The mice in the control group were implanted with a 20 mg testosterone pellet either at early stage (50 days after inoculation) or late stage (92 days after inoculation). Open triangle represent tumors relapsed, while open squares represent tumors disappeared after androgen treatment. Tumor volumes are expressed as the mean ± standard error.

3.3 Molecular mechanism of androgenic suppression

Antiandrogen Casodex (bicalutamide) does not affect proliferation of 104-R1 and 104-R2 cells but blocked androgenic repression of growth as well as androgenic induction of PSA (Kokontis et al 1998). Knockdown of AR expression in CDXR3 cells by shRNA relieved androgenic repression of growth (Kokontis et al 2005). Retroviral overexpression of AR in IS cells restored the androgen-repressed phenotype in these cells (Kokontis et al 2005). These observations confirmed that androgen cause growth inhibition via AR.

Synthetic androgen R1881 increases S phase population in androgen-dependent LNCaP 104-S cells but induces G1 arrest in androgen-independent LNCaP cells (such as 104-R1m 104-R2, CDXR, etc.) within 24 hours of treatment (Joly-Pharaboz et al 2000, Kokontis et al 1994, Kokontis et al 1998, Kokontis et al 2005, Soto et al 1995) (Figure 4). Cell cycle inhibitors p21[wafl/cip1] and p27[Kip1] were induced by androgen in 104-R1 and 104-R2 cells (Kokontis et al 1998a) (Figure 4). In contrast, expression of p21[wafl/cip1] and p27[Kip1] was repressed by androgen in 104-S cells. Androgen down-regulates F-box protein S phase kinase-associated protein 2 (Skp2), a protein mediating the ubiquitination and degradation of p27[Kip1]. Androgen also decreases c-Myc at the protein and mRNA level in hours in 104-R1 cells (Figure 5). Enforced retroviral overexpression of c-Myc blocks androgenic repression of 104-

R1 growth (Kokontis et al 1994). Therefore, androgen regulate cell cycle and proliferation of LNCaP cells via AR, Skp2, c-Myc, and p27^{Kip1}.

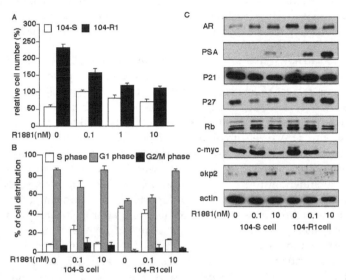

Fig. 4. Effect of androgen on cell proliferation, cell cycle, and cell cycle-related proteins in androgen-dependent 104-S and androgen-independent 104-R1 cells. (A) LNCaP 104-S and 104-R2 cells were treated with increasing concentration of synthetic androgen R1881 for 96 hours. Relative cell number was determined by 96-well proliferation assay and was normalized to cell number of 104-S cells at 0.1 nM R1881. (B) Percentage of 104-S and 104-R1 cells in S phase determined by flow cytometry. LNCaP 104-S and 104-R2 cells were treated with increasing concentration of synthetic androgen R1881 for 96 hours. Values represent the mean +/- Standard Error derived from 5 independent experiments. (C) Protein expression of androgen receptor (AR), prostate specific antigen (PSA), p21^{cip}, p27^{Kip}, retinoblastoma protein (Rb), c-myc, S phase kinase-associated protein 2 (Skp2) were determined by Western bloting assay in 104-S and 104-R1 cells treated 96 hrs with different concentration of R1881. β-actin was used as loading control.

4. Androgen treatment of advanced prostate cancer in clinical

Clinical and basic studies showed that in comparison with continuous androgen ablation (CAB) therapy, intermittent androgen suppression (IAS) therapy substantially prolongs the time to development of castration-resistant prostate cancer (Akakura et al 1993, Mathew 2008, Sato et al 1996, Szmulewitz et al 2009). Intermittent androgen ablation therapy is a strategy to periodically perform and terminate the androgen ablation therapy, allowing the endogenous testosterone level to elevate during the period between ablation therapies. IAS therapy delayed the androgen-independent progression of Shionogi mammary carcinoma (Akakura et al 1993) and LNCaP xenograft (Sato et al 1996). Pether et al. reported in a clinical trial of 102 patients that there is a trend toward extended times to progression and death compared to CAB treatment, and growth of advanced prostate tumors was delayed in ~50% patients treated with IAS (Pether et al 2003). Bruchovsky et al. showed that IAS therapy cause repeated differentiation of tumor with recovery of apoptotic potential, inhibition of tumor growth by rapid restoration of serum testosterone, and restraint of tumor growth by subnormal levels of serum testosterone (Bruchovsky et al 2000). They concluded that IAS is a viable treatment option for men with prostate cancer which affords an improved quality of life as well as reduced toxicity and costs (Bruchovsky et al 2000, Morris et al 2009, Pether et al 2003).

A few studies have shown that androgen is safe and potentially effective for treatment of advanced prostate cancer. Mathew reported that the testosterone level in a prostate cancer patient undergone radical prostatectomy and LH-RH therapy remained at castrated levels and serum PSA was undetectable for 15 years. PSA levels then began to rise and the patient was given testosterone replacement therapy to attain a normal range of serum testosterone. After an initial flare, PSA levels gradually declined over 18 months. After 27 months, PSA level started to increase. When testosterone replacement therapy was discontinued, PSA levels dropped (Mathew 2008). The observation was similar to the transition from 104-R1 to R1Ad phenotype under androgen treatment in our LNCaP progression model (Chuu et al 2005, Kokontis et al 1998). Szmulewitz et al. reported that 15 prostate cancer patients with progressive disease following androgen ablation, anti-androgen therapy, and withdrawal without minimal metastatic disease were randomized to treatment with three doses of transdermal testosterone of 2.5, 5.0, or 7.5 mg/day, resulting in increase of serum testosterone concentrations to 305 ng/dl, 308 ng/dl, and 297 ng/dl, respectively. The conclusion of this study is that testosterone is a feasible and reasonably well-tolerated therapy for men with early hormone-refractory prostate cancer (Szmulewitz et al 2009). Morris et el. performed a phase 1 clinical trial to determine the safety of high-dose exogenous testosterone in patients with castration-resistant metastatic prostate cancer. Cohorts of 3-6 patients with progressive castration-resistant prostate cancer who had been castrated for at least 1 yr received testosterone by skin patch or topical gel for 1 week, 1 month, or until disease progression. No adverse effect was reported. The serum testosterone ranged from 330-870 ng/dl (Morris et al 2009). This study suggested that patients with advanced prostate cancer can be safely treated with exogenous testosterone. Researchers suggested that maximizing testosterone serum levels in selected patients with androgen receptor over-expression may improve the treatment outcome.

5. Liver X receptor (LXR) signaling

5.1 LXRα and LXRβ

Liver X receptors are ligand-activated transcriptional factors that belong to the nuclear receptor superfamily. There are two LXR isoforms, LXRα and LXRβ (Chuu et al 2007). Although LXRα and LXRβ share high similarity in their DNA- and ligand-binding domains, expression of these proteins in various tissues differs. LXRα expression is restricted to liver, kidney, intestine, fat tissue, macrophages, lung, and spleen (Edwards et al 2002, Willy et al 1995). LXRβ is ubiquitously expressed (Song et al 1994). LXRα and LXRβ form heterodimers with the obligate partner 9-cis retinoic acid receptor (RXR) (Chuu et al 2007, Song et al 1994, Willy et al 1995). The LXR/RXR heterodimer can be activated with either an LXR agonist (oxysterols) or a RXR agonist (cis-retinoic acid). Oxysterols are oxygenated derivatives of cholesterol. Oxysterols, such as 22(R)-hydroxycholesterol, 24(S)-hydroxycholesterol, and cholestenoic acid, are natural ligands for LXR (Chuu et al 2007, Forman et al 1997, Janowski et al 1996). A few synthetic LXR agonists have been developed, including non-steroidal LXR agonists T0901317 (Schultz et al 2000) and GW3965 (Collins et al 2002), and steroidal LXR agonists hypocholamide (Song and Liao 2001) and YT-32 (Kaneko et al 2003)].

5.2 Role of LXR signaling in metabolism

LXRs are important regulators of cholesterol, fatty acid, and glucose homeostasis (Chuu et al 2007). Oral administration of an LXR agonist has an overall hypolipidemic effect in hypercholesterolemic rats, mice, and hamsters (Song and Liao 2001). LXRα-/- mice are healthy when fed with a low-cholesterol diet. However, LXRα-/- mice develop enlarged fatty livers, hepatocellular degeneration, high hepatic cholesterol levels, and impaired liver function when fed a high-cholesterol diet (Alberti et al 2001, Edwards et al 2002, Peet et al 1998). LXRβ-/- mice are unaffected by a high-cholesterol diet, suggesting that LXRα and LXRβ have separate roles. LXRα and LXRβ regulate cholesterol transport. LXRs induces expression of the cholesterol transporters ATP-binding cassette transporter A1 and G1 (ABCA1 and ABCG1) (Edwards et al 2002, Nakamura et al 2004, Venkateswaran et al 2000) as well as cholesterol acceptor apolipoprotein E (ApoE) (Chawla et al 2001). Treatment with LXR agonists (hypocholamide, T0901317, or GW3965) lowers the cholesterol level in serum and liver and inhibits the development of atherosclerosis in murine disease models (Blaschke et al 2004, Joseph et al 2002, Song et al 2001, Song and Liao 2001).

LXRs regulate fatty acid synthesis by modulating the expression of sterol regulatory element-binding protein-1c (SREBP-1c) (Repa et al 2000, Yoshikawa et al 2001) and downstream lipogenic genes, including acetyl CoA carboxylase and FAS (Liang et al 2002). LXRs also regulate insulin signaling in liver (Chen et al 2004b, Tobin et al 2002). LXRα-/-LXRβ-/- double knockout mice lack insulin-mediated induction of an entire class of enzymes involved in both fatty acid and cholesterol metabolism (Tobin et al 2002). Treatment with T0901317 stimulates insulin secretion in pancreatic beta cells, reduces plasma glucose, and improves glucose tolerance and insulin resistance in murine and rat obesity models (Cao et al 2003, Efanov et al 2004, Joseph et al 2003).

LXR signaling is important for brain function as well. LXRs regulate lipid homeostasis in the brain. LXRα-/- LXRβ-/- mice develop neurodegenerative changes in brain tissue (Wang et al 2002). Knockout of LXRβ, but not LXRα, results in adult-onset motor neuron degeneration in male mice (Andersson et al 2005), suggesting a different role of LXRβ from LXRα. Treatment with T0901317 decreases amyloidal beta production in an Alzheimer's disease mouse model (Koldamova et al 2005).

6. Anti-cancer effect of LXR agonists

6.1 Anti-proliferative effect of LXR agonists in cancer cells

Based on our recent observations using several prostate cancer cell lines, we discovered that LXR agonists suppress proliferation of human prostate cancer cell lines. Treatment of PC-3, DU-145, and LNCaP sublines (104-S, 104-R1, 104-R2, CDXR, R1Ad, IS) cells with LXR agonists (22(R)-hydroxycholesterol, 24(S)-hydroxycholesterol, or T0901317) suppresses the proliferation of these cells (Chuu and Lin 2010, Fukuchi et al 2004b, Vigushin et al 2004).

LXR agonists treatment causes growth inhibition in prostate cancer cells via induction of G1 cell cycle arrest (Chuu and Lin 2010, Fukuchi et al 2004b). T0901317 decreases the percentage of cells in S-phase and increases the percentage of cells in G1-phase. T0901317 suppresses the expression of Skp2 and causes the accumulation of p27Kip1. Overexpression of Skp2 in PC-3 cells or knockdown of p27Kip1 in LNCaP cells increases the resistance of cells to T0901317 treatment (Chuu and Lin 2010, Fukuchi et al 2004b). Daily oral administration of T0901317 (10 mg/kg) suppresses growth of androgen-dependent LNCaP 104-S prostate tumors in athymic mice, resulting in a 2-fold difference in mean tumor volume between the control and the T0901317 treatment group (Fukuchi et al 2004b) (Figure 5).

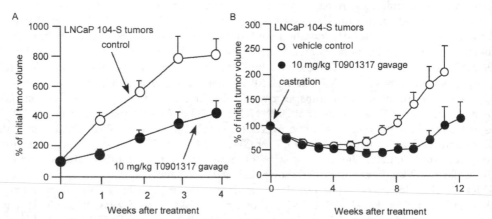

Fig. 5. Inhibition of proliferation and progression of prostate cancer by the LXR agonists T0901317. (A) Mice carrying 104-S tumors were administered 10 mg/kg T0901317 (filled circle, 10 mice with 13 tumors) or vehicle alone (open circle, 10 mice with 15 tumors) by gavage once a day during the experiment period, resulting in a more than 2-fold difference in mean tumor volume between vehicle and T0901317-treated tumors after 4 weeks. Relative tumor volumes were expressed as mean ± SE. (Fukuchi et al 2004b). (B) After castration, mice carrying 104-S tumors were administered 10 mg/kg T0901317 (filled circle, 9 mice with 15 tumors) or vehicle alone (open circles, 9 mice with 13 tumors) by gavage five times a week during the experiment period, resulting in a 4-week delay in time required for development of androgen-independent relapsed tumors between vehicle and T0901317-treated group. Relative tumor volumes were expressed as mean ± SE. See reference 8 for details.

T0901317 and 22(R)-hydroxycholesterol also suppresses the proliferation of several commonly used human cancer cell lines, including breast cancer MCF-7 cells, hepatoma HepG2 cells, non-small lung cancer H1299 cells, cervical cancer HeLa cells, epidermoid carcinoma A431 cells, osteosarcoma saos-2 cells, melanoma MDA-MB-435 cells, squamous carcinoma SCC13 cells, CAOV3 and SKOV3 ovarian cancer cells, as well as T and B cells of chronic lymphoblastic leukemia (CLL) (Chuu and Lin 2010, Fukuchi et al 2004b, Geyeregger et al 2009, Scoles et al 2010, Vedin et al 2009). Expression of LXRα mRNA in these cancer cells correlates with the cancer cells' sensitivity to 22(R)-hydroxycholesterol treatment (Chuu and Lin 2010), suggesting that G1 cell cycle arrest induced by LXR agonists in cancer cells is partially mediated through LXRα gene regulation (Fukuchi et al 2004b).

The EC_{50} for 22(R)-hydroxycholesterol in suppressing the proliferation of cancer cells (Chuu and Lin 2010) is comparable to the concentration required for 22(R)-hydroxycholesterol to activate LXRα (1.5 μM) (Janowski et al 1996), this may explain why the level of LXRα correlates with the sensitivity of different cancer cells to 22(R)-hydroxycholesterol treatment. The effective concentrations for 22(R)-hydroxycholesterol to suppress cancer cell growth is within its known physiological range and is much lower than the concentrations to activate other nuclear receptors (Janowski et al 1996). LXRβ-ABCG1 signaling was reported to regulate sterol metabolism (Bensinger et al 2008). Activation of LXRβ inhibited the proliferation of T-cells but had no effect on cell viability (Bensinger et al 2008). Since T0901317 did not inhibit the proliferation of CAOV3 ovarian cancer cells treated with siRNA against LXRα or LXRβ (Scoles et al 2010), it is possible that 22(R)-hydroxycholesterol inhibited cell proliferation mainly through activation of LXRα, while inhibition of T0901317 may be caused by both LXRα and LXRβ activation. We did not observe T0901317 to cause cancer cell growth inhibition at 300 nM (data not shown). It is unclear why the concentration needed for T0901317 to suppress the proliferation of human cancer cells is 15-fold higher than the effective concentration for T0901317 to activate LXRα (20 nM) (Schultz et al 2000). The concentration of T0901317 observed to cause growth inhibition of ovarian cancer cell lines by Scoles et al. was 10-50 nM when the researchers used 0.1% FBS (Scoles et al 2010). We used 10% FBS in our study, it is possible that some proteins or growth factors in serum may hinder the suppressive effect of T0901317.

6.2 Inhibition of prostate cancer progression by LXR agonists

In our progression model, expression of LXRα and its target gene ABCA1 is higher in androgen-dependent LNCaP 104-S cells than in androgen-independent LNCaP 104-R1 and 104-R2 cells (Fukuchi et al 2004a). Expression of the LXRα, ABCA1, and sterol 27-hydroxylase (CYP27) genes, all target genes of LXRα, decreases during prostate cancer progression towards androgen-independency in athymic mice (Chuu et al 2006). The change in expression of genes involved in LXR signaling suggests a potential role of LXR signaling during prostate cancer progression. LXR agonists treatment on LNCaP sublines suggested that androgen-dependency and expression of AR level did not affect the growth inhibition caused by LXR agonists, thus LXR agonists may inhibit different progression stages of prostate tumors in patients (Chuu and Lin 2010).

We found that suppression of ABCA1 expression by androgen coincided with increased proliferation of androgen-dependent LNCaP 104-S cells (Fukuchi et al 2004a). Thus, under androgen-depleted conditions, ABCA1 levels are high and proliferation of 104-S cells is inhibited. During progression, the surviving androgen-independent relapsed tumor cells appear to escape ABCA1 suppression by down-regulating expression of LXR target genes. T0901317 induces expression of the ABCA1 gene in 104-S tumors in athymic mice (Fukuchi et al 2004b). Compared to the control group, T0901317 treatment delays the development of androgen-independent relapsed tumors for 4 weeks in athymic mice bearing 104-S tumors after castration (Chuu et al 2006) (Figure 5). This result indicates that treatment with an LXR agonist may retard development of androgen-independent prostate cancer.

7. Conclusion

Our LNCaP progression model may provide the molecular explanation for IAS treatment. As most relapsed prostate tumors after androgen ablation therapy express AR and expression of mRNA and protein level of AR are frequently elevated (de Vere White et al 1997, Ford et al 2003, Linja et al 2001), restoration of endogenous testosterone level by IAS treatment or treatment with exogenous testosterone will suppress the proliferation of the AR-rich relapsed prostate cancer cell according, similar to the observations in LNCaP 104-R1, 104-R2, CDXR, and in other relapsed prostate cancer cell models. Patients showed no response to IAS treatment might have tumors with very low or no AR expression. At the beginning of IAS or testosterone treatment, serum PSA level will increase dramatically (Mathew 2008), similar to the stimulated PSA expression in 104-R1, 104-R2, and CDXR cells. The AR-rich relapsed prostate cancer cells will then undergo G1 cell cycle arrest and/or apoptosis, causing the regression of tumor and decrease of serum PSA level. The regression of tumors can continue for weeks or months before the prostate cancer cells adapt to the androgenic suppression, possibly by down-regulating AR. The adapted cells are probably similar to R1Ad cells in patients receiving androgen ablation therapy (LH-RH agonists) or similar to IS cells in patients receiving combined treatment of LH-RH agonists and anti-androgens. The PSA secretion stimulated by androgen in R1Ad or IS cells is very low, so the serum PSA level will remain low until the adapted tumors start to grow, either stimulated by testosterone like R1Ad cells or by androgen-insensitive growth like IS cells. IAS will delay the growth of R1Ad-like but not IS-like tumors, therefore, only the subgroup of patients carrying R1Ad-like tumors will respond to the subsequent cycles of IAS treatment. As 104-R1 cells will progress to 104-R2 cells in androgen-depleted medium and 104-R2 cells, like CDXR cells, will generate IS-like cells following androgen treatment, patients receiving a few cycle of IAS treatment will ultimately develop IS-like tumors which don't respond to further IAS treatment. Alternative therapies, such as green tea catechin epigallocatechin 3-gallate (EGCG) or liver X receptor agonists might be able to suppress growth of these androgen-insensitive prostate tumors.

Patients develop relapsed androgen-independent prostate tumors after androgen ablation therapy should be biopsied for expression level of AR protein in tumors. IAS and/or administration of androgen at a concentration 5-fold higher than the physiologic concentration will benefit patients with AR-rich relapsed tumors by suppressing tumor growth, improving quality of life, and reducing risks for cardiovascular diseases and diabetes. Combined treatment of androgen ablation therapy with anti-androgen may cause a more rapid and irreversible selection of CDXR-like advanced prostate cancer cells, although androgen treatment may cause regression and disappearance of these tumors (Kokontis et al 2005). Androgen deprivation therapy alone, on the other hand, may promote a slow adaptation to androgen-independence. LXR agonists suppress the proliferation of multiple human prostate cancer cell lines via reduction of Skp2 and induction of $p27^{Kip}$, thus cause G1 cell cycle arrest. LXR agonist T0901317 treatment also delays the progression of androgen-dependent LNCaP xenograft towards androgen-independency in castrated nude mice. It is therefore possible to modulate LXR signaling as an adjuvant therapy for treatment of all stages of prostate cancer. In conclusion, manipulating androgen/AR might be a potential therapy for AR-positive advanced prostate cancer, and LXR agonists might be an adjuvant therapy for treatment of advanced prostate cancer.

8. Acknowledgements

This work is supported by CS-100-PP-12 (NHRI), DOH100-TD-C-111-014 (DOH), and NSC 99-2320-B-400-015-MY3 (NSC) in Taiwan for C.-P.Chuu.

9. References

Akakura K, Bruchovsky N, Goldenberg SL, Rennie PS, Buckley AR &Sullivan LD (1993) Effects of intermittent androgen suppression on androgen-dependent tumors. Apoptosis and serum prostate-specific antigen. *Cancer*, Vol.71, No.9, (May 1993), pp.2782-2790, ISSN 0008-543X

Alberti S, Schuster G, Parini P, Feltkamp D, Diczfalusy U, Rudling M, Angelin B, Bjorkhem I, Pettersson S &Gustafsson JA (2001) Hepatic cholesterol metabolism and resistance to dietary cholesterol in LXRbeta-deficient mice. *J Clin Invest*, Vol.107, No.5, (Mar 2001), pp.565-573, ISSN 0021-9738

Anderson KM &Liao S (1968) Selective retention of dihydrotestosterone by prostatic nuclei. *Nature*, Vol.219, No.5151, (Jul 1968), pp.277-279, ISSN 0028-0836

Andersson S, Gustafsson N, Warner M &Gustafsson JA (2005) Inactivation of liver X receptor beta leads to adult-onset motor neuron degeneration in male mice. *Proc Natl Acad Sci U S A*, Vol.102, No.10, (Mar 2005), pp.3857-3862, ISSN 0027-8424

Bensinger SJ, Bradley MN, Joseph SB, Zelcer N, Janssen EM, Hausner MA, Shih R, Parks JS, Edwards PA, Jamieson BD &Tontonoz P (2008) LXR signaling couples sterol metabolism to proliferation in the acquired immune response. *Cell*, Vol.134, No.1, (Jul 2008), pp.97-111, ISSN 1097-4172

Blaschke F, Leppanen O, Takata Y, Caglayan E, Liu J, Fishbein MC, Kappert K, Nakayama KI, Collins AR, Fleck E, Hsueh WA, Law RE &Bruemmer D (2004) Liver X receptor agonists suppress vascular smooth muscle cell proliferation and inhibit neointima formation in balloon-injured rat carotid arteries. *Circ Res*, Vol.95, No.12, (Dec 10,2004), pp.e110-123, ISSN 1524-4571

Bruchovsky N, Klotz LH, Sadar M, Crook JM, Hoffart D, Godwin L, Warkentin M, Gleave ME &Goldenberg SL (2000) Intermittent androgen suppression for prostate cancer: Canadian Prospective Trial and related observations. *Mol Urol*, Vol.4, No.3, (Fall 2000), pp.191-199;discussion 201, ISSN 1091-5362

Bubendorf L, Schopfer A, Wagner U, Sauter G, Moch H, Willi N, Gasser TC &Mihatsch MJ (2000) Metastatic patterns of prostate cancer: an autopsy study of 1,589 patients. *Hum Pathol*, Vol.31, No.5, (May 2000), pp.578-583, ISSN 0046-8177

Cao G, Liang Y, Broderick CL, Oldham BA, Beyer TP, Schmidt RJ, Zhang Y, Stayrook KR, Suen C, Otto KA, Miller AR, Dai J, Foxworthy P, Gao H, Ryan TP, Jiang XC, Burris TP, Eacho PI &Etgen GJ (2003) Antidiabetic action of a liver x receptor agonist mediated by inhibition of hepatic gluconeogenesis. *J Biol Chem*, Vol.278, No.2, (Jan 2003), pp.1131-1136, ISSN 0021-9258

Chang CS, Kokontis J &Liao ST (1988a) Molecular cloning of human and rat complementary DNA encoding androgen receptors. *Science*, Vol.240, No.4850, (Apr 1988), pp.324-326, ISSN 0036-8075

Chang CS, Kokontis J &Liao ST (1988b) Structural analysis of complementary DNA and amino acid sequences of human and rat androgen receptors. *Proc Natl Acad Sci U S A*, Vol.85, No.19, (Oct 1988), pp.7211-7215, ISSN 0027-8424

Chawla A, Boisvert WA, Lee CH, Laffitte BA, Barak Y, Joseph SB, Liao D, Nagy L, Edwards PA, Curtiss LK, Evans RM &Tontonoz P (2001) A PPAR gamma-LXR-ABCA1 pathway in macrophages is involved in cholesterol efflux and atherogenesis. *Mol Cell*, Vol.7, No.1, (Jan 2001), pp.161-171, ISSN 1097-2765

Chen CD, Welsbie DS, Tran C, Baek SH, Chen R, Vessella R, Rosenfeld MG &Sawyers CL
    (2004a) Molecular determinants of resistance to antiandrogen therapy. *Nat Med*,
    Vol.10, No.1, (Jan 2004), pp.33-39, ISSN 1078-8956

Chen G, Liang G, Ou J, Goldstein JL &Brown MS (2004b) Central role for liver X receptor in
    insulin-mediated activation of Srebp-1c transcription and stimulation of fatty acid
    synthesis in liver. *Proc Natl Acad Sci U S A*, Vol.101, No.31, (Aug 2004), pp.11245-
    11250, ISSN 0027-8424

Chuu CP, Hiipakka RA, Fukuchi J, Kokontis JM &Liao S (2005) Androgen causes growth
    suppression and reversion of androgen-independent prostate cancer xenografts to
    an androgen-stimulated phenotype in athymic mice. *Cancer Res*, Vol.65, No.6, (Mar
    2005), pp.2082-2084, ISSN 0008-5472

Chuu CP, Hiipakka RA, Kokontis JM, Fukuchi J, Chen RY &Liao S (2006) Inhibition of
    tumor growth and progression of LNCaP prostate cancer cells in athymic mice by
    androgen and liver X receptor agonist. *Cancer Res*, Vol.66, No.13, (Jul 2006),
    pp.6482-6486, ISSN 0008-5472

Chuu CP, Kokontis JM, Hiipakka RA &Liao S (2007) Modulation of liver X receptor
    signaling as novel therapy for prostate cancer. *J Biomed Sci*, Vol.14, No.5, (Sep 2007),
    pp.543-553, ISSN 1021-7770

Chuu CP, Chen RY, Kokontis JM, Hiipakka RA &Liao S (2009) Suppression of androgen
    receptor signaling and prostate specific antigen expression by (-)-epigallocatechin-
    3-gallate in different progression stages of LNCaP prostate cancer cells. *Cancer Lett*,
    Vol.275, No.1, (Mar 2009), pp.86-92, ISSN 1872-7980

Chuu CP &Lin HP (2010) Antiproliferative effect of LXR agonists T0901317 and 22(R)-
    hydroxycholesterol on multiple human cancer cell lines. *Anticancer Res*, Vol.30,
    No.9, (Sep 2010), pp.3643-3648, ISSN 1791-7530

Collins JL, Fivush AM, Watson MA, Galardi CM, Lewis MC, Moore LB, Parks DJ, Wilson JG,
    Tippin TK, Binz JG, Plunket KD, Morgan DG, Beaudet EJ, Whitney KD, Kliewer SA
    &Willson TM (2002) Identification of a nonsteroidal liver X receptor agonist
    through parallel array synthesis of tertiary amines. *J Med Chem*, Vol.45, No.10, (May
    2002), pp.1963-1966, ISSN 0022-2623

Culig Z, Hoffmann J, Erdel M, Eder IE, Hobisch A, Hittmair A, Bartsch G, Utermann G,
    Schneider MR, Parczyk K &Klocker H (1999) Switch from antagonist to agonist of
    the androgen receptor bicalutamide is associated with prostate tumour progression
    in a new model system. *Br J Cancer*, Vol.81, No.2, (Sep 1999), pp.242-251, ISSN 0007-
    0920

de Vere White R, Meyers F, Chi SG, Chamberlain S, Siders D, Lee F, Stewart S &Gumerlock
    PH (1997) Human androgen receptor expression in prostate cancer following
    androgen ablation. *Eur Urol*, Vol.31, No.1, (1997), pp.1-6, ISSN 0302-2838

Edwards J, Krishna NS, Grigor KM &Bartlett JM (2003) Androgen receptor gene
    amplification and protein expression in hormone refractory prostate cancer. *Br J
    Cancer*, Vol.89, No.3, (Aug 2003), pp.552-556, ISSN 0007-0920

Edwards PA, Kennedy MA &Mak PA (2002) LXRs; oxysterol-activated nuclear receptors
    that regulate genes controlling lipid homeostasis. *Vascul Pharmacol*, Vol.38, No.4,
    (Apr 2002), pp.249-256, ISSN 1537-1891

Efanov AM, Sewing S, Bokvist K &Gromada J (2004) Liver X receptor activation stimulates insulin secretion via modulation of glucose and lipid metabolism in pancreatic beta-cells. *Diabetes*, Vol.53 Suppl 3, (Dec 2004), pp.S75-78, ISSN 0012-1797

Feldman BJ &Feldman D (2001) The development of androgen-independent prostate cancer. *Nat Rev Cancer*, Vol.1, No.1, (Oct 2001), pp.34-45, ISSN 1474-175X

Ford OH, 3rd, Gregory CW, Kim D, Smitherman AB &Mohler JL (2003) Androgen receptor gene amplification and protein expression in recurrent prostate cancer. *J Urol*, Vol.170, No.5, (Nov 2003), pp.1817-1821, ISSN 0022-5347

Forman BM, Ruan B, Chen J, Schroepfer GJ, Jr. &Evans RM (1997) The orphan nuclear receptor LXRalpha is positively and negatively regulated by distinct products of mevalonate metabolism. *Proc Natl Acad Sci U S A*, Vol.94, No.20, (Sep 1997), pp.10588-10593, ISSN 0027-8424

Fowler JE, Jr., Bigler SA, Kolski JM &Yee DT (1998) Early results of a prospective study of hormone therapy for patients with locally advanced prostate carcinoma. *Cancer*, Vol.82, No.6, (Mar 1998), pp.1112-1117, ISSN 0008-543X

Fukuchi J, Hiipakka RA, Kokontis JM, Hsu S, Ko AL, Fitzgerald ML &Liao S (2004a) Androgenic suppression of ATP-binding cassette transporter A1 expression in LNCaP human prostate cancer cells. *Cancer Res*, Vol.64, No.21, (Nov 2004), pp.7682-7685, ISSN 0008-5472

Fukuchi J, Kokontis JM, Hiipakka RA, Chuu CP &Liao S (2004b) Antiproliferative effect of liver X receptor agonists on LNCaP human prostate cancer cells. *Cancer Res*, Vol.64, No.21, (Nov 2004), pp.7686-7689, ISSN 0008-5472

Geyeregger R, Shehata M, Zeyda M, Kiefer FW, Stuhlmeier KM, Porpaczy E, Zlabinger GJ, Jager U &Stulnig TM (2009) Liver X receptors interfere with cytokine-induced proliferation and cell survival in normal and leukemic lymphocytes. *J Leukoc Biol*, Vol.86, No.5, (Nov 2009), pp.1039-1048, ISSN 1938-3673

Gregory CW, Johnson RT, Jr., Mohler JL, French FS &Wilson EM (2001) Androgen receptor stabilization in recurrent prostate cancer is associated with hypersensitivity to low androgen. *Cancer Res*, Vol.61, No.7, (Apr 2001), pp.2892-2898, ISSN 0008-5472

Hara T, Nakamura K, Araki H, Kusaka M &Yamaoka M (2003) Enhanced androgen receptor signaling correlates with the androgen-refractory growth in a newly established MDA PCa 2b-hr human prostate cancer cell subline. *Cancer Res*, Vol.63, No.17, (Sep 2003), pp.5622-5628, ISSN 0008-5472

Heisler LE, Evangelou A, Lew AM, Trachtenberg J, Elsholtz HP &Brown TJ (1997) Androgen-dependent cell cycle arrest and apoptotic death in PC-3 prostatic cell cultures expressing a full-length human androgen receptor. *Mol Cell Endocrinol*, Vol.126, No.1, (Jan 1997), pp.59-73, ISSN 0303-7207

Hellerstedt BA &Pienta KJ (2002) The current state of hormonal therapy for prostate cancer. *CA Cancer J Clin*, Vol.52, No.3, (May-Jun 2002), pp.154-179, ISSN 0007-9235

Hoffman MA, DeWolf WC &Morgentaler A (2000) Is low serum free testosterone a marker for high grade prostate cancer? *J Urol*, Vol.163, No.3, (Mar 2000), pp.824-827, ISSN 0022-5347

Holzbeierlein J, Lal P, LaTulippe E, Smith A, Satagopan J, Zhang L, Ryan C, Smith S, Scher H, Scardino P, Reuter V &Gerald WL (2004) Gene expression analysis of human prostate carcinoma during hormonal therapy identifies androgen-responsive genes and mechanisms of therapy resistance. *Am J Pathol*, Vol.164, No.1, (Jan 2004), pp.217-227, ISSN 0002-9440

Horoszewicz JS, Leong SS, Chu TM, Wajsman ZL, Friedman M, Papsidero L, Kim U, Chai LS, Kakati S, Arya SK &Sandberg AA (1980) The LNCaP cell line--a new model for studies on human prostatic carcinoma. *Prog Clin Biol Res*, Vol.37, (1980), pp.115-132, ISSN 0361-7742

Huggins C SR, Hodges C (1941) Studies on prostatic cancer: II. The effects of castration on advanced carcinoma of the prostate gland. *Arch Surg*, Vol.43, No.2, (1941), pp.15,

Ibrahim T, Flamini E, Mercatali L, Sacanna E, Serra P &Amadori D (2010) Pathogenesis of osteoblastic bone metastases from prostate cancer. *Cancer*, Vol.116, No.6, (Mar 2010), pp.1406-1418, ISSN 0008-543X

Janowski BA, Willy PJ, Devi TR, Falck JR &Mangelsdorf DJ (1996) An oxysterol signalling pathway mediated by the nuclear receptor LXR alpha. *Nature*, Vol.383, No.6602, (Oct 1996), pp.728-731, ISSN 0028-0836

Joly-Pharaboz MO, Soave MC, Nicolas B, Mebarki F, Renaud M, Foury O, Morel Y &Andre JG (1995) Androgens inhibit the proliferation of a variant of the human prostate cancer cell line LNCaP. *J Steroid Biochem Mol Biol*, Vol.55, No.1, (Oct1995), pp.67-76, ISSN 0960-0760

Joly-Pharaboz MO, Ruffion A, Roch A, Michel-Calemard L, Andre J, Chantepie J, Nicolas B &Panaye G (2000) Inhibition of growth and induction of apoptosis by androgens of a variant of LNCaP cell line. *J Steroid Biochem Mol Biol*, Vol.73, No.5, (Jul-Aug 2000), pp.237-249, ISSN 0960-0760

Joseph SB, McKilligin E, Pei L, Watson MA, Collins AR, Laffitte BA, Chen M, Noh G, Goodman J, Hagger GN, Tran J, Tippin TK, Wang X, Lusis AJ, Hsueh WA, Law RE, Collins JL, Willson TM &Tontonoz P (2002) Synthetic LXR ligand inhibits the development of atherosclerosis in mice. *Proc Natl Acad Sci U S A*, Vol.99, No.11, (May 2002), pp.7604-7609, ISSN 0027-8424

Joseph SB, Castrillo A, Laffitte BA, Mangelsdorf DJ &Tontonoz P (2003) Reciprocal regulation of inflammation and lipid metabolism by liver X receptors. *Nat Med*, Vol.9, No.2, (Feb 2003), pp.213-219, ISN 1078-8956

Kaneko E, Matsuda M, Yamada Y, Tachibana Y, Shimomura I &Makishima M (2003) Induction of intestinal ATP-binding cassette transporters by a phytosterol-derived liver X receptor agonist. *J Biol Chem*, Vol.278, No.38, (Sep 2003), pp.36091-36098, ISSN 0021-9258

Keating NL, O'Malley AJ &Smith MR (2006) Diabetes and cardiovascular disease during androgen deprivation therapy for prostate cancer. *J Clin Oncol*, Vol.24, No.27, (Sep 2006), pp.4448-4456, ISSN 1527-7755

Keating NL, O'Malley AJ, Freedland SJ &Smith MR (2010) Diabetes and cardiovascular disease during androgen deprivation therapy: observational study of veterans with prostate cancer. *J Natl Cancer Inst*, Vol.102, No.1, (Jan 2010), pp.39-46, ISSN 1460-2105

Keller ET, Zhang J, Cooper CR, Smith PC, McCauley LK, Pienta KJ &Taichman RS (2001) Prostate carcinoma skeletal metastases: cross-talk between tumor and bone. *Cancer Metastasis Rev*, Vol.20, No.3-4, (2001), pp.333-349, ISSN 0167-7659

Kim D, Gregory CW, French FS, Smith GJ &Mohler JL (2002) Androgen receptor expression and cellular proliferation during transition from androgen-dependent to recurrent growth after castration in the CWR22 prostate cancer xenograft. *Am J Pathol*, Vol.160, No.1, (Jan 2002), pp.219-226, ISSN 0002-9440

Klotz L, Schellhammer P &Carroll K (2004) A re-assessment of the role of combined androgen blockade for advanced prostate cancer. *BJU Int*, Vol.93, No.9, (Jun 2004), pp.1177-1182, ISSN 1464-4096

Kokontis J, Ito K, Hiipakka RA &Liao S (1991) Expression and function of normal and LNCaP androgen receptors in androgen-insensitive human prostatic cancer cells. Altered hormone and antihormone specificity in gene transactivation. *Receptor*, Vol.1, No.4, (1991), pp.271-279, ISSN 1052-8040

Kokontis J, Takakura K, Hay N &Liao S (1994) Increased androgen receptor activity and altered c-myc expression in prostate cancer cells after long-term androgen deprivation. *Cancer Res*, Vol.54, No.6, (Mar 1994), pp.1566-1573, ISSN 0008-5472

Kokontis JM, Hay N &Liao S (1998) Progression of LNCaP prostate tumor cells during androgen deprivation: hormone-independent growth, repression of proliferation by androgen, and role for p27Kip1 in androgen-induced cell cycle arrest. *Mol Endocrinol*, Vol.12, No.7, (Jul 1998), pp.941-953, ISSN 0888-8809

Kokontis JM &Liao S (1999) Molecular action of androgen in the normal and neoplastic prostate. *Vitam Horm*, Vol.55, (1999), pp.219-307, ISSN 0083-6729

Kokontis JM, Hsu S, Chuu CP, Dang M, Fukuchi J, Hiipakka RA &Liao S (2005) Role of androgen receptor in the progression of human prostate tumor cells to androgen independence and insensitivity. *Prostate*, Vol.65, No.4, (Dec 2005), pp.287-298, ISSN 0270-4137

Koldamova RP, Lefterov IM, Staufenbiel M, Wolfe D, Huang S, Glorioso JC, Walter M, Roth MG &Lazo JS (2005) The liver X receptor ligand T0901317 decreases amyloid beta production in vitro and in a mouse model of Alzheimer's disease. *J Biol Chem*, Vol.280, No.6, (Feb 2005), pp.4079-4088, ISSN 0021-9258

Lane BR, Stephenson AJ, Magi-Galluzzi C, Lakin MM &Klein EA (2008) Low testosterone and risk of biochemical recurrence and poorly differentiated prostate cancer at radical prostatectomy. *Urology*, Vol.72, No.6, (Dec 2008), pp.1240-1245, ISSN 1527-9995

Liang G, Yang J, Horton JD, Hammer RE, Goldstein JL &Brown MS (2002) Diminished hepatic response to fasting/refeeding and liver X receptor agonists in mice with selective deficiency of sterol regulatory element-binding protein-1c. *J Biol Chem*, Vol.277, No.11, (Mar 2002), pp.9520-9528, ISSN 0021-9258

Liang T &Liao S (1992) Inhibition of steroid 5 alpha-reductase by specific aliphatic unsaturated fatty acids. *Biochem J*, Vol.285 (Pt 2), (Jul 1992), pp.557-562, ISSN 0264-6021

Liao S, Umekita Y, Guo J, Kokontis JM &Hiipakka RA (1995) Growth inhibition and regression of human prostate and breast tumors in athymic mice by tea epigallocatechin gallate. *Cancer Lett*, Vol.96, No.2, (Sep 1995), pp.239-243, ISSN 0304-3835

Liao S, Kokontis JM, Chuu CP, Hsu S, Fukuchi J, Dang MT &Hiipakka RA (2005). Four stages of prostate cancer: suppression and eradication by androgen and green tea epigallocatechin gallate. In: Li JJ, Li SA (eds). *Hormonal Carcinogenesis IV*. Springer: New York. pp 211-220. ISBN 038-7237-83-6

Linja MJ, Savinainen KJ, Saramaki OR, Tammela TL, Vessella RL &Visakorpi T (2001) Amplification and overexpression of androgen receptor gene in hormone-refractory prostate cancer. *Cancer Res*, Vol.61, No.9, (May 2001), pp.3550-3555, ISSN 0008-5472

Litvinov IV, Antony L &Isaacs JT (2004) Molecular characterization of an improved vector for evaluation of the tumor suppressor versus oncogene abilities of the androgen receptor. *Prostate*, Vol.61, No.4, (Dec 2004), pp.299-304, ISSN 0270-4137

Mathew P (2008) Prolonged control of progressive castration-resistant metastatic prostate cancer with testosterone replacement therapy: the case for a prospective trial. *Ann Oncol*, Vol.19, No.2, (Feb 2008), pp.395-396, ISSN 1569-8041

Morgentaler A &Rhoden EL (2006) Prevalence of prostate cancer among hypogonadal men with prostate-specific antigen levels of 4.0 ng/mL or less. *Urology*, Vol.68, No.6, (Dec 2006), pp.1263-1267, ISSN 1527-9995

Morris MJ, Huang D, Kelly WK, Slovin SF, Stephenson RD, Eicher C, Delacruz A, Curley T, Schwartz LH &Scher HI (2009) Phase 1 trial of high-dose exogenous testosterone in patients with castration-resistant metastatic prostate cancer. *Eur Urol*, Vol.56, No.2, (Aug 2009), pp.237-244, ISSN 1873-7560

Nakamura K, Kennedy MA, Baldan A, Bojanic DD, Lyons K &Edwards PA (2004) Expression and regulation of multiple murine ATP-binding cassette transporter G1 mRNAs/isoforms that stimulate cellular cholesterol efflux to high density lipoprotein. *J Biol Chem*, Vol.279, No.44, (Oct 2004), pp.45980-45989, ISSN 0021-9258

Peet DJ, Turley SD, Ma W, Janowski BA, Lobaccaro JM, Hammer RE &Mangelsdorf DJ (1998) Cholesterol and bile acid metabolism are impaired in mice lacking the nuclear oxysterol receptor LXR alpha. *Cell*, Vol.93, No.5, (May 1998), pp.693-704, ISSN 0092-8674

Pether M, Goldenberg SL, Bhagirath K &Gleave M (2003) Intermittent androgen suppression in prostate cancer: an update of the Vancouver experience. *Can J Urol*, Vol.10, No.2, (Apr 2003), pp.1809-1814, ISSN 1195-9479

Repa JJ, Liang G, Ou J, Bashmakov Y, Lobaccaro JM, Shimomura I, Shan B, Brown MS, Goldstein JL &Mangelsdorf DJ (2000) Regulation of mouse sterol regulatory element-binding protein-1c gene (SREBP-1c) by oxysterol receptors, LXRalpha and LXRbeta. *Genes Dev*, Vol.14, No.22, (Nov 2000), pp.2819-2830, ISSN 0890-9369

Sadar MD (2011) Small molecule inhibitors targeting the "achilles' heel" of androgen receptor activity. *Cancer Res*, Vol.71, No.4, (Feb 2011), pp.1208-1213, ISSN 1538-7445

Saigal CS, Gore JL, Krupski TL, Hanley J, Schonlau M &Litwin MS (2007) Androgen deprivation therapy increases cardiovascular morbidity in men with prostate cancer. *Cancer*, Vol.110, No.7, (Oct 2007), pp.1493-1500, ISSN 0008-543X

Sato N, Gleave ME, Bruchovsky N, Rennie PS, Goldenberg SL, Lange PH &Sullivan LD (1996) Intermittent androgen suppression delays progression to androgen-independent regulation of prostate-specific antigen gene in the LNCaP prostate tumour model. *J Steroid Biochem Mol Biol*, Vol.58, No.2, (May 1996), pp.139-146, ISSN 0960-0760

Schultz JR, Tu H, Luk A, Repa JJ, Medina JC, Li L, Schwendner S, Wang S, Thoolen M, Mangelsdorf DJ, Lustig KD &Shan B (2000) Role of LXRs in control of lipogenesis. *Genes Dev*, Vol.14, No.22, (Nov 2000), pp.2831-2838, ISSN 0890-9369

Scoles DR, Xu X, Wang H, Tran H, Taylor-Harding B, Li A &Karlan BY (2010) Liver X receptor agonist inhibits proliferation of ovarian carcinoma cells stimulated by oxidized low density lipoprotein. *Gynecol Oncol*, Vol.116, No.1, (Jan 2010), pp.109-116, ISSN 1095-6859

Seruga B &Tannock IF (2008) Intermittent androgen blockade should be regarded as standard therapy in prostate cancer. *Nat Clin Pract Oncol*, Vol.5, No.10, (Oct 2008), pp.574-576, ISSN 1743-4262

Shi XB, Ma AH, Tepper CG, Xia L, Gregg JP, Gandour-Edwards R, Mack PC, Kung HJ &deVere White RW (2004) Molecular alterations associated with LNCaP cell progression to androgen independence. *Prostate*, Vol.60, No.3, (Aug 2004), pp.257-271, ISSN 0270-4137

Singh SS, Qaqish B, Johnson JL, Ford OH, 3rd, Foley JF, Maygarden SJ &Mohler JL (2004) Sampling strategy for prostate tissue microarrays for Ki-67 and androgen receptor biomarkers. *Anal Quant Cytol Histol*, Vol.26, No.4, (Aug,2004), pp.194-200, ISSN 0884-6812

Song C, Kokontis JM, Hiipakka RA &Liao S (1994) Ubiquitous receptor: a receptor that modulates gene activation by retinoic acid and thyroid hormone receptors. *Proc Natl Acad Sci U S A*, Vol.91, No.23, (Nov 8,1994), pp.10809-10813, ISSN 0027-8424

Song C, Hiipakka RA &Liao S (2001) Auto-oxidized cholesterol sulfates are antagonistic ligands of liver X receptors: implications for the development and treatment of atherosclerosis. *Steroids*, Vol.66, No.6, (Jun 2001), pp.473-479, ISSN 0039-128X

Song C &Liao S (2001) Hypolipidemic effects of selective liver X receptor alpha agonists. *Steroids*, Vol.66, No.9, (Sep 2001), pp.673-681, ISSN ISSN 0039-128X

Soto AM, Lin TM, Sakabe K, Olea N, Damassa DA &Sonnenschein C (1995) Variants of the human prostate LNCaP cell line as tools to study discrete components of the androgen-mediated proliferative response. *Oncol Res*, Vol.7, No.10-11, (1995), pp.545-558, ISSN 0965-0407

Szmulewitz R, Mohile S, Posadas E, Kunnavakkam R, Karrison T, Manchen E &Stadler WM (2009) A randomized phase 1 study of testosterone replacement for patients with low-risk castration-resistant prostate cancer. *Eur Urol*, Vol.56, No.1, (Jul 2009), pp.97-103, ISSN 1873-7560

Tobin KA, Ulven SM, Schuster GU, Steineger HH, Andresen SM, Gustafsson JA &Nebb HI (2002) Liver X receptors as insulin-mediating factors in fatty acid and cholesterol biosynthesis. *J Biol Chem*, Vol.277, No.12, (Mar 2002), pp.10691-10697, ISSN 0021-9258

Umekita Y, Hiipakka RA, Kokontis JM &Liao S (1996) Human prostate tumor growth in athymic mice: inhibition by androgens and stimulation by finasteride. *Proc Natl Acad Sci U S A*, Vol.93, No.21, (Oct 1996), pp.11802-11807, ISSN 0027-8424

Vedin LL, Lewandowski SA, Parini P, Gustafsson JA &Steffensen KR (2009) The oxysterol receptor LXR inhibits proliferation of human breast cancer cells. *Carcinogenesis*, Vol.30, No.4, (Apr 2009), pp.575-579, ISSN 1460-2180

Veldscholte J, Ris-Stalpers C, Kuiper GG, Jenster G, Berrevoets C, Claassen E, van Rooij HC, Trapman J, Brinkmann AO &Mulder E (1990) A mutation in the ligand binding domain of the androgen receptor of human LNCaP cells affects steroid binding characteristics and response to anti-androgens. *Biochem Biophys Res Commun*, Vol.173, No.2, (Dec 1990), pp.534-540, ISSN 0006-291X

Venkateswaran A, Laffitte BA, Joseph SB, Mak PA, Wilpitz DC, Edwards PA &Tontonoz P (2000) Control of cellular cholesterol efflux by the nuclear oxysterol receptor LXR alpha. *Proc Natl Acad Sci U S A*, Vol.97, No.22, (Oct 2000), pp.12097-12102, ISSN 0027-8424

Vermeulen A, Oddens, B.J. (1996) Declining Androgens with Age: An Overview. *Androgens and the Aging Male*, (1996), pp.3-14, ISBN 185-0707-63-4

Vigushin DM, Dong Y, Inman L, Peyvandi N, Alao JP, Sun C, Ali S, Niesor EJ, Bentzen CL &Coombes RC (2004) The nuclear oxysterol receptor LXRalpha is expressed in the normal human breast and in breast cancer. *Med Oncol*, Vol.21, No.2, (2004), pp.123-131, ISSN 1357-0560

Visakorpi T, Hyytinen E, Koivisto P, Tanner M, Keinanen R, Palmberg C, Palotie A, Tammela T, Isola J &Kallioniemi OP (1995) In vivo amplification of the androgen receptor gene and progression of human prostate cancer. *Nat Genet*, Vol.9, No.4, (Apr 1995), pp.401-406, ISSN 1061-4036

Wang L, Schuster GU, Hultenby K, Zhang Q, Andersson S &Gustafsson JA (2002) Liver X receptors in the central nervous system: from lipid homeostasis to neuronal degeneration. *Proc Natl Acad Sci U S A*, Vol.99, No.21, (Oct 2002), pp.13878-13883, ISSN 0027-8424

Wang LG, Ossowski L &Ferrari AC (2001) Overexpressed androgen receptor linked to p21WAF1 silencing may be responsible for androgen independence and resistance to apoptosis of a prostate cancer cell line. *Cancer Res*, Vol.61, No.20, (Oct 2001), pp.7544-7551, ISSN 0008-5472

Willy PJ, Umesono K, Ong ES, Evans RM, Heyman RA &Mangelsdorf DJ (1995) LXR, a nuclear receptor that defines a distinct retinoid response pathway. *Genes Dev*, Vol.9, No.9, (May 1995), pp.1033-1045, ISSN 0890-9369

Yoshikawa T, Shimano H, Amemiya-Kudo M, Yahagi N, Hasty AH, Matsuzaka T, Okazaki H, Tamura Y, Iizuka Y, Ohashi K, Osuga J, Harada K, Gotoda T, Kimura S, Ishibashi S &Yamada N (2001) Identification of liver X receptor-retinoid X receptor as an activator of the sterol regulatory element-binding protein 1c gene promoter. *Mol Cell Biol*, Vol.21, No.9, (May 2001), pp.2991-3000, ISSN 0270-7306

Yuan S, Trachtenberg J, Mills GB, Brown TJ, Xu F &Keating A (1993) Androgen-induced inhibition of cell proliferation in an androgen-insensitive prostate cancer cell line (PC-3) transfected with a human androgen receptor complementary DNA. *Cancer Res*, Vol.53, No.6, (Mar 1993), pp.1304-1311, ISSN 0008-5472

Zhang L, Johnson M, Le KH, Sato M, Ilagan R, Iyer M, Gambhir SS, Wu L &Carey M (2003) Interrogating androgen receptor function in recurrent prostate cancer. *Cancer Res*, Vol.63, No.15, (Aug 2003), pp.4552-4560, ISSN 0008-5472

Zhau HY, Chang SM, Chen BQ, Wang Y, Zhang H, Kao C, Sang QA, Pathak SJ &Chung LW (1996) Androgen-repressed phenotype in human prostate cancer. *Proc Natl Acad Sci U S A*, Vol.93, No.26, (Dec 1996), pp.15152-15157, ISSN 0027-8424

14

New Botanical Materials with Anti-Androgenic Activity

Tomoyuki Koyama
Tokyo University of Marine Science and Technology
Japan

1. Introduction

Enlargement of prostate, which affects 50% of men aged 60 and 90% of men by age 80, is commonly referred to as benign prostate hyperplasia (BPH) (Russell & Wilson, 1994). BPH is a slow, progressive enlargement of the fibromuscular and epithelial structures of the prostate gland (Cristoni et al., 2000). Substantial evidence indicates that the androgens testosterone (T) and dihydrotestosterone (DHT) contribute to the production of BPH (Lowe et al., 2003). The principal serum androgen T is converted by 5alpha-reductase (5aR) to DHT. DHT binds to androgen receptor (AR) in the prostate, where it initiates DNA synthesis (Marks, 2004). This action, in turn induces protein synthesis and abnormal growth of prostate. Current clinical evidence indicates that either the inhibition of 5aR or the inhibition of the binding of DHT to AR reverses the symptoms of BPH in human males.

The effective drugs, finasteride as a 5aR inhibitor and flutamide as a binding inhibitor to AR are utiliezed clinically for treatment of BPH. Alternatively functional foods are eclectic selection as dietary approaches to prevent BPH in middle-aged men. Natural products are frequently used to care BPH in preference to therapeutic agents that can cause severe side-effects. Plant extracts such as the lipid extracts of saw palmetto berry extract (SPE) have also been found to reduce the conversion of testosterone (T) to dihydrotestosterone (DHT) by inhibiting 5alpha-reductase (5aR) both in vitro and in vivo (Elliot, 2001). However, few products of natural origin besides SPE are believed to be effective against enlargement of the prostate. The scientifically-proven food materials are expected to be of benefit for prevention of BPH.

In our preliminary study, the suppressive effects of natural food materials have been found in BHT model mice. We introduce here the suppressive effects against BHT of two materials, i.e., "banana peel" and "leaf of *Houttuynia cordata*". The effects of these materials in the androgen-responsive LNCaP human prostate cancer cell line and in effects of BHT model mice were examined. These data presented here demonstrate that these materials inhibit the growth of the prostate and HCE has anti-androgenic activity.

2. Experimental

2.1 Drugs and chemicals

The chemicals used and their sources were as follows: testosterone propionate and dihydrotestosterone from Wako Pure Chemical Industries (Osaka, Japan); flutamide from

Sigma–Aldrich Japan (Tokyo); finasteride from LKT Labs. (St. Paul, MN); and pentobarbital from Dainippon Sumitomo Pharma (Osaka, Japan). Other chemicals were of analytical grade.

2.2 Animal experiments

Male ddY mice (6-8 weeks of age) were purchased from SLC Inc., Shizuoka, Japan. The room was maintained at 24±1°C and 50±10% humidity under a 12 h light/dark cycle (lights on from 8:00 AM to 8:00 PM), and the animals had free access to water and food. Animal studies were conducted according to the 2006 guidelines entitled Notification No. 88 of the Ministry of the Environment in Japan and Guidelines for Animal Experimentation of Tokyo University of Marine Science and Technology with the approval of the Animal Care and Use Committee of Tokyo University of Marine Science and Technology.

2.3 Growth suppression of mouse prostates and seminal vesicles in testosterone-induced BPH model mice

Assay of growth suppression in castrated mouse prostates and seminal vesicles was performed based on the OECD protocol. (Yamasaki et al., 2003) The testes of ddY mice were removed at 7 weeks of age under anesthesia by intraperitoneal injection of pentobarbital (50 mg/ml/kg). After 1 d, testosterone propionate (TP) was injected intraperitoneally into the mice once daily for 10 d. Enlargement of the reproductive organs in the mice was demonstrated dose-dependently due to TP in our preliminary studies as shown in Fig. 1A. The growth of these organs is androgen-dependent (Franck-Lissbrant et al., 1998).

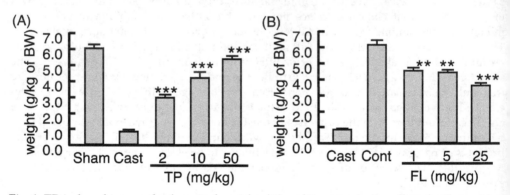

Fig. 1. TP-induced regrowth of seminal vesicles (A) and its suppressive effects by flutamide (B) in castrated mice

Testosterone propionate (TP; 2, 10, and 50 mg/kg) was injected i.p. into castrated mice (7-weeks-old) once daily for 10 days. Flutamide (1, 5, and 25 mg/kg) suspended in 1% ethanol and orally administered once daily. The seminal vesicles were removed and weighed and compared with castrated mice as a control. Cast: castrated control, Cont: control (TP-treated), and FL: flutamide. Each value represents the mean ± S.E., $n=5$. **: $p<0.01$,***: $p<0.005$ vs control.

To evaluate the effects on reproductive organs, each of various doses of sample extract was suspended in 1% ethanol and orally administered to the BPH model mice once daily. After 10 d, the mice were weighed, and sacrificed by cervical dislocation. The lengths of the short and long axes of the prostates were then measured with vernier calipers, and the seminal vesicles were removed and weighed. In particular, the weights of the seminal vesicles were sensitive to androgenic effects in our mice model. Finasteride (FI, 2 mg/kg) and flutamide (FL, 10 mg /kg) were used as positive control for the assay system. As shown in Fig. 1B, orally administration of flutamide suppressed weight of the seminal vesicles in BPH model mice with dose dependent manner (1-25 mg/kg/day) for 10 d.

2.4 Cell culture and growth studies of human prostate cancer cells
The LNCaP human prostate cancer cell line is a well-established androgen-dependent cell line. (Goldman et al., 2004) AR-positive human prostate cancer LNCaP cells were obtained from the Riken BRC Cell Bank (Tsukuba, Japan). The cells were plated onto a 96-well plate at a density of 2×10^5 /well and supplemented with 10% charcoal stripped fetal bovine serum (CSFBS) obtained from Invitrogen Japan (Tokyo). Twenty-four h later, the cells were treated with either vehicle control or androgens (T or DHT) in the presence and the absence of each concentration of assessed samples for another 3 d. Sample was dissolved in ethanol and added to the cells after further dilution so that the final volume of ethanol was 1% or less. After culture, cell proliferation was determined to measure cell viability by 3-[4,5-dimethyl thiazol-2-yl]-2,5-diphenyl tetrazolium bromide (MTT) assay. (Hamid et al., 2004) The cells were treated with 1 mg/ml of MTT for 2 h, and precipitated dye was dissolved into dimethylsulfoxide. The absorbance of each well was measured at 570 nm.

2.5 Statistical analysis
Data were analyzed statistically by Student's t-test to determine significant differences in the data among the groups. The p values less than 0.05 were considered significant. The values were expressed as mean $\pm$ S.E.

3. Banana peel

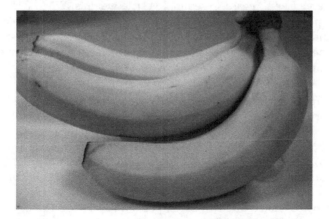

Fig. 2. Banana peel extract (BPEx) prepared from fresh peel part from organically-cultivated bananas showed suppressive effects for enlargement of prostate in BPH model mice

3.1 Source material

The common banana (Musa spp.) is a tropical fruit that grows in the western hemisphere. Primarily viewed as a food source, the banana has a fleshy inside portion surrounded by an outer typically yellow peel (Fig. 2). The fleshy inside portion, or pulp, is edible when raw, and the peel is usually discarded. When ripe, bananas have a deep yellow rind with brown spots, and a creamy pulp, which is easily digested. Bananas are rich in carbohydrates and contain relatively large amounts of vitamins A, B and C and the minerals potassium and phosphorous (Proteggente et al., 2002; Blades et al., 2003). However, banana peel has not been studied nutritionally and pharmaceutically as a source of bioactive compounds. In this report, we examined the effects of banana peel extract (BPEx) on androgen-induced enlargement of accessory reproductive organs in castrated mice. To elucidate the mechanisms of action, the effects of BPEx on the androgen-responsive LNCaP human prostate cancer cell line were investigated. The data presented here indicate that BPEx inhibits growth of the prostate and that BPEx has anti-androgenic activity through inhibition of 5aR.

Fresh banana peel (2.4 kg) of organically-cultivated bananas were cut and extracted with methanol at room temperature for 2 days. The extracts were filtered, concentrated under a vacuum, and freeze-dried. BPEx (56 g) was stored in a refrigerator before assay.

3.2 Suppressive effect of benign prostate hyperplasia in mouse

Our research group has been shown that BPEx treatment (10 d of administration at 0, 50, 100, and 200 mg/kg per orally) dose-dependently reduced the prostate size and the weights of seminal vesicles in the BPH model mice. Then, the effects of BPEx on the growth of mouse prostates and seminal vesicles were studied as compared with those of flutamide and finasteride in the BPH model mice for 10 d. The short and long axes of the ventral prostates and the weights of the seminal vesicles were severely reduced, and when TP (2 mg/kg i.p.) was injected, significant growth of prostates and seminal vesicles was induced. BPEx (200 mg/kg) produced a reduction in prostate weight. Finasteride (2 mg/kg) and flutamide (10 mg/kg), well-known anti-androgens, showed larger reductions in prostate weight. Similar results were observed with regard to seminal vesicle weights. When DHT (6 mg/kg, i.p.) was injected in place of T, significant growth of the prostate and seminal vesicles was induced. BPEx did not inhibit these effects of DHT (Akamine, 2009). These results indicate that orally treatment of BPEx suppress the action of testosterone against enlargement of the reproductive organs in vivo.

3.3 Effects of parts of banana fruit on mouse prostate and seminal vesicles

Testosterone propionate (TP, 2 mg/kg, i.p.) and sample solution (p.o.) were treated to castrated mice once daily for 10 d (Fig. 3). The lengths of the long axes (A) of the prostates of mice were measured vernier calipers, and seminal vesicles (B) were removed and weighed. Cast, castration only; Cont, control; Pe, banana peel (200 mg/kg); Ed, edible part (200 mg/kg). Each value represents the mean ± S.E., n=5. *: p<0.05; **: p<0.01 $vs.$ control (TP-treated without samples).

Fresh banana fruits separated into two parts, peel and edible part to evaluate suppressive effects of the extracts ("Pe" and "Ed", respectively) on BPH model mice. The inhibitory effects of BPEx on the growth of mouse prostates and seminal vesicles were estimated after 10 d of administration. BPEx dose-dependently reduced the prostate size and the weights of seminal vesicles, and showed almost maximal effect at 200 mg/kg. These results indicate that some components in banana peel will be required to suppress prostate enlargement in this model.

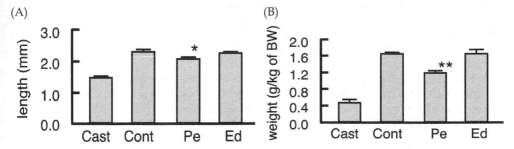

Fig. 3. Effects of extracts of peel (Pe) and edible part (Ed) of banana fruit on TP-induced regrowth of prostates and seminal vesicles in castrated mice

3.4 Inhibitory effects of BPEx on prostate cancer cells

The effects of BPEx on the proliferation of prostate cancer cells (LNCaP cells) were investigated. LNCaP cells show most of the characteristics of human prostatic carcinoma, such as dependence on androgens, the presence of ARs, and the production of acid phosphatase and prostate-specific antigen. The LNCaP cell line is used as an attractive model for in vitro studies of the biology of human prostate cancer. LNCaP cells were incubated with different concentrations of BPEx (3.13–100 μg/ml) with and without T or DHT for 3 d. In the absence of BPEx, T alone stimulated LNCaP cell number about $20.5 \pm 0.5 \times 10^5$ /well, and DHT alone stimulated LNCaP cell numbers to about $30.4 \pm 2.1 \times 10^5$ /well.

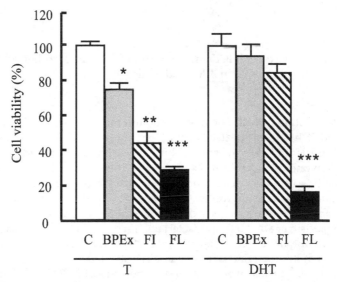

Fig. 4. Inhibitory effects of BPEx on the proliferation of LNCaP cells induced by testosterone (T) or dihydrotestosterone (DHT)

Treatment of LNCaP cells with BPEx in the presence of T resulted in dose-dependent inhibition of cell growth. In the presence of T, both finasteride and flutamide inhibited cell proliferation. However, in the presence of DHT, while flutamide inhibited cell proliferation, finasteride did not. These results indicate that BPEx will suppress on T did not affect on DHT in vivo and in vitro experiments. Fig. 4 showed the inhibitory effects of anti-androgenic samples at 25 µg/ml on LNCaP cells. Scince BPEx showed similar profile with that of FI and not FL, BPEx was estimate to inhibit BPH by its inhibitory activity against 5aR.

Proliferation of prostate cancer cells (LNCaP) were evaluated cell viability (% of control) by MTT assay after 3 days incubation with or without samples at 25 µg/ml in the presence of testosterone (T: 10 mg/ml) or dihydrotestosterone (DHT: 10 mg/ml). BPEx: banana peel extract; FI: finasteride; FI: flutamide. Each data presents as mean±S.E. (n=4).

4. Leaf of *Houttuynia cordata*

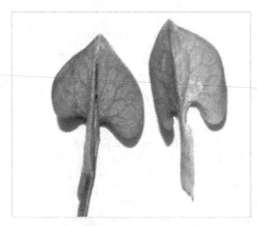

Fig. 5. *Houttuynia cordata* extract (HCE) prepared from fresh leaf part showed suppressive effects for enlargement of prostate in BPH model mice

4.1 Source material

Houttuynia cordata Thunb., which is called dokudami in Japanese, is widely distributed in eastern Asia, and it has a thin leafstalk and heart-shaped leaf (Fig. 5). It is used in folk medicine for diuresis and detoxification. Thus far, it has been reported that *H. cordata* contains many flavonoids (quercitrin, isoquercitrin, rutin, etc.), alkaloids (aristolactam B, norcepharadione B, splendidine, etc.), and volatile components of essential oils (methyl-n-nonyl ketone, lauraldehyde, β-myrcene, etc.) (Meng et al., 2005; Kim et al., 2001; Xu et al., 2005). The extracts and components exhibit diuretic, anti-obesity (Miyata et al., 2009), antioxidative (Kusirisin et al., 2009), antibacterial (Kim et al., 2008), anti-inflammatory (Lu et al., 2006), and apoptotic effects (Tang et al., 2009). The effects for benign prostate hyperplasia (BPH) of this material have been not investigated.

The fresh *Houttuynia cordata* were cut and extracted with 99.5% methanol at room temperature for 2 days. The extract were filtered, and concentrated under a vacuum. The extract was stored in the refrigerator before assay.

We examined the effects of *H. cordata* extract (HCE) in the androgen-responsive effects in BPH model mice and LNCaP human prostate cancer cell line. The data presented here demonstrate that HCE inhibits the growth of the prostate with anti-androgenic activity.

4.2 Suppressive effect of benign prostate hyperplasia in mouse

Testosterone propionate (TP, 2 mg/kg, i.p.) and sample solution (p.o.) were treated to castrated mice once daily for 10 d. The seminal vesicles were removed and weighed. Cast, castration only; Cont, TP treated control; HCE: *Houttuynia cordata* extract (20, 100, and 500 mg/kg). Each data presents as mean±S.E., *n*=6, *: *p*<0.05, **: *p*<0.01, ***: *p*<0.005 vs control (Cont) as shown in Fig. 6.

The suppressive effects of HCE on reproductive organs were investigated in testosterone-induced BPH model mice. The assay to evaluate the effects of HCE on castrated mice prostates and seminal vesicles was performed based on the Hershberger assay as a mean of rapidly developing in vivo. The testes of ddY mice were removed at 7 weeks of age under anesthesia with intraperitoneal injection of pentobarbital (50 mg/ml/kg). After one day of orchiectmy, testosterone propionate (TP) 2 mg/kg was injected intraperitoneally (i.p.) into the mice once daily for 10 days. HCE was administered once daily. After 10 days, mice were weighted and sacrificed by cervical dislocation. The lengths of the long axes of prostate were measured by vernier calipers, and seminal vesicles were removed and weighed.

As shown in Fig. 6, HCE suppress prostates and seminal in a dose-dependent manner at 20, 100, and 500 mg/kg.

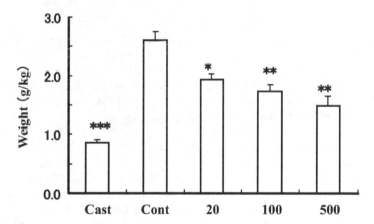

Fig. 6. Effects of extracts of HCE on TP-induced regrowth of prostates and seminal vesicles in castrated mice

In the further experiments, the suppressive effects of HCE were compared with flutamide (FL, 10 mg/kg/day) and finasteride (FI, 2 mg/kg/day) in BPH model mice. As shown in Fig. 7, the size of long-axis length of prostates (A) and the weight of seminal vesicles (B) were severely reduced by HCE ingestion, and when T was injected, a significant growth of prostates and seminal vesicles was induced. Flutamide and finasteride are well known anti-androgen drugs, showed a larger reduction in prostate and seminal vesicle. HCE showed suppressive effect on reproductive organs as same as these medicine at these experimental conditions.

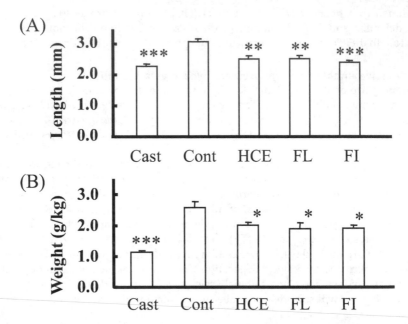

Fig. 7. Evaluation of HCE on T-induced regrowth in castrated mouse prostates and seminal vesicles. (A) long-axis length of prostates, (B) weight of seminal vesicles.

Testosterone propionate (TP, 2 mg/kg, i.p.) and sample solution (p.o.) were treated to castrated mice once daily for 10 d. The lengths of the long axes (A) of the prostates of mice were measured vernier calipers, and seminal vesicles (B) were removed and weighed. Cast: Castration without T-treatment (50 mg/kg, i.p.), Cont: Control, HCE: *H. cordata* extract (100 mg/kg), FI : Finasteride 2 mg/kg, FL: Flutamide 10 mg/kg. Each value represents the means±S.E., n=5. *:$p<0.05$, **:$p<0.01$, ***:$p<0.005$ vs Control.

4.3 Inhibitory effects of HCE on LNCaP cells

The effects of HCE on the proliferation of prostate cancer cells (LNCaP cells) were investigated. After incubation, the cell numbers in T-treated and DHT-treated groups were defined as 100%. As shown in Fig. 8 finasteride, 5aR inhibitor, showed dose-dependent inhibition in T-treated and DHT-treated LNCaP cells. However, its inhibitory effects on DHT-treated group are relatively weak. In contrast, flutamide, androgen receptor antagonist, showed inhibition both in T alone and DHT alone groups at the similar concentrations. On the other hand, the treatment of HCE to LNCaP cells in the presence of T and DHT resulted in the concentration-dependent inhibition of cell proliferation at the same concentrations as same as case of flutamide treatment. These results indicate that HCE suppress enlargement of prostate with a different mechanism with finasteride, 5aR inhibitor. Proliferation of prostate cancer cells (LNCaP) were evaluated cell viability (% of control) by MTT assay after 3 days incubation with or without samples at 6.25, 25, 100 µg/ml in the presence of testosterone (T: 10 mg/ml) or dihydrotestosterone (DHT: 10 mg/ml). HCE: *Houttuynia cordata* extract; FI: finasteride; FI: flutamide. Each data presents as mean±S.E. (n=4).

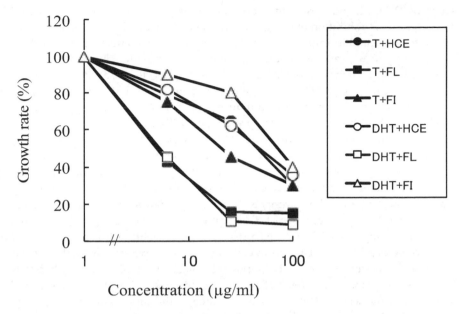

Fig. 8. Inhibitory effects of HCE, Flutamide (FL), and Finasteride (FI) on LNCaP cell proliferation in the presence of testosterone (T) or dihydrotestosterone (DHT). Each point shows the mean of the separated duplicate experiments.

5. Discussion

We studied the in vivo potency of BPEx and HCE, as new botanical materials in immature castrated mice. We evaluated these biological effects in the androgen-responsive LNCaP human prostate cancer cell line and in effects of BHT model mice.

BPEx inhibited TP-induced growth of prostates and seminal vesicles in castrated mice, although it was less potent than finasteride at the same doses. While BPEx inhibited the action of TP, it did not inhibit DHT-induced organ growth. In addition, BPEx inhibited cell proliferation in the presence of T, but not in the presence of DHT. These results suggest that BPEx suppressed the growth of prostates and seminal vesicles by inhibiting the conversion of T to DHT, rather than by blocking the binding of androgen and its receptor. BPEx may have reduced prostate size and seminal vesicle weight by inhibiting 5aR. In further study, we found that treatment of LNCaP cells with BPEx inhibited T-induced cell proliferation (Akamine et al., 2009). The inhibition of this effect of T might have be due, at least in part, to inhibition of 5aR or to antagonism of androgen binding to the AR (Lazier et al., 2004). Since 25 µg/ml of BPEx inhibited 5aR activity by about 30%, we expected to find that this dose would inhibit T action. Similar results have been found with finasteride, a well-known inhibitor of 5aR (McConnell et al., 1992; Sudduth & Koronkowski, 1993), at doses above 25 µg/ml. Similar results were also found with flutamide, an antagonist of androgen binding to the AR (Bergman, & Eriksson, 1996; Sundblad et al., 2005). On the other hand, treatment of LNCaP cells with BPEx in the presence of DHT did not result in a dose-dependent inhibition of cell growth. These results suggest that inhibition of cell growth in the presence of BPEx was not the result of a cell cytotoxic effect, but rather was due to an anti-androgen effect, such as inhibition of 5aR. According to a previous report describing discrimination between cytotoxic and cytostatic effects of integrants on LNCaP cells (Romijn et al., 1988), cytotoxic effects are detectable as a decrease in MTT conversion to a level below that of the starting cells. In our experiment, growth of androgen-induced LNCaP cells was suppressed without decreasing from the starting level in the presence of BPEx during the experimental period. Therefore, a cytostatical effect was estimated for suppression of BPEx on LNCaP cell growth. However, since no index markers related to apoptotic signaling were measured in our experiments, the possibility of a non-cytostatical effect should be considered and confirmed in further detailed investigation. There are generally two ways to suppress prostate regrowth in animal experiments: by inhibiting 5aR activity, and through the use of an androgen receptor antagonist (Imperato-McGinley et al., 1992). An androgen antagonist can suppress DHT-induced prostate and seminal vesicle regrowth (Geller et al., 1981) Therefore, blocking DHT from binding to androgen receptors in the prostate and seminal vesicle is considered to be a possible mechanism of action (other than 5aR inhibition) (Nakayama et al., 1997). To examine this possibility, the effects of BPEx on prostate growth induced by DHT were investigated. If the suppression of prostate growth is caused only by inhibition of 5aR, DHT-induced prostatic regrowth should not be suppressed. Ten d after castration, the weights of mouse prostates were markedly reduced, and prostate size was restored by i.p. injections of TP or DHT. BPEx had no effect on the sizes of the prostate and seminal vesicle of castrated mice that received DHT, whereas flutamide, an androgen receptor antagonist, significantly reduced prostate weight (Fig. 3). In our study, blood levels of testosterone and samples were not measured, but in vivo and in vitro experiments gave mutually correlated results with regard with their mechanism of action. These results suggest that BPEx inhibited prostate growth by inhibiting 5aR activity rather than by exerting a direct effect on the androgen receptor, although the detailed mechanism including bioavailability remains unclear. Recently, there is research reports on components of the banana peel: dietary fiber and pectin (Happi Emaga et al., 2008), and phytosterol from unripe pulp and peel (Oliveira et al., 2008) have been reported. In particular, phytosterols are able to be the active principle in BPEx, due to their anti-androgen activity based on structural similarity. Investigation to elucidate the active components in banana peel is in progress. In this study, we found that BPEx can have anti-androgenic activities through in vitro 5aR inhibitory activity and in vivo growth suppression of prostates and seminal vesicles from castrated mice.

In this study, we have shown that HCE inhibited the T-induced growth of prostates and seminal vesicles in castrated mice and that HCE inhibited T- and DHT-induced cell proliferation in NLCaP cells at the same concentration. The inhibition of this effect of T may be due, at least in part, to the inhibition of 5aR or to antagonism of androgen binding to the AR. And treatment of LNCaP cells with HCE in the presence of DHT result in the dose-dependent inhibition of cell growth. These results were seen with flutamide, which is an antagonist of androgen binding to the AR. These results suggested that the inhibition of cell proliferation in the presence HCE was not the result of a cell cytotoxic effect, but rather was due to an anti-androgen effect, such as inhibition of AR. These results suggest that HCE suppressed the growth of prostates and seminal vesicles by blocking the binding to AR, rather then by conversion of T to DHT. HCE may have reduced prostate size and seminal vesicle weight by blocking the binding of androgen and its receptor.

There are generally two ways to suppress prostate regrowth in animal experiments: by inhibiting 5aR activity and by blocking the binding of androgen and its receptor. An androgen antagonist can suppress DHT-induced prostate and seminal vesicle regrowth. Therefore, blocking DHT from binding to androgen receptors in the prostate and seminal vesicle was considered to be possible mechanism of action (other than 5aR inhibition) of the extract of HCE. To examine this possibility, the effects of HCE on LNCaP cells growth induced by DHT were investigated. These results suggest that HCE inhibited prostate growth by inhibiting androgen receptor rather than by having a direct effect on the 5aR, although the detailed mechanism unclear. In this study, we found that HCE may have anti-androgenic activities through in vitro androgen binding to the AR and in vivo growth suppression of prostate and seminal vesicles from castrated mice. Active compounds showing anti-androgen activity in HCE are of scientific interest. Since, the clinical implications of this activity are currently unknown, further research is needed before is needed before HCE can for the treatment of BPH.

For several years, SPEx has been used as a popular phytotherapeutic agent in the treatment of BPH, but its active component and mechanism of action have not been fully elucidated (Hill & Kyprianou, 2004). Banana peel is usually considered useless and is discarded, but the anti-androgenic activity of BPEx might be useful in the treatment of BPH patients. And leaf of H. cordata have been used as folk medicine, however, never used for treatment BPH with suppressive effect of androgenic functions. Since the clinical implications of this activity are currently unknown, further research is needed before BPEx can be used in the treatment of BPH.

6. Conclusion

In this chapter, the androgen-responsive effects of the two natural extracts from banana peel extract (BPEx) and leaf of *H. cordata* extract (HCE) were shown in BPH model mice and LNCaP human prostate cancer cell line. The data presented here revealed that BPEx was estimated to inhibit the growth of the prostate in BPH model mice by its inhibitory activity against 5-alpha reductase (5aR). And HCE was estimated to inhibit BPH in mice by its anti-androgenic activity different from 5aR inhibition. Therefore, these new botanical materials can be promising most likely candidates as potential material for preventing benign prostate hyperplasia, and it is able to continue to be one of the best preventive medicinal foods to keep our good health in the future.

7. References

Akamine, K.; Koyama, T. & Yazawa, K. (2009) Banana peel extract suppresses prostate gland enlargement in testosterone-treated mice. *Biosci. Biotech. Biochem.* Vol. 73, No. 9, pp. 1911-1914, ISSN: 0916-8451

Bergman, L. & Eriksson, E. (1996) Marked symptom reduction in two women with bulimia nervosa treated with the testosterone receptor antagonist flutamide. *Acta Psychiatrica Scandinavica*, Vol. 94, pp. 137-139, ISSN: 0001-690X

Blades, B. L.; Dufficy, L.; Englberger, L.; Daniells, J. W.; Coyne, T.; Hamill, S. & Wills, R. L. (2003) Bananas and plantains as a source of provitamin A. *Asia Pac J Clin Nutr.*, Vol. 12, pp. S36, ISSN: 0964-7058

Cristoni A.; Di Pierro F. & Bombardelli E. (2000). Botanical derivatives for the prostate. *Fitoterapia*, Vol. 71, pp. S21-S28, ISSN: 0367-326X

Elliot, F. & Franklin, C. L. (2001) Saw Palmetto Berry as a Treatment for BPH. *Rev Urol.*, Vol. 3, pp. 134-138, ISSN: 1523-6161

Franck-Lissbrant, I.; Haggstom, S.; Damber, J. E. & Bergh, A. (1998) Testosterone stimulates angiogenesis and vascular regrowth in the ventral prostate in castrated adult rats. *Endocrinology*, Vol. 139, pp. 451-456, ISSN: 0013-7227

Geller, J.; Albert, J. & Nachtsheim, D. A. (1981) The effects of flutamide on total DHT and nuclear DHT levels in the human prostate. *Prostate*, Vol. 2, pp. 309-314, ISSN: 0270-4137

Goldman, W. H.; Sharma, A. L.; Currier, S. J.; Johnston, P. D.; Rana, A. & Sharma, C. P. (2004) Saw palmetto berry extract inhibits cell growth and Cox-2 expression in prostatic cancer cells. *Cell Biol Int.*, Vol. 25, pp. 1117-1124, ISSN:1065-6995

Happi Emaga, T.; Robert, C.; Ronkart, S. N.; Wathelet, B. & Paquot, M. (2008) Dietary fibre components and pectin chemical features of peels during ripening in banana and plantain varieties. *Bioresour Technol.*, Vol. 99, pp. 4346-4354, ISSN: 0960-8524

Hamid, R.; Rotshteyn, Y.; Rabadi, L.; Parikh, R. & Bullock, P. (2004) Comparison of alamar blue and MTT assays for high through-put screening. *Toxicology in Vitro*, Vol. 18, pp. 703-710, ISSN: 0887-2333

Hill, B. & Kyprianou, N. (2004) Effect of permixon on human prostate cell growth: Lack of apoptotic action. *Prostate*, Vol. 61, pp. 73-80, ISSN: 0270-4137

Imperato-McGinley, J.; Sanchez, R. S.; Spencer, J. R.; Yee, B. & Vaughan, E. D. (1992) Comparison of the effects of the 5 alpha-reductase inhibitor finasteride and the antiandrogen flutamide on prostate and genital differentiation: dose-response studies. *Endocrinology*, Vol. 131, pp. 1149-1156, ISSN: 0013-7227

Kim, G. S.; Kim, D. H., Lim, J. J., Lee, J. J.; Han, D. Y.; Lee, W. M.; Jung, W. C.; Min, W. G., Won, C. G.; Rhee, M. H.; Lee, H. J. & Kim, S. (2008). Biological and antibacterial activities of the natural herb *Houttuynia cordata* water extract against the intracellular bacterial pathogen salmonella within the RAW 264.7 macrophage. *Biol Pharm Bull*, Vol. 31, 2012-2017, ISSN: 0918-6158

Kim, S. K.; Ryu, S. Y.; No, J.; Choi, S. U.; & Kim, Y. S. (2001). Cytotoxic alkaloids from *Houttuynia cordata*. *Arch Pharm Res*, Vol. 24, 518-521, ISSN: 0253-6269

Kusirisin, W; Srichairatanakool, S.; Lerttrakarnnon, P.; Lailerd, N.; Suttajit, M.; Jaikang, C. & Chaiyasut, C. (2009). Antioxidative activity, polyphenolic content and anti-glycation effect of some Thai medicinal plants traditionally used in diabetic patients. *Med Chem*, Vol. 5, No. 2, pp. 139-147, ISSN: 1573-4064

Lu, H. M.; Liang, Y. Z.; Yi, L. Z.; Wu, X. J. (2006). Anti-inflammatory effect of *Houttuynia cordata* injection. *J Ethnopharmacol*, Vol. 104, 245-249, ISSN: 0378-8741

Lazier, C. B.; Thomas, L. N.; Douglas, R. C.; Vessey, J. P. & Rittmaster, R. S. (2004) Dutasteride, the dual 5 alpha-reductase inhibitor, inhibits androgen action and promotes cell death in the LNCaP prostate cancer cell line *Prostate*, Vol. 58, pp. 130-144, ISSN: 0270-4137

Lowe, F. C.; McConnell, J. D.; Hudson, P. B.; Romas, N.A.; Boake, R.; Lieber, M.; Elhilali, M.; Geller, J.; Imperto-McGinely, J.; Andriole, G. L.; Bruskewitz, R. C.; Walsh, P. C.; Bartsch, G.; Nacey, J. N.; Shah, A.; Pappas F.; Ko, A.; Cook, T.; Stoner, E. & Waldstreicher, J. (2003) Long-term 6-year experience with finasteride in patients with benign prostatic hyperplasia. *Urology* Vol. 61, pp. 791-796. ISSN: 0090-4295

Marks. L. S. (2004) 5alpha-reductase: history and clinical importance. *Rev Urol.* Vol. 6, pp. S11-S21, ISSN: 1523-6161

McConnell, J. D.; Wilson, J. D.; George, F. W.; Geller, J.; Pappas, F.; Stoner, E. (1992) Finasteride, an inhibitor of 5 alpha-reductase, suppresses prostatic dihydrotestosterone in men with benign prostatic hyperplasia. *Journal of Clinical Endocrinology and Metabolism*, Vol. 74, No. 3, 505-508, ISSN: 0021-972X

Meng, J.; Leung, K. S.; Jiang, Z.; Dong, X.; Zhao, Z. & Xu, L. J. (2005). Establishment of HPLC-DAD-MS fingerprint of fresh *Houttuynia cordata. Chem Pharm Bull*, Vol. 53, 1604-1609, ISSN:

Miyata, M.; Koyama, T. & Yazawa, K. (2010). Water extract of *Houttuynia cordata* Thunb. leaves exerts anti-obesity effects by inhibiting fatty acid and glycerol absorption. *J Nutr Sci Vitaminol*, Vol. 56, No. 2, 150-156, ISSN: 0301-4800

Nakayama, O.; Hirosumi, J.; Chida, N.; Takahashi, S.; Sawada, K.; Kojo, H. & Notsu, Y. (1997) FR146687, a novel steroid 5 alpha-reductase inhibitor: In vitro and in vivo effects on prostates. *Prostate*, Vol. 31, pp. 241-249, ISSN: 0270-4137

Oliveira, L.; Freire, C.S.; Silvestre, A. J. & Cordeiro, N. (2008) Lipophilic extracts from banana fruit residues: a source of valuable phytosterols. *J Agric Food Chem.* Vol. 56, pp. 9520-9524, ISSN: 0021-8561

Proteggente, A. R.; Pannala, A. S.; Paganga, G.; Van Buren, L.; Wagner, E.; Wiseman, S.; Van De Put, F.; Dacombe, C. & Rice-Evans, C. A. (2002) The antioxidant activity of regularly consumed fruit and vegetables reflects their phenolic and vitamin C composition. *Free Radic Res.*, Vol. 36, pp. 217-233, ISSN: 1071-5762

Romijn, J. C.; Verkoelen, C. F. & Schroeder, F. H. (1988) Application of the MTT assay to human prostate cancer cell lines in vitro: establishment of test conditions and assessment of hormone-stimulated growth and drug-induced cytostatic and cytotoxic effects. *Prostate*, Vol. 12, pp. 99-110, ISSN: 0270-4137

Russell, D. W. & Wilson J. D. (1994). Steroid 5 alpha-reductase: two genes/two enzymes. *Annual Review of Clinical Biochemistry*, Vol 63, pp. 25-61, PMID: 7979239

Sudduth, S. L. & Koronkowski, M. J. (1993) Finasteride- The first 5-alpha-reductase inhibitor. *Pharmacotherapy*, Vol. 13, pp. 309-329, ISSN 0277-0008

Sundblad, C.; Landen, M.; Eriksson, T.; Bergman, L. & Eriksson, E. (2005) Effects of the androgen antagonist flutamide and the serotonin reuptake inhibitor citalopram in bulimia nervosa: a placebo-controlled pilot study. *Journal of Clinical Psychopharmacology*, Vol. 25, pp. 85-88, ISSN: 0271-0749

Tang, Y. J.; Yang, J. S.; Lin, C. F.; Shyu, W. C.; Tsuzuki, M.; Lu, C. C.; Chen, Y. F. & Lai, K. C. (2009). *Houttuynia cordata* Thunb extract induces apoptosis through mitochondrial-dependent pathway in HT-29 human colon adenocarcinoma cells. *Oncol Rep*, Vol. 22, 1051-1056, ISSN: 1523-3790

Xu, C. J.; Liang, Y. Z.; Chau, F. T. (2005). Identification of essential components of *Houttuynia cordata* by gas chromatography/mass spectrometry and the integrated chemometric approach. *Talanta*, Vol. 68, 108-115, ISSN: 0039-9140

Yamasaki, K.; Sawaki, M.; Ohta, R.; Okuda, H.; Katayama, S.; Yamada, T.; Ohta, T.; Kosaka,
    T. & Owens, W. (2003) OECD validation of the Hershberger assay in Japan: Phase 2
    dose response of methyltestosterone, vinclozolin, and *p,p'*-DDE. *Environ Health
    Perspect*, Vol. 111, pp. 1912-1919, ISSN: 0091-6765

Permissions

The contributors of this book come from diverse backgrounds, making this book a truly international effort. This book will bring forth new frontiers with its revolutionizing research information and detailed analysis of the nascent developments around the world.

We would like to thank Philippe E. Spiess, for lending his expertise to make the book truly unique. He has played a crucial role in the development of this book. Without his invaluable contribution this book wouldn't have been possible. He has made vital efforts to compile up to date information on the varied aspects of this subject to make this book a valuable addition to the collection of many professionals and students.

This book was conceptualized with the vision of imparting up-to-date information and advanced data in this field. To ensure the same, a matchless editorial board was set up. Every individual on the board went through rigorous rounds of assessment to prove their worth. After which they invested a large part of their time researching and compiling the most relevant data for our readers. Conferences and sessions were held from time to time between the editorial board and the contributing authors to present the data in the most comprehensible form. The editorial team has worked tirelessly to provide valuable and valid information to help people across the globe.

Every chapter published in this book has been scrutinized by our experts. Their significance has been extensively debated. The topics covered herein carry significant findings which will fuel the growth of the discipline. They may even be implemented as practical applications or may be referred to as a beginning point for another development. Chapters in this book were first published by InTech; hereby published with permission under the Creative Commons Attribution License or equivalent.

The editorial board has been involved in producing this book since its inception. They have spent rigorous hours researching and exploring the diverse topics which have resulted in the successful publishing of this book. They have passed on their knowledge of decades through this book. To expedite this challenging task, the publisher supported the team at every step. A small team of assistant editors was also appointed to further simplify the editing procedure and attain best results for the readers.

Our editorial team has been hand-picked from every corner of the world. Their multi-ethnicity adds dynamic inputs to the discussions which result in innovative outcomes. These outcomes are then further discussed with the researchers and contributors who give their valuable feedback and opinion regarding the same. The feedback is then collaborated with the researches and they are edited in a comprehensive manner to aid the understanding of the subject.

Apart from the editorial board, the designing team has also invested a significant amount of their time in understanding the subject and creating the most relevant covers. They scrutinized every image to scout for the most suitable representation of the subject and create an appropriate cover for the book.

The publishing team has been involved in this book since its early stages. They were actively engaged in every process, be it collecting the data, connecting with the contributors or procuring relevant information. The team has been an ardent support to the editorial, designing and production team. Their endless efforts to recruit the best for this project, has resulted in the accomplishment of this book. They are a veteran in the field of academics and their pool of knowledge is as vast as their experience in printing. Their expertise and guidance has proved useful at every step. Their uncompromising quality standards have made this book an exceptional effort. Their encouragement from time to time has been an inspiration for everyone.

The publisher and the editorial board hope that this book will prove to be a valuable piece of knowledge for researchers, students, practitioners and scholars across the globe.

List of Contributors

Volker Winkler and Heiko Becher
Institute of Public Health, University of Heidelberg, Germany

Yuanyuan Mi
Department of Urology, The First Affiliated Hospital of Nanjing Medical University, Nanjing, China
Department of Urology, Third Affiliated Hospital of Nantong University, Wuxi, China

Lijie Zhu
Department of Urology, Third Affiliated Hospital of Nantong University, Wuxi, China

Ninghan Feng
Department of Urology, The First Affiliated Hospital of Nanjing Medical University, Nanjing, China

Daniel Djakiew
Georgetown University Medical School, USA

Sanjay Kumar Saxena and Ashutosh Dash
Radiopharmaceuticals Division, Bhabha Atomic Research Centre, Trombay, Mumbai, India

L. Terraneo, E. Finati, E. Virgili, G. Demartini, L. De Angelis, R. Dall'Aglio, F. Fraschini, M. Samaja and R. Paroni
University of Milan, Milan, Italy

Noemí Cárdenas-Rodríguez and Esaú Floriano-Sánchez
Sección de Posgrado e Investigación, Instituto Politécnico Nacional Laboratorio de Bioquímica y Biología Molecular, Escuela Médico Militar Laboratorio de Neuroquímica, Instituto Nacional de Pediatría México, D.F.

Selvalingam S., Leong A.C., Natarajan C. and Sundram M.
Department of Urology, General Hospital Kuala Lumpur, Malaysia

Yunus R.
Department of Pathology, General Hospital Kuala Lumpur, Malaysia

K. Stamatiou
Urology department Tzaneion General Hospital of Pireas, Greece

Sabrina Bouatmane
Département d'Electronique, Faculté des Sciences de l'Ingénieur, Université de Jijel, Jijel, Algérie

Ahmed Bouridane
Department of Computer Science, King Saud University, Riyadh, Saudi Arabia
School of Computing, Engineering and Information Sciences, Northumbria University at Newcastle, Pandon Building, UK

Mohamed Ali Roula
Faculty of Advanced Technology, University of Glamorgan, Pontypridd, UK

Somaya Al-Maadeed
Department of Computer Science & Engineering Qatar University, Doha, Qatar

Carmen Sanmartín, Juan Antonio Palop, Beatriz Romano and Daniel Plano
Department of Organic and Pharmaceutical Chemistry, University of Navarra, Spain

Taku Suzuki and Hideki Mukai
Toho University, Medical Center, Ohashi Hospital, Department of Dermatology, Japan

Yao Tang, Mohammad A. Khan, Bin Zhang and Arif Hussain
University of Maryland School of Medicine and Baltimore VA Medical Center, USA

Chih-Pin Chuu, Hui-Ping Lin, Ching-Yu Lin and Liang-Cheng Su
Affiliated University, Institute of Cellular and System Medicine, Taiwan
Translational Center for Glandular Malignancies, National Health Research Institutes, Taiwan

Chiech Huo
Affiliated University, Institute of Cellular and System Medicine, Taiwan
Translational Center for Glandular Malignancies, National Health Research Institutes, Taiwan
Department of Life Sciences, National Central University, Taiwan

Tomoyuki Koyama
Tokyo University of Marine Science and Technology, Japan

Printed in the USA
CPSIA information can be obtained
at www.ICGtesting.com
JSHW011423221024
72173JS00004B/653

9 781632 413307

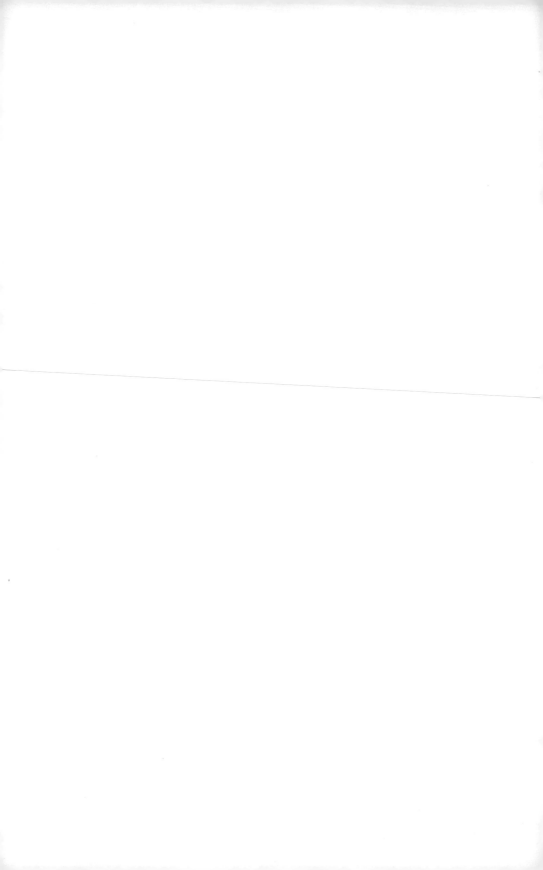